Emerging Virus Infections in Adverse Pregnancy Outcomes

Emerging Virus Infections in Adverse Pregnancy Outcomes

Editors

David Baud
Léo Pomar

MDPI • Basel • Beijing • Wuhan • Barcelona • Belgrade • Manchester • Tokyo • Cluj • Tianjin

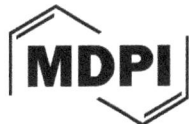

Editors
David Baud
Département
femme-mère-enfant
Lausanne University Hospital
Lausanne
Switzerland

Léo Pomar
Département
femme-mère-enfant
Lausanne University Hospital
Lausanne
Switzerland

Editorial Office
MDPI
St. Alban-Anlage 66
4052 Basel, Switzerland

This is a reprint of articles from the Special Issue published online in the open access journal *Viruses* (ISSN 1999-4915) (available at: www.mdpi.com/journal/viruses/special_issues/Virus_Pregnancy).

For citation purposes, cite each article independently as indicated on the article page online and as indicated below:

LastName, A.A.; LastName, B.B.; LastName, C.C. Article Title. *Journal Name* **Year**, *Volume Number*, Page Range.

ISBN 978-3-0365-5274-3 (Hbk)
ISBN 978-3-0365-5273-6 (PDF)

Cover image courtesy of Léo Pomar

© 2022 by the authors. Articles in this book are Open Access and distributed under the Creative Commons Attribution (CC BY) license, which allows users to download, copy and build upon published articles, as long as the author and publisher are properly credited, which ensures maximum dissemination and a wider impact of our publications.

The book as a whole is distributed by MDPI under the terms and conditions of the Creative Commons license CC BY-NC-ND.

Contents

About the Editors vii

Preface to "Polymer Materials in Sensors, Actuators and Energy Conversion" ix

Léo Pomar and David Baud
Special Issue "Emerging Virus Infections in Adverse Pregnancy Outcomes"
Reprinted from: *Viruses* **2022**, *14*, 285, doi:10.3390/v14020285 1

Manon Vouga, Léo Pomar, Antoni Soriano-Arandes, Carlota Rodó, Anna Goncé and Eduard Gratacos et al.
Maternal Infection and Adverse Pregnancy Outcomes among Pregnant Travellers: Results of the International Zika Virus in Pregnancy Registry
Reprinted from: *Viruses* **2021**, *13*, 341, doi:10.3390/v13020341 3

Eri Nakayama, Yasuhiro Kawai, Satoshi Taniguchi, Jessamine E. Hazlewood, Ken-ichi Shibasaki and Kenta Takahashi et al.
Embryonic Stage of Congenital Zika Virus Infection Determines Fetal and Postnatal Outcomes in Mice
Reprinted from: *Viruses* **2021**, *13*, 1807, doi:10.3390/v13091807 17

Theodoros Kalampokas, Anna Rapani, Maria Papageorgiou, Sokratis Grigoriadis, Evangelos Maziotis and George Anifandis et al.
The Current Evidence Regarding COVID-19 and Pregnancy: Where Are We Now and Where Should We Head to Next?
Reprinted from: *Viruses* **2021**, *13*, 2000, doi:10.3390/v13102000 35

Maria de Lourdes Benamor Teixeira, Orlando da Costa Ferreira Júnior, Esaú João, Trevon Fuller, Juliana Silva Esteves and Wallace Mendes-Silva et al.
Maternal and Neonatal Outcomes of SARS-CoV-2 Infection in a Cohort of Pregnant Women with Comorbid Disorders
Reprinted from: *Viruses* **2021**, *13*, 1277, doi:10.3390/v13071277 57

Sara Cruz Melguizo, María Luisa de la Cruz Conty, Paola Carmona Payán, Alejandra Abascal-Saiz, Pilar Pintando Recarte and Laura González Rodríguez et al.
Pregnancy Outcomes and SARS-CoV-2 Infection: The Spanish Obstetric Emergency Group Study
Reprinted from: *Viruses* **2021**, *13*, 853, doi:10.3390/v13050853 67

Salvador Espino-y-Sosa, Raigam Jafet Martinez-Portilla, Johnatan Torres-Torres, Juan Mario Solis-Paredes, Guadalupe Estrada-Gutierrez and Jose Antonio Hernandez-Pacheco et al.
Novel Ratio Soluble Fms-like Tyrosine Kinase-1/Angiotensin-II (sFlt-1/ANG-II) in Pregnant Women Is Associated with Critical Illness in COVID-19
Reprinted from: *Viruses* **2021**, *13*, 1906, doi:10.3390/v13101906 79

Valentina Giardini, Sara Ornaghi, Eleonora Acampora, Maria Viola Vasarri, Francesca Arienti and Carlo Gambacorti-Passerini et al.
Letter to the Editor: SFlt-1 and PlGF Levels in Pregnancies Complicated by SARS-CoV-2 Infection
Reprinted from: *Viruses* **2021**, *13*, 2377, doi:10.3390/v13122377 91

Johnatan Torres-Torres, Raigam Jafet Martinez-Portilla, Salvador Espino y Sosa, Juan Mario Solis-Paredes, Jose Antonio Hernández-Pacheco and Paloma Mateu-Rogell et al.
Maternal Death by COVID-19 Associated with Elevated Troponin T Levels
Reprinted from: *Viruses* **2022**, *14*, 271, doi:10.3390/v14020271 . . . . **97**

Guillaume Favre, Sara Mazzetti, Carole Gengler, Claire Bertelli, Juliane Schneider and Bernard Laubscher et al.
Decreased Fetal Movements: A Sign of Placental SARS-CoV-2 Infection with Perinatal Brain Injury
Reprinted from: *Viruses* **2021**, *13*, 2517, doi:10.3390/v13122517 . . . . **107**

Gennady Sukhikh, Ulyana Petrova, Andrey Prikhodko, Natalia Starodubtseva, Konstantin Chingin and Huanwen Chen et al.
Vertical Transmission of SARS-CoV-2 in Second Trimester Associated with Severe Neonatal Pathology
Reprinted from: *Viruses* **2021**, *13*, 447, doi:10.3390/v13030447 . . . . **119**

Leonardo Resta, Antonella Vimercati, Sara Sablone, Andrea Marzullo, Gerardo Cazzato and Giuseppe Ingravallo et al.
Is the First of the Two Born Saved? A Rare and Dramatic Case of Double Placental Damage from SARS-CoV-2
Reprinted from: *Viruses* **2021**, *13*, 995, doi:10.3390/v13060995 . . . . **131**

Leonardo Resta, Antonella Vimercati, Gerardo Cazzato, Giulia Mazzia, Ettore Cicinelli and Anna Colagrande et al.
SARS-CoV-2 and Placenta: New Insights and Perspectives
Reprinted from: *Viruses* **2021**, *13*, 723, doi:10.3390/v13050723 . . . . **139**

Sarah Stuckelberger, Guillaume Favre, Michael Ceulemans, Hedvig Nordeng, Eva Gerbier and Valentine Lambelet et al.
SARS-CoV-2 Vaccine Willingness among Pregnant and Breastfeeding Women during the First Pandemic Wave: A Cross-Sectional Study in Switzerland
Reprinted from: *Viruses* **2021**, *13*, 1199, doi:10.3390/v13071199 . . . . **153**

Serge Stroobandt and Roland Stroobandt
Data of the COVID-19 mRNA-Vaccine V-Safe Surveillance System and Pregnancy Registry Reveals Poor Embryonic and Second Trimester Fetal Survival Rate. Comment on Stuckelberger et al. SARS-CoV-2 Vaccine Willingness among Pregnant and Breastfeeding Women during the First Pandemic Wave: A Cross-Sectional Study in Switzerland. *Viruses* 2021, 13, 1199
Reprinted from: *Viruses* **2021**, *13*, 1545, doi:10.3390/v13081545 . . . . **167**

Sarah Stuckelberger, Guillaume Favre, Michael Ceulemans, Eva Gerbier, Valentine Lambelet and Milos Stojanov et al.
Current Data on COVID-19 mRNA-Vaccine Safety during Pregnancy Might Be Subject to Selection Bias. Reply to Stroobandt, S.; Stroobandt, R. Data of the COVID-19 mRNA-Vaccine V-Safe Surveillance System and Pregnancy Registry Reveals Poor Embryonic and Second Trimester Fetal Survival Rate. Comment on "Stuckelberger et al. SARS-CoV-2 Vaccine Willingness among Pregnant and Breastfeeding Women during the First Pandemic Wave: A Cross-Sectional Study in Switzerland. *Viruses* 2021, 13, 1199"
Reprinted from: *Viruses* **2021**, *13*, 1546, doi:10.3390/v13081546 . . . . **169**

About the Editors

David Baud

David Baud is an obstetrician specialized in maternal–fetal medicine. His main topics of interest are fetal therapy and infectious diseases during pregnancy. He is a Full Professor at the University of Lausanne, and head of the obstetrics department of the Lausanne University Hospital.

Léo Pomar

Léo Pomar is a midwife specialized in ultrasound and fetal medicine, with a PhD degree in biology. His main topics of interest are fetal brain imaging and infectious diseases during pregnancy. In addition to his clinical work, he is an associate Professor at the School of Health Sciences in Lausanne.

Preface to "Emerging Virus Infections in Adverse Pregnancy Outcomes"

Viruses that have emerged over recent decades, such as arboviruses and SARS coronaviruses, are increasingly being recognized as potential risk factors for adverse pregnancy outcomes.

On the fetal side, arboviruses have proved their ability to cross the placental barrier at different stages of pregnancy, and have been associated with fetal losses, fetal malformations (Zika, West Nile, and Venezuelan equine encephalitis viruses) and adverse neonatal outcomes (Dengue and Chikungunya viruses). SARS-COV-2 has also be associated with rare maternal–fetal transmission and placental affection, leading to fetal losses.

On the maternal side, SARS-COV-2 can compromise maternal health, and risk factors for severe COVID-19 during pregnancy need to be investigated.

In this Special Issue of *Viruses*, we present original research, reviews and commentaries that contribute to improving our understanding of the viral infection of placenta and fetal cells, or that report on the maternal and fetal outcomes after an emerging viral infection during pregnancy.

David Baud and Léo Pomar
Editors

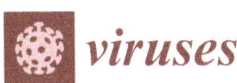

Editorial

Special Issue "Emerging Virus Infections in Adverse Pregnancy Outcomes"

Léo Pomar [1,2,*] and David Baud [1,*]

1. Materno-Fetal and Obstetrics Research Unit, Department Woman-Mother-Child, Lausanne University Hospital, University of Lausanne, 1011 Lausanne, Switzerland
2. School of Health Sciences (HESAV), University of Applied Sciences and Arts Western Switzerland, 1011 Lausanne, Switzerland
* Correspondence: leo.pomar@chuv.ch (L.P.); david.baud@chuv.ch (D.B.)

Dear contributors and readers,

In this 2021 edition of the Special Issue "Emerging Virus Infections in Adverse Pregnancy Outcomes", we have received and published some very relevant studies on these topics. Regarding congenital Zika infections, a mouse model confirmed that the embryological stage at the time of congenital infection was a determining factor for adverse outcomes in infected fetuses and that maternal neutralizing antibodies could protect the offspring from neonatal death after congenital infection. The results of the International Zika Virus in Pregnancy Registry showed that the risk of infection was lower among pregnant women who travelled in endemic areas compared to residents and was related to the presence of ongoing outbreaks and stay duration. In this registry, adverse perinatal outcomes were observed in 8.3% of infected travelers and 12.7% of infected residents.

We also received several high-quality papers on SARS-CoV-2 infections during pregnancy. Rare but dramatic cases of placental and fetal infection, resulting in fetal or neonatal death or severe neonatal morbidity, were reported. The analysis of infected placentas revealed extensive and multifocal chronic intervillositis, as well as malperfusion, potentially causing leucomalacia in neonates. Fetal and early neonatal infections were also confirmed in several cases published in this issue, and a decrease in fetal movements was described as a warning sign for adverse perinatal outcomes following maternal SARS-CoV-2 infection. Concerning maternal outcomes, a cohort study from the Spanish Obstetric Emergency Group and a Brazilian cohort of pregnant individuals with high rates of comorbidities presented the risks of maternal and obstetrical adverse outcomes related to COVID-19 during pregnancy: death, pneumonia, ICU admission, iatrogenic prematurity, venous thrombotic events, severe pre-eclampsia, fetal, and neonatal death. We are also very grateful for a study based on a cohort in Mexico that analyzed the endothelial response to COVID-19 during pregnancy through the modification of the Soluble Fms-like Tyrosine Kinase-1/Angiotensin-II ratio. Finally, a Swiss study investigated the willingness of pregnant individuals to receive the SARS-CoV-2 vaccine and potential barriers to their immunization.

Overall, we would like to thank all the researchers and clinicians who contributed to this Special Issue, and we hope to work with them again for future editions. We will continue this Special Issue with a 2022 edition on the same topics, in which we would also like to give more space to other emerging and endemic viruses that can complicate pregnancies.

Conflicts of Interest: The authors declare no conflict of interest.

Citation: Pomar, L.; Baud, D. Special Issue "Emerging Virus Infections in Adverse Pregnancy Outcomes". *Viruses* 2022, *14*, 285. https://doi.org/10.3390/v14020285

Received: 26 January 2022
Accepted: 27 January 2022
Published: 29 January 2022

Publisher's Note: MDPI stays neutral with regard to jurisdictional claims in published maps and institutional affiliations.

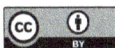

Copyright: © 2022 by the authors. Licensee MDPI, Basel, Switzerland. This article is an open access article distributed under the terms and conditions of the Creative Commons Attribution (CC BY) license (https://creativecommons.org/licenses/by/4.0/).

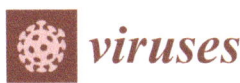

Article

Maternal Infection and Adverse Pregnancy Outcomes among Pregnant Travellers: Results of the International Zika Virus in Pregnancy Registry

Manon Vouga [1], Léo Pomar [1,2], Antoni Soriano-Arandes [3], Carlota Rodó [4], Anna Goncé [5], Eduard Gratacos [5], Audrey Merriam [6], Isabelle Eperon [7], Begoña Martinez De Tejada [7,8], Béatrice Eggel [9], Sophie Masmejan [1], Laurence Rochat [10], Blaise Genton [10], Tim Van Mieghem [11], Véronique Lambert [2], Denis Malvy [12], Patrick Gérardin [13], David Baud [1,*] and Alice Panchaud [14,15,16]

1. Materno-Fetal and Obstetrics Research Unit, Department "Woman-Mother-Child", Lausanne University Hospital, University of Lausanne, 1011 Lausanne, Switzerland; manon.vouga@chuv.ch (M.V.); leo.pomar@chuv.ch (L.P.); Sophie.Masmejan@chuv.ch (S.M.)
2. Department of Obstetrics and Gynecology, Centre Hospitalier-Franck Joly, 97393 Saint-Laurent du Maroni, French Guiana; v.lambert@ch-ouestguyane.fr
3. Paediatric Infectious Diseases and Immunodeficiencies Unit, Hospital Universitari Vall d'Hebron, 08035 Barcelona, Spain; tsorianoarandes@gmail.com
4. Maternal-Fetal Medicine Unit, Department of Obstetrics, Hospital Universitari Vall d'Hebron, 08035 Barcelona, Spain; carlotarodo@gmail.com
5. Institut Clínic de Ginecología, Obstetricia i Neonatologia and BCNatal (Barcelona Center for Maternal-Fetal and Neonatal Medicine), Hospital Clínic and Hospital Sant Joan de Deu, Institut d'Investigacions Biomèdiques August Pi i Sunyer, Universitat de Barcelona, Center for Biomedical Research on Rare Diseases (CIBERER), 08028 Barcelona, Spain; agonce@clinic.cat (A.G.); egratacos@ub.edu (E.G.)
6. Department of Obstetrics and Gynecology, New York Presbyterian Hospital Columbia University, New York, NY 10032, USA; aamerr02@gmail.com
7. Department of Obstetrics and Gynecology, University Hospitals of Geneva, 1205 Geneva, Switzerland; isabelle.eperon@gmail.com (I.E.); begona.martinezdetejada@hcuge.ch (B.M.D.T.)
8. Faculty of Medicine, University of Geneva, 1205 Geneva, Switzerland
9. Obstetrics and Gynecology Department, Centre Hospitalier du Centre Valais (CHCVs), 1950 Sion, Switzerland; Beatrice.Eggel-Hort@hopitalvs.ch
10. Center for Primary Care and Public Health, University of Lausanne, 1011 Lausanne, Switzerland; Laurence.rochat@huv.ch (L.R.); blaise.genton@unisante.ch (B.G.)
11. Maternal-Fetal Medicine Unit, Department of Obstetrics and Gynecology, Mount Sinai Hospital and University of Toronto, Toronto, ON M5G 1X5, Canada; Tim.vanmieghem@sinaihealth.ca
12. Department for Infectious and Tropical Diseases, CHU Hôpitaux de Bordeaux and Inserm 1219, University of Bordeaux, 33000 Bordeaux, France; denis.malvy@chu-bordeaux.fr
13. INSERM CIC1410 Clinical Epidemiology, Centre Hospitalier Universitaire de la Réunion, 97410 Saint Pierre La Réunion, France; patrick.gerardin@chu-reunion.fr
14. School of Pharmaceutical Sciences, Geneva University and Service of Pharmacy, Lausanne University Hospital, 1011 Lausanne, Switzerland; alice.panchaud@chuv.ch
15. Service of Pharmacy, Lausanne University Hospital, University of Lausanne, 1011 Lausanne, Switzerland
16. Institute of Primary Health Care (BIHAM), University of Bern, 3012 Bern, Switzerland
* Correspondence: david.baud@chuv.ch

Abstract: In this multicentre cohort study, we evaluated the risks of maternal ZIKV infections and adverse pregnancy outcomes among exposed travellers compared to women living in areas with ZIKV circulation (residents). The risk of maternal infection was lower among travellers compared to residents: 25.0% (*n* = 36/144) versus 42.9% (*n* = 309/721); aRR 0.6; 95% CI 0.5–0.8. Risk factors associated with maternal infection among travellers were travelling during the epidemic period (i.e., June 2015 to December 2016) (aOR 29.4; 95% CI 3.7–228.1), travelling to the Caribbean Islands (aOR 3.2; 95% CI 1.2–8.7) and stay duration >2 weeks (aOR 8.7; 95% CI 1.1–71.5). Adverse pregnancy outcomes were observed in 8.3% (*n* = 3/36) of infected travellers and 12.7% (*n* = 39/309) of infected residents. Overall, the risk of maternal infections is lower among travellers compared to residents and related to the presence of ongoing outbreaks and stay duration, with stays <2 weeks associated with minimal risk in the absence of ongoing outbreaks.

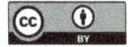

Keywords: Zika; congenital Zika syndrome; pregnancy; travelers

1. Introduction

Zika virus (ZIKV) has emerged as an arthropod-borne infection associated with adverse pregnancy outcomes [1]. The risks associated with intrauterine ZIKV infection have been well documented among women living in areas with active ZIKV circulation where the overall risk of severe adverse pregnancy outcomes for exposed foetuses was estimated to range between 5 to 13% [2–4]. However, the risks for pregnant travellers with brief exposures remain poorly described. Though transmission has now declined all over the world, epidemic clusters are still being reported [5] with the possibility of emergence/re-emergence in all areas where competent vectors are found [1]. Given the known sexual transmission and the risk for maternal infection at an early stage of pregnancy, several international agencies [6,7] continue to recommend a 2 to 3-month delay prior to attempting conception after returning from areas with ongoing or past ZIKV circulation. As these regions encompass most tropical areas, and represent popular travel destinations, it appears imperative to accurately assess the risk of infection in order to establish appropriate guidelines for pregnant travellers.

We launched an international web registry [8] in January 2016 to allow structured collection of data regarding pregnant women and their foetuses exposed to ZIKV. In this article, we present risk assessments for maternal ZIKV infections and adverse pregnancy outcomes among exposed travellers compared to women living in areas with ZIKV circulation using this dataset.

2. Materials and Methods

2.1. Study Population and Data Collection

This study utilized the Zika international registry in pregnancy dataset [8]. Health facilities with an antenatal obstetric clinic willing to participate in this international data sharing initiative (available at the time of the study at https://ispso.unige.ch/zika-in-pregnancy-registry/ from 9 March 2017) were invited to systematically enroll all pregnant women attending their clinic that were screened for ZIKV infection at any stage of pregnancy regardless of their infectious status and type of exposure (i.e., exposure through mosquito bites, unprotected sexual intercourse or other). Details regarding participating countries can be found in Annex 1; participating centres have at least one contributing authors in the present paper. All pregnant women exposed to ZIKV at any stage of gestation or prior to gestation were eligible for inclusion in this multicentre study. Exclusion criteria were age <18 years and the inability to consent due to inadequate comprehension of the study purposes. Oral and written information available in English, French, Spanish, Italian and German were provided by the investigators at each centre and oral or written consent obtained. Pregnant women enrolled in the International Zika in Pregnancy registry with an unreported type of exposure or who had not travelled but were exposed through potential sexual transmission were excluded from this analysis. Pregnant women with unreported follow-up after 14 weeks gestation (WG) were also excluded.

Deidentified data were prospectively recorded by each centre using the REDCap (Research Electronic Data Capture) electronic data capture tool [9,10]. Details regarding data collection and validation procedures as well as the collected information can be found in Annex 2. At inclusion (i.e., at the time of ZIKV screening), the following data were recorded: socio-demographic characteristics, obstetrical history and ZIKV exposure. Pregnancies were monitored as clinically indicated according to the local recommendations. After delivery, the following data were collected within 4 weeks: results of maternal testing (ZIKV and/or other infectious pathogens), pregnancy outcomes and neonatal outcomes.

The study was approved by both the Swiss Ethical Board (CER-VD-2016-00801) and local Ethical boards from the different participating centres. The study was conducted from January 2016 to July 2019.

2.2. Study Group and Exposure Definition

Pregnant women living in areas with ZIKV circulation (residents) were defined as pregnant women whose pregnancy was monitored or who had stayed >6 months in areas where past or active ZIKV circulation had been described according to the Centers for Disease Control and Prevention (CDC) map [7]. Pregnant travellers were defined as pregnant women whose pregnancy was monitored in areas without past or current ZIKV circulation and who had stayed in the above-mentioned areas 6 months.

2.3. Definition of Outcomes

1. Primary outcome: Absolute risk (%) of maternal ZIKV infection. Exposed women were tested for ZIKV infection according to local recommendations, through serological and molecular testing (RT-PCR). A recent maternal infection was defined by one of the following results: a positive RT-PCR performed either on urine, blood or saliva, or the presence of specific IgM antibodies confirmed by a Plaque reduction neutralization test (PRNT).
2. Secondary outcome: Absolute risk (%) of severe adverse pregnancy outcomes. Foetal and neonatal outcomes were defined as previously described [2,11]. A scoring congenital ZIKV syndrome (CZS) system was created (Table S1). For multiple gestations, the analysis considered the whole pregnancy. Foetal loss was defined as a spontaneous antepartum foetal death > 14 weeks' gestation (WG) (i.e., late miscarriages (14–24 WG) and stillbirths (foetal demise >24 WG). Severe adverse pregnancy outcomes were defined as either [1] severely affected foetuses/new-borns and/or [2] foetal loss.

Among exposed foetuses/new-borns, a congenital ZIKV infection was defined either by ZIKV RNA amplification by RT-PCR from at least one foetal/neonatal specimen (placenta, amniotic fluid, cerebrospinal fluid, urine or blood) or identification of ZIKV specific IgM antibodies in the umbilical cord/neonatal blood or in cerebrospinal fluid.

2.4. Statistical Analysis

Absolute risks and the 95% confidence intervals (95% CIs) were estimated using the binomial Wilson score and compared as risk differences (RD) with the relevant 95% CIs. To assess whether travelling was associated with in increased risk of maternal infection, relative risks (RR) were assessed using multivariate Poisson regression models for dichotomous outcomes with robust variance options to estimate the adjusted RR with 95% CIs while controlling for known potential confounding factors and major discrepancies between the study groups. The following variables were included in the model maternal age, maternal comorbidities, aneuploidy and abnormal antenatal screening (defined as an abnormal serology or and non-invasive prenatal testing (NIPT)/amniocentesis).

Risk factors for maternal infection among pregnant travellers were evaluated in a nested case control study comparing infected pregnant travellers, considered as cases, to non-infected pregnant travellers, taken as controls. Odds ratios were calculated for travelling to South America and the Caribbean Islands compared to other regions (reference group), duration of stay > 2 weeks, > 3 weeks or > 4 weeks compared to those 2 weeks, 3 weeks and 4 weeks, respectively (reference groups) and timing of travel during the epidemic period compared to outside of the epidemic period (reference group). The epidemic period was defined between June 2015 and December 2016, based on the following facts: the first confirmed autochthonous ZIKV case reported in Brazil occurred in early May 2015, the peak of the epidemic in South America occurred during the first half of 2016 [12,13], while in the Caribbean, the epidemic occurred from January 2016 to October 2016 [14]. The end of epidemiological emergency was declared in November 2016.

To better assess the general impact of each risk factor on the risk of maternal infection, we performed a multivariate analysis. Adjusted odds ratios were adjusted for missing values and for significant risk factors identified in the univariate analysis: travelling during the epidemic (yes/no), dichotomized length of stay and dichotomized region of travel. Except when assessing OR associated with travelling to South America, travelling to the Caribbean Islands was used in the model. Similarly, stays > 2 weeks were used in the model except when assessing longer stays. Collinearity between the variables were assessed using pairwise correlation coefficient. The following relations were assessed: length of stay and travelling during the epidemic, length of stay and travelling to the Caribbean Islands, travelling during the epidemic and travelling to the Caribbean Islands.

Analysis were performed using Stata 14 (Stata Corporation, College Station, TX, USA). A P value inferior of 0.05 was considered as statistically significant.

Missing values: Maternal comorbidities were considered as negative if not reported, based on the assumption that severe comorbidities are normally well documented. Missing risk of aneuploidy was estimated based on maternal age [15,16]. Based on the hypothesis of missing variables completely at random (MCAR), multiple imputations were performed to increase the power of comparisons and estimate the risks while taking into account missing data on the length of stay, region of travel and period of travel. As significant heterogeneities exist between national standards for prenatal screening, in particular serologies performed during antenatal care, only abnormal serology results were considered.

Sensitivity analysis: We conducted a sensitivity analysis using a broader definition for the diagnosis of a maternal infection: (1) All possible ZIKV infection was defined by one of the following positive results: a positive RT-PCR performed either in urine, blood or saliva, or the presence of specific IgM antibodies confirmed by the PRNT assay and also included pregnant women with only neutralizing antibodies to ZIKV, identified through PRNT assay, without specific IgM antibodies: (2) An active ZIKV infection was defined by a positive RT-PCR performed either in urine, blood or saliva.

3. Results

From January 2016 to July 2019, 973 pregnant women were enrolled in the registry and a total of 865 patients were included in the final analysis (Figure 1). Socio-demographic characteristics are presented in Table 1.

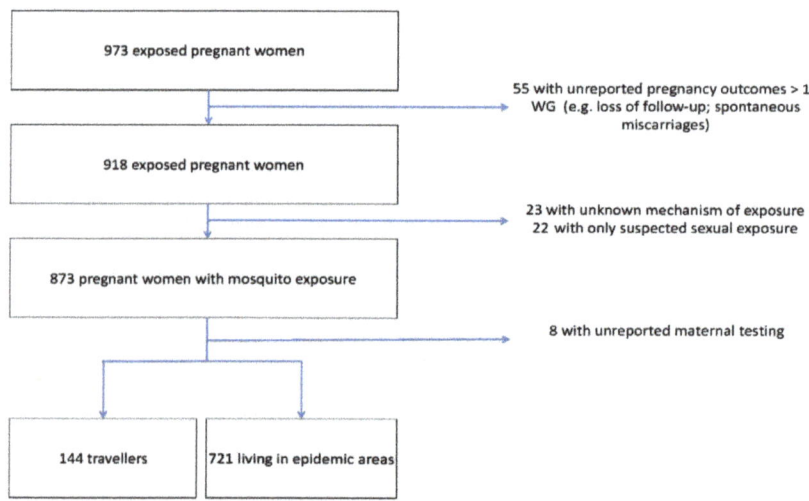

Figure 1. Flow chart. Abbreviations: WG, weeks' gestation; ZIKV, Zika virus.

Table 1. Maternal characteristics within the cohort. Abbreviations: DS, Down syndrome; HTD, Hypertensive disorders; IQR, interquartile range; NIPT, Non-Invasive Prenatal Testing; y.o., years old; ZIKV, Zika Virus.

Socio-Demographic Factors	Pregnant Travellers			Pregnant Women Living in Endemic Areas			
	n = 144			n = 721			
	All Pregnant Travellers	Recent Maternal ZIKV Infection	Negative ZIKV Infection	All Pregnant Women Living in Endemic Areas	Recent Maternal ZIKV Infection	Negative ZIKV Infection	
	n = 144	n = 36	n = 108	n = 721	n = 309	n = 412	
Maternal age							
Median—y.o. (IQR)	31 (27–35)	28.5 (24–31.5)	32 (28–35)	28 (23–34)	27.1 (22.4–32.7)	28.3 (23.6–34.0)	
Age > 35 y.o.—no (%)	38 (26.4)	5 (13.9)	33 (30.6)	193 (26.8)	52 (16.8)	141 (34.2)	
Ethnicity							
Caucasian	29 (20.1)	2 (5.6)	27 (25.0)	1 (0.1)	0 (0.0)	1 (0.2)	
Hispanic or latino-american	47 (32.6)	16 (44.4)	31 (28.7)	644 (89.3)	300 (97.1)	344 (83.5)	
Afro-american	5 (3.5)	0 (0.0)	5 (4.6)	2 (0.3)	0 (0.0)	2 (0.5)	
Asian or Pacific Islands	8 (5.6)	1 (2.8)	7 (6.5)	2 (0.3)	0 (0.0)	2 (0.5)	
Other	3 (2.1)	0 (0.0)	3 (2.8)	0 (0.0)	0 (0.0)	0 (0.0)	
Unknown	52 (36.1)	17 (47.2)	35 (32.4)	72 (10.0)	9 (2.9)	63 (15.3)	
Previous pregnancies—no (IQR)							
Nulliparous—no (%)	76 (52.8)	18 (50.0)	58 (53.7)	307 (42.6)	105 (34.0)	202 (49.0)	
Multiparous	68 (47.2)	18 (50.0)	50 (46.3)	414 (57.4)	204 (66.0)	210 (51.0)	
Multiparous ≥ 3	5 (3.5)	2 (5.6)	3 (2.8)	296 (41.1)	141 (45.6)	155 (37.6)	
Previous adverse pregnancy outcomes—no (%)							
Stillbirths	11 (7.6)	0 (0.0)	11 (10.2)	27 (3.8)	10 (3.2)	17 (4.1)	
Spontaneous abortions	44 (30.6)	11 (30.6)	33 (30.6)	147 (20.4)	45 (14.6)	102 (24.8)	
Maternal comorbidities—no (%)							
All maternal comorbidities	50 (34.7)	10 (27.8)	40 (37.0)	292 (40.5)	125 (40.4)	167 (40.5)	
Diabetes (previous or gestational)							
Previous	1 (0.7)	0 (0.0)	1 (0.9)	7 (1)	3 (1.0)	4 (1.0)	
Gestational	6 (4.2)	1 (2.8)	5 (4.6)	29 (4.0)	11 (3.6)	18 (4.4)	
unknown	45 (31.3)	20 (55.6)	25 (23.1)	80 (11.1)	17 (5.5)	63 (1.5)	
Thyroid dysfunction							
Hypothyroidism	7 (4.9)	1 (2.8)	6 (5.6)	3 (0.4)	1 (0.3)	2 (0.5)	
Hyperthyroidism	0 (0.0)	0 (0.0)	0 (0.0)	0 (0.0)	0 (0.0)	0 (0.0)	
Unknown	56 (38.9)	20 (55.6)	36 (33.3)	693 (96.1)	293 (94.8)	400 (97.1)	

Table 1. Cont.

Socio-Demographic Factors		Pregnant Travellers		Pregnant Women Living in Endemic Areas	
Vascular pathologies					
	Pre-existing HTA	1 (0.7)	1 (2.8)	0 (0.0)	9 (1.3)	5 (1.6)	4 (1.0)
	Gestational/pre-eclampsia	3 (2.1)	0 (0.0)	7 (6.5)	34 (4.7)	17 (5.5)	17 (4.1)
	Unknown	15 (10.4)	10 (27.8)	5 (4.6)	12 (1.7)	10 (3.2)	2 (0.5)
Drugs					
	Cigarettes	6 (4.2)	0 (0.0)	6 (5.6)	1 (0.1)	0 (0.0)	1 (0.2)
	Alcool	5 (3.5)	0 (0.0)	5 (4.6)	12 (1.7)	6 (1.9)	6 (1.5)
	Unknown	48 (33.3)	20 (55.6)	28 (25.9)	81 (11.2)	18 (5.8)	63 (1.5)
Antenatal screening					
Aneuploidy screening					
	Risk of T21 > 1/1000	6 (4.2)	1 (2.8)	5 (4.6)	108 (15.0)	26 (8.4)	82 (19.9)
	Unknown T21 risk	82 (56.8)	29 (80.6)	53 (49.1)	273 (37.9)	146 (47.3)	127 (30.8)
Genetic screening (NIPT/Amniocentesis)					
	Abnormal	1 (0.7)	0 (0)	1 (0.9)	1 (0.1)	1 (0.3)	0 (0)
Serologies screening					
	Abnormal	0 (0)	0 (0)	0 (0)	3 (0.4)	0 (0)	3 (0.7)

3.1. Risk of Maternal ZIKV Infection

3.1.1. Absolute and Relative Risk (RR) of Maternal Infection among Pregnant Travellers Compared to Pregnant Residents

The risk of maternal infection was significantly lower among travellers compared to residents 25.0% ($n = 36/144$) versus 42.9% ($n = 309/721$); crude RR 0.6, 95% CI 0.4–0.8; this remained significant after adjustment for potential confounding factors aRR 0.6, 95% CI 0.4–0.8 (Table 2). Among infected pregnant women, 61.1% ($n = 22/36$) of travellers presented with symptoms compatible with a ZIKV infection compared to 19.4% ($n = 60/309$) of residents (Table 2).

Table 2. Risk of maternal infection. Abbreviations: aRR, adjusted risk ratio; CI; Confidence interval; RD, Risk difference; RR, Risk ratio; ZIKV, Zika virus. * adjusted for missing values length of stay, region of travel and travelling during the epidemic.

	Pregnant Travellers $n = 144$		Pregnant Residents $n = 721$		RD (95% CI)	Crude RR (95% CI)	p Value	aRR (95% CI)	p Value
	n (%)	95% CI	n (%)	95% CI					
Maternal infection									
Recent Maternal infection	36 (25.0)	18.2–32.9	309 (42.9)	39.2–46.6	17.9 (25.8–1.0)	0.6 (0.4–0.8)	0.0001	0.6 (0.4–0.8)	0.0001
Symptomatic infection	22 (61.1)	43.5–76.9	60 (19.4)	15.2–24.3	41.7 (25.2–58.2)	3.1 (2.2–4.4)	<0.0001	3.0 (2.1–4.3)	<0.0001

* adjusted for maternal age (>35 y.o. cat), maternal comorbidities (yes/no), risk of aneuploidy (yes/no) and abnormal prenatal screening (yes/no).

In a sensitivity analysis accounting for different definitions for maternal ZIKV infection, the risk of all possible ZIKV infection remained significantly lower among travellers compared to residents 36.8% ($n = 53/144$) versus 48.1% ($n = 347/721$); RD 11.3%, 95% CI 2.6%–20.0%; crude RR 0.8, 95% CI 0.6–0.9; aRR 0.8, 95% CI 0.6–0.9. When considering active ZIKV infections, there was no difference between travellers compared to residents 16.3% ($n = 14/86$) versus 10.7% (9/84); RD 5.6%, 95% CI 4.7%–15.8%; crude RR 1.5, 95% CI 0.7–3.3; aRR 1.4, 95% CI 0.6–3.3). This subgroup was small, given RT-PCR results were only available for 11.6% of residents ($n = 84/721$) compared to 59.7% of travellers ($n = 86/144$).

3.1.2. Risk Factors for Maternal Infection among Pregnant Travelers

We performed a nested case control study to evaluate potential risk factors for maternal infections (Table 3). Travelling during the epidemic [crude OR 46.4, 95% CI 7.0–1916.5] and travelling to the Caribbean islands compared to other regions [crude OR 5.0, 95% CI 2.0–12.6] were associated with an increased risk of maternal infection. Similarly, a duration of stay >2 weeks [crude OR 12.8, 95% CI 1.9–541.3] and a duration of stay > 3 weeks [crude OR 2.9, 95% CI 1.0–8.9] compared to those $\leq$ 2 weeks or $\leq$ 3 weeks, respectively, were both associated with an increased risk for maternal infection. Similar findings were also observed when considering all possible ZIKV infections or active ZIKV infections, except that a duration of stay > 4 weeks compared to those $\leq$ 4 weeks was also associated with an increased risk of possible ZIKV infections.

Table 3. Risk factors for maternal infection among pregnant travellers. Abbreviations: aOR, adjusted odds ratio; CI, Confidence interval; OR, Odds Ratio; ZIKV, Zika virus; n.a., not applicable; * adjusted for missing values "length of stay", "region of travel" and "travelling during the epidemic".

Exposition	Pregnant Travellers							
	Recent Maternal ZIKV Infection n = 36		Negative Maternal ZIKV Infection n = 108		Crude OR (95% CI)	p Value	aOR (95% CI)	p Value
	n (%)	95% CI	n (%)	95% CI				
Region of travelling								
Known								
South America	35 (97.2)	85.8–99.5	102 (94.4)	88.4–97.4				
Carribean	11 (31.4)	18.6–48.0	46 (45.1)	35.8–54.8	0.6 (0.2–1.4)	0.1705	0.4 (0.2–1.1)	0.087
South East Asia	24 (68.6)	52.0–81.4	31 (30.4)	22.3–39.8	5.0 (2.0–12.6)	0.0001	3.2 (1.2–8.7)	0.023
Africa	0 (0)	0–9.8	12 (11.8)	6.9–19.4				
Other	0 (0)	0–9.8	7 (6.9)	3.4–13.5				
	0 (0)	0–9.8	6 (5.9)	2.7–12.2				
Unknown	1 (2.8)	0.5–14.2	6 (5.6)	2.6–11.6				
Length of stay								
Known								
≤2 weeks	27 (75.0)	58.9–86.2	91 (84.3)	76.3–89.9				
≤3 weeks	1 (3.7)	6.5–18.3	30 (33.0)	24.2–43.1	12.8 (1.9–541.3)	0.0021	8.7 (1.1–71.5)	0.0041
≤4 weeks	7 (25.9)	13.2–44.7	46 (50.6)	40.5–60.6	2.9 (1.0–8.9)	0.0284	1.5 (0.5–4.5)	0.471
>4 weeks	12 (44.4)	27.6–62.7	51 (56.0)	45.8–65.8	1.6 (0.6–4.2)	0.3801	0.8 (0.3–2.3)	0.752
	15 (55.6)	37.3–72.4	40 (44.0)	34.2–54.2				
Unknown	9 (25.0)	13.8–41.0	17 (15.7)	10.1–23.8				
Period of exposure								
Known	34 (94.4)	81.9–98.5	101 (93.5)	87.2–96.8				
During the epidemic peak	33 (97.1)	85.1–99.5	42 (41.6)	32.5–51.3	46.4 (7.0–1916.5)	<0.0001	29.4 (3.7–228.1)	0.001
July–Dec 2015	1 (3.0)	0.5–15.3	1 (2.3)	0.4–12.3				
Jan–June 2016	25 (75.8)	59.0–87.2	20 (47.6)	33.4–62.3				
July–Dec 2016	7 (21.2)	10.7–37.8	21 (50.0)	35.5–64.5				
Outside of the epidemic peak	1 (2.9)	0.5–14.9	59 (58.4)	48.7–67.5				
Prior to June 2015	0 (0)	n.a.	1 (1.7)	0.3–9.0				
2017	1 (100)	n.a.	55 (93.2)	83.8–97.3				
2018	0 (0)	n.a.	3 (5.1)	1.7–13.9				
Unknown	2 (5.6)	1.5–18.1	7 (6.5)	3.2–12.8				
Use of mosquitoes' repellent								
Known	10 (27.8)	15.8–44.0	52 (48.1)	39.0–57.5				
Use of repellent	8 (80.0)	49.0–94.3	28 (53.8)	40.5–66.6	3.5 (0.6–35.5)	0.1705	1.1 (0.1–7.9)	0.925
Unknown	26 (72.2)	56.0–84.2	56 (51.9)	42.5–61.0				

* adjusted for missing values length of stay, region of travel, and travelling during the epidemic.

In a multivariate analysis accounting for missing values through multiple imputation, travelling during the epidemic period, travelling to the Caribbean Islands and a duration of stay > 2 weeks were independently associated with the risk of maternal infection [aOR 29.4, 95% CI 3.7–228.1 for travelling during the epidemic period, aOR 3.2, 95% CI 1.2–8.7 for travelling to the Caribbean Islands and aOR 8.7, 95% CI 1.1–71.5 for stays abroad >2 weeks, respectively] when compared to travelling outside of the epidemic, to other regions or stays ≤ 2 weeks, respectively (Table 3). In contrast, a duration of stay >3 weeks compared to ≤ 3 weeks was not associated with a significant increased risk of maternal infection [aOR 1.5, 95% CI 0.5–4.5] (Table 3). When considering all possible ZIKV infection, these associations remained significant. In addition, a duration of stay >3 weeks was also associated with an increased risk of possible ZIKV maternal infections when compared to ≤3 weeks [aOR 3.5, 95% CI 1.2–10.0], but a duration of stay >4 weeks was not associated with an increased risk compared to ≤ 4 weeks [aOR 1.9, 95% CI 0.7–5.1]. Active ZIKV infections were not tested because the sample size was considered too limited.

3.2. Risk of Adverse Pregnancy Outcomes

3.2.1. Absolute and Relative Risk for Adverse Pregnancy Outcomes among Exposed Pregnant Travellers Compared to Pregnant Residents

Overall, the risk of severe adverse pregnancy outcomes within the cohort was 7.8% (n = 67/865), including 8.3% (n = 3/36) among travellers and 12.7% (n = 39/309) among residents. (Table 4). Asymptomatic new-borns were more frequently observed among travellers with a recent maternal ZIKV infection compared to infected residents [91.7% (n = 33/36) *versus* 76.7% (n = 237/309)] (Table 4).

Table 4. Adverse pregnancy outcomes among infected pregnant travellers compared to infected pregnant residents. Abbreviations: CI; Confidence interval; ZIKV, Zika virus.

	Positive Recent Maternal ZIKV Infection			
	Pregnant Travellers n = 36		Pregnant Residents n = 309	
	n (%)	95% CI	n (%)	95% CI
Foetal/Neonatal outcomes				
Asymptomatic	33 (91.7)	78.2–97.1	237 (76.7)	71.7–81.1
Severe adverse pregnancy outcomes	3 (8.3)	2.9–21.8	39 (12.6)	9.4–16.8
Foetal/neonatal testing				
Known	23 (63.9)	47.6–77.5	293 (94.8)	91.7–96.8
Positive	5 (21.7)	9.7–41.0	76 (25.9)	21.3–31.2
Negative	18 (78.3)	58.1–90.3	217 (70.2)	64.9–75.1
Unknown	13 (36.1)	22.5–52.4	16 (5.2)	3.2–8.2

Results of foetal/neonatal testing were available in 20.1% (n = 29/144) of travellers and 87.8% residents (n = 633/721). A congenital infection was confirmed in 17.2% [(n = 5/29), 95% CI 7.6%–34.5%)] of foetuses/new-borns among travellers with available testing and 12.2% [(n = 77/633), 95% CI 9.8%–14.9%] among residents (Supplementary Table S2). Interestingly, one confirmed congenital infection among residents occurred in a woman with negative ZIKV testing. This woman was identified to be IgG positive with positive PRNT testing and was therefore considered as a possible ZIKV infection. The new-born was asymptomatic at birth and specific IgM antibodies were detected. Among infected pregnant women, materno-foetal transmission rate was 21.7% (n = 5/23) among travellers and 25.9% (n = 76/293) among residents (Table 4).

3.2.2. Absolute Risk of Adverse Pregnancy Outcomes among Infected Travellers Compared to Non-Infected Pregnant Travellers

Adverse pregnancy outcomes were observed in 8.3% (n = 3/36) of infected travellers *versus* 3.7% (4/108) among non-infected travellers. Findings of cases with severe adverse pregnancy outcomes among travellers are presented in Table 5. Of five cases with a confirmed foetal infection (Supplementary Tables S2 and S3), three cases had severe adverse pregnancy outcomes. All women with severe adverse pregnancy outcomes were exposed during the first trimester of pregnancy and had travelled more than 2 weeks, during the recent epidemic; of note, two patients experienced symptoms. Among negative mothers, four severe adverse pregnancy outcomes were recorded, one of which occurred in a mother with a *possible ZIKV infection* (Supplementary Table S3). The new-born presented with isolated macular anomalies; he was unfortunately not tested for ZIKV infection.

Table 5. Adverse pregnancy outcomes among infected pregnant travellers compared to non-infected pregnant travellers within a nested case-control study. The risk of severe adverse pregnancy outcomes associated with a recent maternal ZIKV infection among pregnant travellers was evaluated in a nested case control study comparing infected pregnant travellers, considered as cases, to non-infected pregnant travellers, taken as controls. Abbreviations: ZIKV, Zika virus.

	Travellers			
	Positive Recent Maternal ZIKV Infection *n* = 36		Negative Recent Maternal ZIKV Infection *n* = 108	
	n (%)	95% CI	*n* (%)	95% CI
Foetal/Neonatal outcomes				
Asymptomatic	33 (91.7)	78.2–97.1	103 (95.4)	89.6–98.0
Severe adverse pregnancy outcomes	3 (8.3)	2.9–21.8	4 (3.7)	1.4–9.1
Foetal/neonatal testing				
Known	23 (63.9)	47.6–77.5	6 (5.6)	2.6–11.6
Positive	5 (21.7)	9.7–41.0	0 (0.0)	n.a.
Negative	18 (78.3)	58.1–90.3	6 (100.0)	61.0–100.0
Unknown	13 (36.1)	22.5–52.4	102 (94.4)	88.4–97.4

4. Discussion

We present here the first prospective study assessing the risks of maternal ZIKV infection and adverse pregnancy outcomes among travellers compared to residents. The absolute risk of maternal infection was significantly lower for travellers, with a 25% absolute risk over the study period. Importantly, the risk of maternal infection was related to the presence of an ongoing outbreak and the length of stay abroad, as well as the region of travel. Although the numbers were low limiting the generalization of the result, when considering only pregnant travellers that travelled outside the epidemic period or less than 2 weeks, the risk was reduced to 1.7% (1/60) and 3.2% (1/31), respectively. No maternal infections were recorded among pregnant travellers outside the epidemic period and with a length of stay abroad less than two weeks.

Two studies performed in Spain in 2016-2017 observed an incidence of recent/confirmed maternal infection of 1.3% (14/1057) [17] and 3.5% (9/254), respectively [18], while during the 2009–2018 period, Norman et al. observed a 3.8% incidence of arboviral infections among 861 returning travellers, of which 12% were caused by ZIKV [19]. The higher proportion of maternal infection in our study might be related to the inclusion of a majority of women exposed during the recent epidemic and a high detection rate, as all patients were tested. Interestingly, Norman et al. found no association with the length of stay. In their study, most patients had a length of stay > 2 weeks with a median length of stay of 23 days (interquartile range 15 to 55 days) [19]. Travelling to the Caribbean Islands was associated with an increased risk of maternal infection. This association might be explained by the relative homogeneity of the Caribbean region in terms of factors contributing to the cycle of ZIKV vectoral transmission (i.e., climate and Aedes spp. distribution, population densities) compared to South America, where significant socio-ecological variations are observed. As such, the incidence of ZIKV infections in Brazil between 2015–2016 was highly variable depending on the region, with the southern parts of the country, including urban areas of Sao Paulo, being spared [1].

We observed an incidence of severe adverse pregnancy outcomes similar to what has been reported previously. In the US territories, the incidence of severe foetal/neonatal anomalies observed among infected patients ranged from 4% to 8% depending on the gestational trimester of suspected maternal infection [3], while in the Caribbean region, severe adverse outcomes were reported in 8.1% of foetuses [20]. This highlights that the majority of exposed foetuses (>90%) will remain asymptomatic or pauci-symptomatic, even in the case of a confirmed foetal infection [2].

Our study has limitations. First, the diagnosis of a recent ZIKV infection is challenging. We used criteria based on both nucleic acid amplification testing (NAAT) and serology. NAAT are limited by the transient character of the ZIKV viremia [21]. On the other hand, serology is poorly reliable, especially in secondary flavivirus infections. Re-infections are associated with cross-reactions of both specific IgM and neutralizing antibodies. Moreover, secondary stimulations may suppress the production of specific antibodies [22]. In that context, a negative IgM testing does not necessarily exclude a recent infection, as observed in two of our cases, in which congenital ZIKV infection was confirmed by the identification of specific IgM in one of the new-borns, while in the other, severe macular anomalies compatible with ZIKV were observed. To overcome this limitation, we performed a sensitivity analysis including different definitions of exposure, possible ZIKV infections versus active infections (positive viremia). The first strategy supported our findings, while risk estimates using the active infection definition lost their statistical significance owing to the small sample size. These aspects further highlight the difficulties related to the diagnosis of ZIKV infection in pregnant women and further argue against routine screening of exposed women [1].

Second, our study is limited by the small number of cases with adverse pregnancy outcomes among travellers. Though, it allowed us to correctly assess risk factors for maternal infection, our study was not powered to detect differences in pregnancy outcomes between infected and non-infected pregnant travellers and to assess potential contributing factors (e.g., timing of maternal infection, persistent viremia). Furthermore, our study did not assess long term outcomes among new-borns, which may lead to an underestimation of the consequences of congenital infection. In addition, we were not able to capture miscarriages in a systematic way. To avoid underreporting or misclassification, we excluded all pregnant women with unreported outcomes after 14WG. This might have underestimated the rate of adverse outcomes related to ZIKV infection in early pregnancy. Exact rates of miscarriage are difficult to assess, due to the high frequency of unreported early-stage pregnancy loss and might be as high as 30 to 40 % [23]. As to whether maternal ZIKV infection increases this risk remains unclear.

Finally, our study is based on a registry and not systematic sampling. As such, we observed an overrepresentation of symptomatic women among travellers, as asymptomatic women may not have sought medical care. Nevertheless, as symptoms have not been correlated to worse foetal outcomes, the impact of this bias on our results seems limited. Furthermore, although we develop a user-friendly system to collect data in a systematic way, as with all observational studies missing data are inevitable. To account for this we performed multiple imputations, allowing us an acceptable evaluation.

Our study focused on pregnant women. Nevertheless, we believe that our conclusions may be extended to young couples trying to conceive. Although, we did not assess the risks associated with sexual transmission, the probability for a male to subsequently infect his partner is related to his initial risk of infection. Several agencies, including the WHO, CDC and National Travel Health Network and Centre (NaTHNaC) recommend waiting 2 months for women and 3 months for men before getting pregnant after travelling to areas with both current and past outbreaks [6,7,24]. These recommendations might be overly cautious. Based on the present finding of relatively low risk, it seems reasonable not to advise any delay for patients travelling to areas without any current outbreaks who are staying 2 weeks; as supported by the Swiss public health institute [25]. Precaution to avoid mosquitoes bites should nevertheless be strictly applied. Furthermore, recommendations for travelling pregnant women should also take into additional exposure to other infections pathogens. Most areas with ZIKV circulation are also endemic for DENV, CHIKV or malaria. Growing evidence suggests a negative impact of DENV and CHIKV on pregnant women and their offspring [26,27], while Malaria remains a major cause of stillbirth in endemic countries [28].

5. Conclusions

We provided a reliable assessment of the risks of maternal ZIKV infection and associated risk of adverse pregnancy outcomes among travellers. Our findings suggest the risk of maternal infection among travellers is lower to what is observed for pregnant residents. The specific risk of maternal infection for travellers is related to the presence of ongoing outbreaks and stay duration, with stays < 2 weeks associated with a low risk in the absence of ongoing outbreaks.

Supplementary Materials: The following are available online at https://www.mdpi.com/1999-4915/13/2/341/s1, Table S1: Criteria used to diagnose the severity of congenital Zika virus, Table S2: Adverse pregnancy outcomes according to results of foetal/neonatal ZIKV testing among pregnant travellers compared to pregnant residents, Table S3: Description of pregnant travellers presenting with severe adverse pregnancy outcomes.

Author Contributions: M.V., L.P., P.G., D.B. and A.P. conceived and designed the study. L.P., D.B., M.V. and A.P. interpreted the results. L.P., A.S.-A., C.R., A.G., E.G., A.M., I.E., B.M.D.T., B.E., S.M., L.R., B.G., T.V.M., V.L., D.M. and D.B. provided care to the mothers and collected the data. M.V. and A.P. wrote the first version of the report and did the literature review. All authors have read and agreed to the published version of the manuscript.

Funding: This research received no external funding.

Institutional Review Board Statement: The study was conducted according to the guidelines of the Declaration of Helsinki, and approved by both the Swiss Ethical Board (CER-VD-2016-00801) and local Ethical boards from the different participating centres.

Informed Consent Statement: Informed consent was obtained from all subjects involved in the study.

Data Availability Statement: The data presented in this study are available on request from the corresponding author.

Acknowledgments: We gratefully thank all of the clinical staff and research members that participated in the Zika registry by taking care of the patients and filling the data in the registry.

Conflicts of Interest: The authors declare no conflict of interest.

Abbreviations

aOR	adjusted odds ratio
aRR	adjusted risk ratio
CI	Confidence interval
CHIKV	Chikungunya virus
CZS	congenital ZIKV syndrome
DENV	Dengue virus
DS	Down syndrome
HTD	Hypertensive disorders
IQR	interquartile range
MCAR	missing variables completely at random
NAAT	nucleic acid amplification testing
NIPT	non-invasive prenatal testing
OR	odds ratio
PRNT	Plaque reduction neutralization test
RD	Risk difference
RR	Risk ratio
WG	Weeks' gestation
y.o.	years old
ZIKV	Zika virus

References

1. Musso, D.; Ko, A.I.; Baud, D. Zika Virus Infection—After the Pandemic. *N. Engl. J. Med.* **2019**, *381*, 1444–1457. [CrossRef] [PubMed]
2. Pomar, L.; Vouga, M.; Lambert, V.; Pomar, C.; Hcini, N.; Jolivet, A.; Benoist, G.; Rousset, D.; Matheus, S.; Malinger, G.; et al. Maternal-fetal transmission and adverse perinatal outcomes in pregnant women infected with Zika virus: Prospective cohort study in French Guiana. *BMJ* **2018**, *363*, k4431. [CrossRef]
3. Shapiro-Mendoza, C.K.; Rice, M.E.; Galang, R.R.; Fulton, A.C.; VanMaldeghem, K.; Prado, M.V.; Ellis, E.; Anesi, M.S.; Simeone, R.M.; Petersen, E.E.; et al. Pregnancy Outcomes After Maternal Zika Virus Infection During Pregnancy-U.S. Territories, January 1, 2016-April 25, 2017. *MMWR Morb. Mortal. Wkly. Rep.* **2017**, *66*, 615–621. [CrossRef] [PubMed]
4. Honein, M.A.; Dawson, A.L.; Petersen, E.E.; Jones, A.M.; Lee, E.H.; Yazdy, M.M.; Ahmad, N.; Macdonald, J.; Evert, N.; Bingham, A.; et al. Birth Defects Among Fetuses and Infants of US Women with Evidence of Possible Zika Virus Infection During Pregnancy. *JAMA* **2017**, *317*, 59–68. [CrossRef]
5. Biswas, A.; Kodan, P.; Gupta, N.; Soneja, M.; Baruah, K.; Sharma, K.K.; Meena, S. Zika outbreak in India in 2018. *J. Travel Med.* **2020**, *27*, taaa001. Available online: https://academic.oup.com/jtm/advance-article/doi/10.1093/jtm/taaa001/5733644 (accessed on 2 April 2020). [CrossRef] [PubMed]
6. WHO. WHO Guidelines for the Prevention of Sexual Transmission of Zika Virus: Executive Summary. 2019. Available online: https://apps.who.int/iris/bitstream/handle/10665/311026/WHO-RHR-19.4-eng.pdf?ua=1 (accessed on 5 June 2019).
7. Centers for Disease Control and Prevention. Zika Travel Information. Available online: https://wwwnc.cdc.gov/travel/page/zika-information (accessed on 11 February 2020).
8. Panchaud, A.; Vouga, M.; Musso, D.; Baud, D. An international registry for women exposed to Zika virus during pregnancy: Time for answers. *Lancet Infect. Dis.* **2016**, *16*, 995–996. [CrossRef]
9. Harris, P.A.; Taylor, R.; Thielke, R.; Payne, J.; Gonzalez, N.; Conde, J.G. Research electronic data capture (REDCap)—A metadata-driven methodology and workflow process for providing translational research informatics support. *J. Biomed. Inform.* **2009**, *42*, 377–381. [CrossRef]
10. Harris, P.A.; Taylor, R.; Minor, B.L.; Elliott, V.; Fernandez, M.; O'Neal, L.; McLeod, L.; Delacqua, G.; Delacqua, F.; Kirby, J.; et al. The REDCap consortium: Building an international community of software platform partners. *J. Biomed. Inform.* **2019**, *95*, 103208. [CrossRef]
11. Pomar, L.; Musso, D.; Malinger, G.; Vouga, M.; Panchaud, A.; Baud, D. Zika virus during pregnancy: From maternal exposure to congenital Zika virus syndrome. *Prenat. Diagn.* **2019**, *39*, 420–430. [CrossRef] [PubMed]
12. World Health Organization. ZIKA EPIDEMIOLOGY UPDATE. 2019 July. Available online: https://www.who.int/emergencies/diseases/zika/zika-epidemiology-update-july-2019.pdf?ua=1 (accessed on 21 February 2021).
13. Pan American Health Organization/World Health Organization. Timeline of Emergence of Zika virus in the Americas. 2016 Apr. Available online: https://www.paho.org/hq/index.php?option=com_content&view=article&id=11959:timeline-of-emergence-of-zika-virus-in-the-americas&Itemid=41711&lang=en (accessed on 21 February 2021).
14. Cire Antilles Guyane. Surveillance du virus Zika aux Antilles Guyane, Situation épidémiologique, Point au 10 Novembre 2016. Santé Publique France. 2016. Available online: http://invs.santepubliquefrance.fr/fr/Publications-et-outils/Points-epidemiologiques/Tous-les-numeros/Antilles-Guyane/2016/Situation-epidemiologique-du-virus-Zika-aux-Antilles-Guyane.-Point-au-10-novembre-2016 (accessed on 17 January 2017).
15. Hook, E.B.; Cross, P.K.; Schreinemachers, D.M. Chromosomal abnormality rates at amniocentesis and in live-born infants. *JAMA* **1983**, *249*, 2034–2038. [CrossRef]
16. Hartwig, T.S.; Sørensen, S.; Jørgensen, F.S. The maternal age-related first trimester risks for trisomy 21, 18 and 13 based on Danish first trimester data from 2005 to 2014. *Prenat. Diagn.* **2016**, *36*, 643–649. [CrossRef]
17. Sulleiro, E.; Rando, A.; Alejo, I.; Suy, A.; Gonce, A.; Rodó, C.; Torner, N.; Bardají, A.; Fumadó, V.; Soriano-Arandes, A.; et al. Screening for Zika virus infection in 1057 potentially exposed pregnant women, Catalonia (northeastern Spain). *Travel Med. Infect. Dis.* **2019**, *29*, 69–71. [CrossRef] [PubMed]
18. Rodó, C.; Suy, A.; Sulleiro, E.; Soriano-Arandes, A.; Maiz, N.; García-Ruiz, I.; Arévalo, S.; Rando, A.; Anton, A.; Vázquez Méndez, É.; et al. Pregnancy outcomes after maternal Zika virus infection in a non-endemic region: Prospective cohort study. *Clin. Microbiol. Infect.* **2019**, *25*, 633.e5–633.e9. [CrossRef]
19. Norman, F.F.; Henríquez-Camacho, C.; Díaz-Menendez, M.; Chamorro, S.; Pou, D.; Molina, I.; Goikoetxea, J.; Rodríguez-Guardado, A.; Calabuig, E.; Crespillo, C.; et al. Imported Arbovirus Infections in Spain, 2009–2018. *Emerg. Infect. Dis.* **2020**, *26*, 658–666. [CrossRef] [PubMed]
20. Hoen, B.; Schaub, B.; Funk, A.L.; Ardillon, V.; Boullard, M.; Cabié, A.; Callier, C.; Carles, G.; Cassadou, S.; Césaire, R.; et al. Pregnancy Outcomes after ZIKV Infection in French Territories in the Americas. *N. Engl. J. Med.* **2018**, *378*, 985–994. [CrossRef]
21. Landry, M.L.; George, K.S. Laboratory Diagnosis of Zika Virus Infection. *Arch. Pathol. Lab. Med.* **2016**, *141*, 60–67. [CrossRef]
22. Barzon, L.; Pacenti, M.; Franchin, E.; Lavezzo, E.; Trevisan, M.; Sgarabotto, D.; Palù, G. Infection dynamics in a traveller with persistent shedding of Zika virus RNA in semen for six months after returning from Haiti to Italy, January 2016. *Eurosurveillance* **2016**, *21*. [CrossRef]
23. Wilcox, A.J.; Weinberg, C.R.; O'Connor, J.F.; Baird, D.D.; Schlatterer, J.P.; Canfield, R.E.; Armstrong, E.G.; Nisula, B.C. Incidence of Early Loss of Pregnancy. *N. Engl. J. Med.* **1988**, *319*, 189–194. [CrossRef]

24. NaTHNaC. Zika—Risk Assessment. Available online: https://travelhealthpro.org.uk/factsheet/5/zika--risk-assessment (accessed on 27 February 2019).
25. Swiss Tropical and Public Health Institue. Zika Virus Information and Recommendations of the Swiss Expert Committee for Travel Medicine (ECTM)* (Update April 2019). 23 April 2019. Available online: https://www.swisstph.ch/en/travelclinic/zika-info/ (accessed on 5 June 2019).
26. Vouga, M.; Chiu, Y.-C.; Pomar, L.; De Meyer, S.V.; Masmejan, S.; Genton, B.; Musso, D.; Baud, D.; Stojanov, M. Dengue, Zika and chikungunya during pregnancy: Pre- and post-travel advice and clinical management. *J. Travel Med.* **2019**, *26*. [CrossRef] [PubMed]
27. Paixao, E.S.; Harron, K.; Campbell, O.; Teixeira, M.G.; Costa, M.D.C.N.; Barreto, M.L.; Rodrigues, L.C. Dengue in pregnancy and maternal mortality: A cohort analysis using routine data. *Sci. Rep.* **2018**, *8*, 1–6. [CrossRef] [PubMed]
28. Desai, M.; O ter Kuile, F.; Nosten, F.; McGready, R.; Asamoa, K.; Brabin, B.; Newman, R.D. Epidemiology and burden of malaria in pregnancy. *Lancet Infect. Dis.* **2007**, *7*, 93–104. [CrossRef]

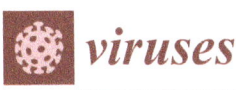

Article

Embryonic Stage of Congenital Zika Virus Infection Determines Fetal and Postnatal Outcomes in Mice

Eri Nakayama [1,*], Yasuhiro Kawai [2,†], Satoshi Taniguchi [1,†], Jessamine E. Hazlewood [3,†], Ken-ichi Shibasaki [1], Kenta Takahashi [4], Yuko Sato [4], Bing Tang [3], Kexin Yan [3], Naoko Katsuta [1], Shigeru Tajima [1], Chang Kweng Lim [1], Tadaki Suzuki [4], Andreas Suhrbier [3] and Masayuki Saijo [1]

1 Department of Virology I, National Institute of Infectious Diseases, Tokyo 162-8640, Japan; rei-tani@nih.go.jp (S.T.); shi-k@nih.go.jp (K.-i.S.); nkatsuta@nih.go.jp (N.K.); stajima@nih.go.jp (S.T.); ck@nih.go.jp (C.K.L.); msaijo@nih.go.jp (M.S.)
2 Management Department of Biosafety and Laboratory Animal, Division of Biosafety Control and Research, National Institute of Infectious Diseases, Tokyo 162-8640, Japan; kaya@nih.go.jp
3 Inflammation Biology Group, QIMR Berghofer Medical Research Institute, Brisbane, QLD 4029, Australia; Jessamine.Hazlewood@qimrberghofer.edu.au (J.E.H.); Bing.Tang@qimrberghofer.edu.au (B.T.); Kexin.Yan@qimrberghofer.edu.au (K.Y.); Andreas.Suhrbier@qimrberghofer.edu.au (A.S.)
4 Department of Pathology, National Institute of Infectious Diseases, Tokyo 162-8640, Japan; tkenta@niid.go.jp (K.T.); kiyonaga@nih.go.jp (Y.S.); tksuzuki@niid.go.jp (T.S.)
* Correspondence: nakayama@nih.go.jp; Tel.: +81-3-5285-1111
† These authors contributed equally to the work and should be considered as second authors.

Abstract: Zika virus (ZIKV) infection during pregnancy causes a wide spectrum of congenital abnormalities and postnatal developmental sequelae such as fetal loss, intrauterine growth restriction (IUGR), microcephaly, or motor and neurodevelopmental disorders. Here, we investigated whether a mouse pregnancy model recapitulated a wide range of symptoms after congenital ZIKV infection, and whether the embryonic age of congenital infection changed the fetal or postnatal outcomes. Infection with ZIKV strain PRVABC59 from embryonic day 6.5 (E6.5) to E8.5, corresponding to the mid-first trimester in humans, caused fetal death, fetal resorption, or severe IUGR, whereas infection from E9.5 to E14.5, corresponding to the late-first to second trimester in humans, caused stillbirth, neonatal death, microcephaly, and postnatal growth deficiency. Furthermore, 4-week-old offspring born to dams infected at E12.5 showed abnormalities in neuropsychiatric state, motor behavior, autonomic function, or reflex and sensory function. Thus, our model recapitulated the multiple symptoms seen in human cases, and the embryonic age of congenital infection was one of the determinant factors of offspring outcomes in mice. Furthermore, maternal neutralizing antibodies protected the offspring from neonatal death after congenital infection at E9.5, suggesting that neonatal death in our model could serve as criteria for screening of vaccine candidates.

Keywords: Zika virus; congenital Zika syndrome; SHIRPA; microcephaly; sequelae; trimester; mouse model

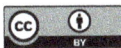

1. Introduction

The World Health Organization declared the outbreak of Zika virus (ZIKV) infection in the American continent as a public health emergency of international concern in 2016. ZIKV causes a spectrum of congenital abnormalities including fetal loss, intrauterine growth restriction (IUGR), neonatal death, and microcephaly, together termed congenital Zika syndrome (CZS), which is likely associated with complex and life-long disabilities in children born to women infected with ZIKV during pregnancy [1–6]. Postnatal developmental sequelae, such as gross motor impairment, delayed neurodevelopment, cognitive impairment, auditory abnormalities, and/or ophthalmological abnormalities have also been recognized after congenital ZIKV infection, [7–16]. Some children who were asymptomatic with normal head circumferences at birth also developed postnatal symptoms [7,8,14,17,18].

CZS or developmental sequelae was recognized regardless of the trimesters in which the pregnant mothers were infected [1,7,18–20], although ZIKV infection in the first trimester has been thought to be a risk factor for severe CZS [21–25]. In line with this, a series of murine pregnancy models have been established [26–37]; however, each model recapitulated only some of the fetal or postnatal symptoms seen in human cases (Supplemental Table S1). Moreover, the embryonic ages of congenital ZIKV infection and inspection of offspring, virus strain, infection dose, or route of infection were not consistent in the mouse models (Supplemental Table S1), and how these differences affect the outcomes remains elusive. In this study, IFNα/β receptor knockout (IFNAR$^{-/-}$) dams that were crossed with wild-type sires were infected subcutaneously (s.c.) with ZIKV at various embryonic days, and a series of fetal and postnatal outcomes were comprehensively evaluated.

2. Materials and Methods

2.1. Ethics Statement

All mouse experiments were conducted in accordance with the Guidelines for Animal Experiments performed at the National Institute of Infectious Diseases (NIID) or the Australian Code for Care and Use of Animals for Scientific Purposes, as outlined by the National Health and Medical Research Council of Australia. Animal experiments were approved by the Animal Welfare and Animal Care Committee of NIID (Ethics numbers: 116123 and 119155) or the QIMR Berghofer Medical Research Institute Animal Ethics Committee (Ethics number: A1604-611M). All mice were bred and housed under specific pathogen-free conditions.

2.2. Cell and Virus Stocks

Vero (strain 9013, JCRB9013, the Japanese Collection of Research Bioresources Cell Bank, Osaka, Japan) and C6/36 cells (CRL1660, the American Type Culture Collection Manassas, VA, USA) were maintained in Eagle's minimum essential medium (MEM) supplemented with 10% fetal bovine serum (FBS) and 100 µg/mL penicillin-streptomycin (Life Technologies, Carlsbad, CA, USA). Vero cells and C6/36 cells were cultured at 37 °C and 28 °C, respectively, in a 5% CO_2 atmosphere. ZIKV strain PRVABC59 (GenBank accession no. KU501215), which was isolated from a patient in Puerto Rico in 2015 [38], was kindly provided by Dr. Beth Bell of the US Center for Disease Control and Prevention. E protein amino acid position 330 of PRVABC59 was a mixture of V and L, as previously reported [39,40]. Natal RGN strain (GenBank accession no. KU527068) was isolated from human fetal autopsy cases with microcephaly in Brazil and prepared as previously described [26,41,42]. ZIKV stocks were tittered by plaque assay on Vero cells, as described previously [43,44].

2.3. Virus Titration

Indicated tissues and serum obtained from the blood of the tail vein were collected at the specified time points and stored at -80 °C until analysis. The tissues were homogenized in MEM containing 2% FBS (2MEM) using a tissue homogenizer and beads (Bio Medical Science, Tokyo, Japan) according to the manufacturer's instructions. The 50% cell culture infective dose ($CCID_{50}$) assays for serum and supernatants from homogenized tissues were performed as described previously [26,40–43,45,46].

2.4. Reverse Transcription Quantitative PCR (qRT-PCR)

qRT-PCR was performed as described previously [40,42,45,46]. Briefly, tissues were placed in RNAlater (Ambion, Austin, TX, USA), and RNA was extracted with TRIzol (Life Technologies, Carlsbad, CA, USA) from homogenized tissues prepared by bead homogenization. cDNA was generated using an iScript cDNA Synthesis Kit (Bio-Rad, Hercules, CA, USA). qPCR was performed using iTaq Universal SYBR Green Supermix (Bio-Rad) and the following primers: ZIKV E-Forward, 5'-CCGCTGCCCAACACAAG-3'; ZIKV E-Reverse, 5'-CCACTAACGTTCTTTTGCAGACAT-3'; ZIKV prM-Forward, TTGGTCAT

GATACTGCTGATTGC-3'; and ZIKV prM-Reverse, 5'-CCTTCCACAAAGTCCCTATTGC-3' [47]. Values were normalized using the housekeeping gene mouse RPL13A (Forward, 5'-GAGGTCGGGTGGAAGTACCA-3'; Reverse, 5'-TGCATCTTGGCCTTTTCCTT-3') [48,49].

2.5. Histology and Immunohistochemistry (IHC)

Tissue samples were fixed in 10% phosphate-buffered formalin, embedded in paraffin, sectioned, and stained with hematoxylin and eosin (H&E). IHC was performed using an anti-ZIKV NS1 antibody (C01886G, Meridian Bioscience, Cincinnati, OH, USA) as the primary antibody [40,43]. Specific antigen-antibody reactions were visualized by 3,3-diaminobenzidine tetrahydrochloride staining using a VECTASTAIN ABC HRP system (Vector Laboratories, Burlingame, CA, USA).

2.6. Mice

IFNAR$^{-/-}$ mice on a C57BL/6J background were bred in-house at NIID [40,43]. Female IFNAR$^{-/-}$ mice (>7 weeks old) were paired with C57BL/6J mice (>8 weeks old) purchased from SLC Ltd. (Shizuoka, Japan), as described previously [29]. When a plug was detected, this was deemed embryonic day 0.5 (E0.5). Pregnancy was confirmed by weight gain. At the indicated time points, dams were infected s.c. with 1×10^4 plaque-forming unit (PFU) of PRVABC59, euthanized at the indicated time points, and their fetuses and indicated tissues were harvested. The fetal crown rump body length (CRL), head length from the tip of the nose to the occiput, head width, and body weight were measured. For postnatal analyses, the dams were infected s.c. with 1×10^4 PFU of PRVABC59 and monitored until offspring were born. The offspring were monitored every day for 14 days after birth (P14), and their body weights and head diameters were measured from P3 to P11.

For the SmithKline Beecham, Harwell, Imperial College, Royal London Hospital, phenotype assessment (SHIRPA) primary screen [50,51], dams were infected s.c. with 1×10^4 PFU of PRVABC59 at E12.5, and their offspring were monitored until SHIRPA screening was performed at the indicated time points. Offspring born to PRVABC59-infected or uninfected dams were weighed at P7 or P8 to confirm their growth; they were otherwise left alone to avoid excessive handling, which may modulate the fear, anxiety, or stress response after development [52,53]. The SHIRPA primary screen was performed as previously described [51] with modifications. Briefly, each mouse was placed in a transparent cylindrical viewing jar (15 cm diameter, 11 cm height) for 5 min to observe rearing, grooming, respiration rate, and tremor. Subsequently, the mouse was transferred to an arena (33 cm wide × 55 cm long × 18 cm height) that consisted of 15 evenly spaced squares (11 cm × 11 cm) to evaluate transfer arousal and motor behavior; thereafter, palpebral closure, piloerection, gait, pelvic elevation, and tail elevation were observed in the arena. A sequence of manipulations was performed to evaluate touch escape, positional passivity, trunk curl, limb grasping and visual placing, grip strength, body tone, pinna reflex, corneal reflex, tow pinch, and wire maneuver. To complete the assessment, the mice were restrained in a supine position to record autonomic behaviors prior to measurement of the righting reflex, contact righting reflex, and negative geotaxis. Throughout the procedure, vocalization, fear, irritability, and aggression were recorded. All behaviors were scored as previously described [51]. The individual parameters assessed by SHIRPA were grouped into five functional categories: neuropsychiatric state, motor behavior, autonomic function, muscle tone and strength, and reflex and sensory function [54,55]. The neuropsychiatric state includes spontaneous activity, transfer arousal, touch escape, positional passivity, biting, fear, irritability, aggression, and vocalization. Motor behavior includes body position, tremor, locomotor activity, pelvic elevation, tail elevation, gait, trunk curl, limb grasping, wire maneuver, and negative geotaxis. Autonomic function includes respiration rate, palpebral closure, piloerection, skin color, heart rate, lacrimation, salivation, and body temperature. Muscle tone and strength include grip strength, body tone, limb tone, and abdominal tone. Reflex and sensory functions include visual placement, pinna reflex, corneal reflex, toe pinch, and righting reflex.

To induce neutralizing antibodies against ZIKV, seven female mice (Group A) and three female mice (Group B) were infected s.c. with 1×10^4 PFU of PRVABC59 40 days before mating. Four female mice (Group C) or one female mouse (Group D) were infected s.c. with 1×10^4 PFU of PRVABC59 twice at a 57–60 days interval before mating. Ten female mice in Group E were inoculated s.c. with 2MEM twice at a 57–60 day interval before mating. After plugging, the mice were bled and the neutralizing antibody titer was determined by the standard 50% plaque reduction neutralization (PRNT$_{50}$) assay [56,57]. Dams in Groups A, C, and E were infected s.c. with 1×10^4 PFU of PRVABC59 at E9.5, and dams in Groups B and D were inoculated s.c. with 2MEM at E9.5. The offspring were monitored from P1 to P21. For the uninfected control, seven female mice were left without any treatment before mating and during pregnancy.

2.7. Statistical Analyses

The Student's t-test was performed for normally distributed data sets where differences in variance were <4, skewness was >−2, and kurtosis was <2. The Kolmogorov–Smirnov test was used for non-parametric data where differences in variance were >4, skewness was <−2, and kurtosis was >2. The log-rank test was used for the statistical analysis of survival rates. Repeated-measures ANOVA was used to determine differences in postnatal growth over time. Pearson or Spearman correlation analyses were performed for normally distributed data or non-parametric data, respectively. Statistical significance was set at $p < 0.05$. Statistical analysis of the experimental data was performed using JMP 13 software (SAS Institute, Inc., Cary, NC, USA).

3. Results and Discussion

3.1. Fetal Outcomes

To assess fetal outcomes after congenital ZIKV infection, dams were s.c. infected with PRVABC59 at E6.5, E7.5, E8.5, E9.5, E10.5, E11.5, E12.5, E13.5, and E14.5, and the fetuses were visually inspected at 6 days post-infection (dpi; Figure 1A). Most of the fetuses infected at E6.5, E7.5, and E8.5 (100%, 100%, and 75%, respectively) showed abnormalities (IUGR, deformed fetal/placental masses, or fetal death). The number of infected embryonic days was inversely correlated with the prevalence of IUGR or deformed masses (Figure 1B,C). The CRL (Figure 1D insert), head length from the tip of the nose to the occiput (Figure 1E insert), and weight of infected fetuses were significantly smaller than those of uninfected fetuses (Figure 1D–F). The fetal CRL and head length from the tip of the nose to the occiput were measured to provide evidence for IUGR and to predict fetal cranium growth, respectively [37,58]. The lower prevalence of fetuses with gross abnormalities after infection at or after E9.5 (Figure 1A–C) was confirmed by visual inspection at 2 and 4 dpi at E9.5 and E13.5 (Figure 1G). In addition, intracranial hemorrhage (Figure 1H) and ocular malformation (Figure 1I), which were similar to those observed in human neonates with CZS [59–62], were observed in fetuses after infection at E13.5. Thus, ZIKV infection during early pregnancy between E6.5–E8.5, corresponding to the first trimester in humans [63], was a significant risk factor for severe fetal outcomes, such as fetal death, resorption (observed as deformed fetal/placental masses), and severe IUGR, whereas infection at or after E9.5 caused relatively mild outcomes (Figure 1D–F), but did not enhance fetal lethality (Figure 1A). Thus, the embryonic timing of congenital ZIKV infection affects the severity of fetal outcomes.

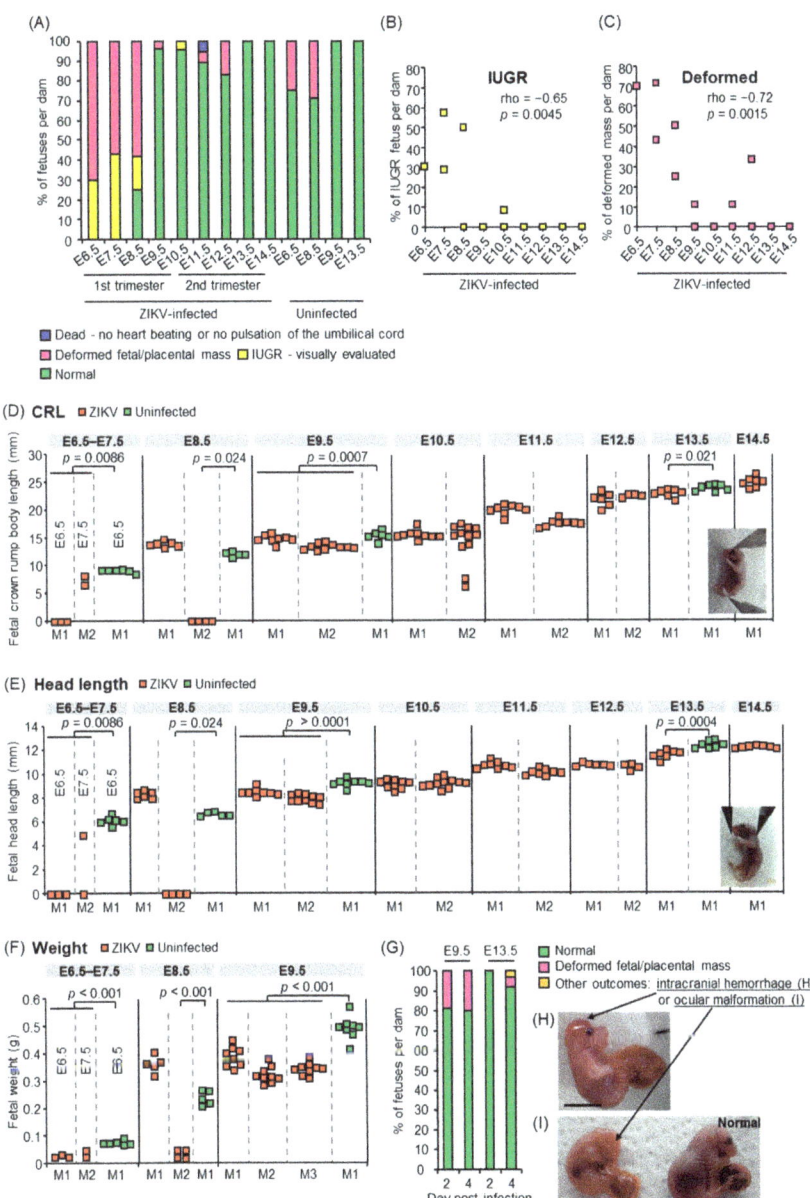

Figure 1. Fetal outcomes. (**A**) Percentages of each fetal outcome: fetuses that died in utero, were deformed, showed IUGR, or appeared normal at 6 days after congenital ZIKV infection. Survival of fetuses was confirmed by heartbeat or pulsation of the umbilical cord as observed under a microscope. The x-axis shows the embryonic days of ZIKV infection or 2MEM inoculation for uninfected controls. The ZIKV-infected group consisted of 10 fetuses from 1 dam infected at E6.5, 14 fetuses from 2 dams infected at E7.5, 22 fetuses from 3 dams infected at E8.5, 28 fetuses from 3 dams infected at E9.5, 21 fetuses from 2 dams infected at E10.5, 17 fetuses from 2 dams infected at E11.5, 13 fetuses from 2 dams infected at E12.5, and 7 fetuses from 1 dam infected at E13.5 or E14.5. The uninfected group consisted of 8 fetuses from 1 dam at E6.5 or E9.5 and 7 fetuses from 1 dam at E8.5 or E13.5. (**B**) Inverse correlation between IUGR prevalence at 6 dpi and infected embryonic days. The x-axis shows ZIKV-infected embryonic days. Significance was determined by Spearman's correlation

test. (**C**) Inverse correlation between the prevalence of deformed masses at 6 dpi and infected embryonic days. The *x*-axis shows ZIKV-infected embryonic days. Significance was determined by Spearman's correlation test. (**D**) Fetal CRL at 6 dpi. Dams were infected with ZIKV or inoculated with 2MEM (uninfected) at the indicated embryonic days. Individual dams are indicated on the *x*-axis; each square represents one fetus. Vertical dashed gray lines separate litters from each dam. If the fetal heads were indistinguishable from the body, their CRL was considered as zero (below the detection limit). Significance was determined by *t*-test or Kolmogorov–Smirnov test. (**E**) Fetal head length at 6 dpi. Data are from the same fetuses as described for panel C. If the fetal heads were indistinguishable from the body, their head length was considered as zero (below the detection limit). Significance was determined by *t*-test or Kolmogorov–Smirnov test. (**F**) Fetal weights at 6 dpi. Dams were infected with ZIKV or inoculated with 2MEM (uninfected) at the indicated embryonic days. Individual dams are indicated on the *x*-axis; each square represents one fetus. Vertical dashed gray lines separate litters from each dam. Significance was determined by *t*-test. (**G**) Percentages of each fetal outcome at 2 or 4 dpi. Dams were infected with ZIKV at E9.5 or E13.5, and fetuses were visually inspected at 2 or 4 dpi. The data include 18 fetuses from 2 litters at 2 dpi at E9.5, 10 fetuses from 1 litter at 4 dpi at E9.5, 4 fetuses from 1 litter at 2 dpi at E13.5, or 75 fetuses from 8 litters at 4 dpi at E13.5. (**H**) The fetus with intracranial hemorrhage at 4 dpi at E13.5. Scale bar = 1 cm. (**I**) The fetus with ocular malformation and an apparently normal littermate. Scale bar = 1 cm.

3.2. Fetal and Placental Infection

To confirm the vertical transmission of ZIKV, viral titers in the placentas, fetal whole bodies, and deformed masses at 6 dpi were determined by $CCID_{50}$ assays. Most placentas were infected irrespective of the infected embryonic days, whereas the titer of most fetuses was lower than the detection limit at 6 dpi (Figure 2A). To assess whether ZIKV did not transmit to fetuses or did not replicate in fetal tissues, or whether active virus replication decreased to undetectable levels before 6 dpi, the placentas and fetal tissues were collected at 2 or 4 dpi at E9.5–E10.5 (first trimester in humans) or E12.5 (second trimester in humans) and tissue virus titers determined. The fetal heads were titrated rather than the whole body, except for fetal samples collected at 2 dpi at E9.5, as the fetal heads were indistinguishable from the body. A total of 60% and 100% of fetuses in each dam infected at E9.5 and 60%, 20%, and 16.7% of fetuses in each dam infected at E12.5 were infected at 2 dpi; all fetuses were infected by 4 dpi with a similar titer after infection at E9.5–E10.5 and E12.5 ($p = 0.97$, Figure 2B). The virus titers were similar in each tissue of dams infected at E9.5–E10.5 and E12.5 (Supplemental Figure S1), showing that the dams were equally susceptible to ZIKV infection irrespective of embryonic days, as previously reported [64]. The placental virus titers were not different after infection at E9.5–E10.5 and E12.5 (Figure 2B, $p = 0.053$ for 2 dpi, $p = 0.13$ for 4 dpi), with no correlation in virus titers between the fetal heads and corresponding placentas (Figure 2C, $p = 0.47$ for 2 dpi, $p = 0.17$ for 4 dpi). The placentas at 6 dpi at E8.5, E9.5, or E13.5 were smaller than uninfected placentas (Figure 2D) as previously reported [29]. However, histological abnormality was not observed in placentas from infected dams (Figure 2E,F,I,J). In addition, viral antigens were found only in the histologically normal decidual cells in the peripheral area of placentas by IHC with anti-NS1 antibody (Figure 2G,H,K,L). The mouse placenta forms a definitive structure and becomes functional around E10.5–E11.5 [65,66]. The infection of fetal heads after E12.5 infection suggests that ZIKV crossed the placental barrier. Taken together, fetuses were infected congenitally, irrespective of gross abnormalities (Figure 1) or embryonic days of congenital infection. The former observation is partially consistent with previous work in which ZIKV RNA was detected in the fetal heads with only mild IUGR after infection at E6.5 or E7.5 [29].

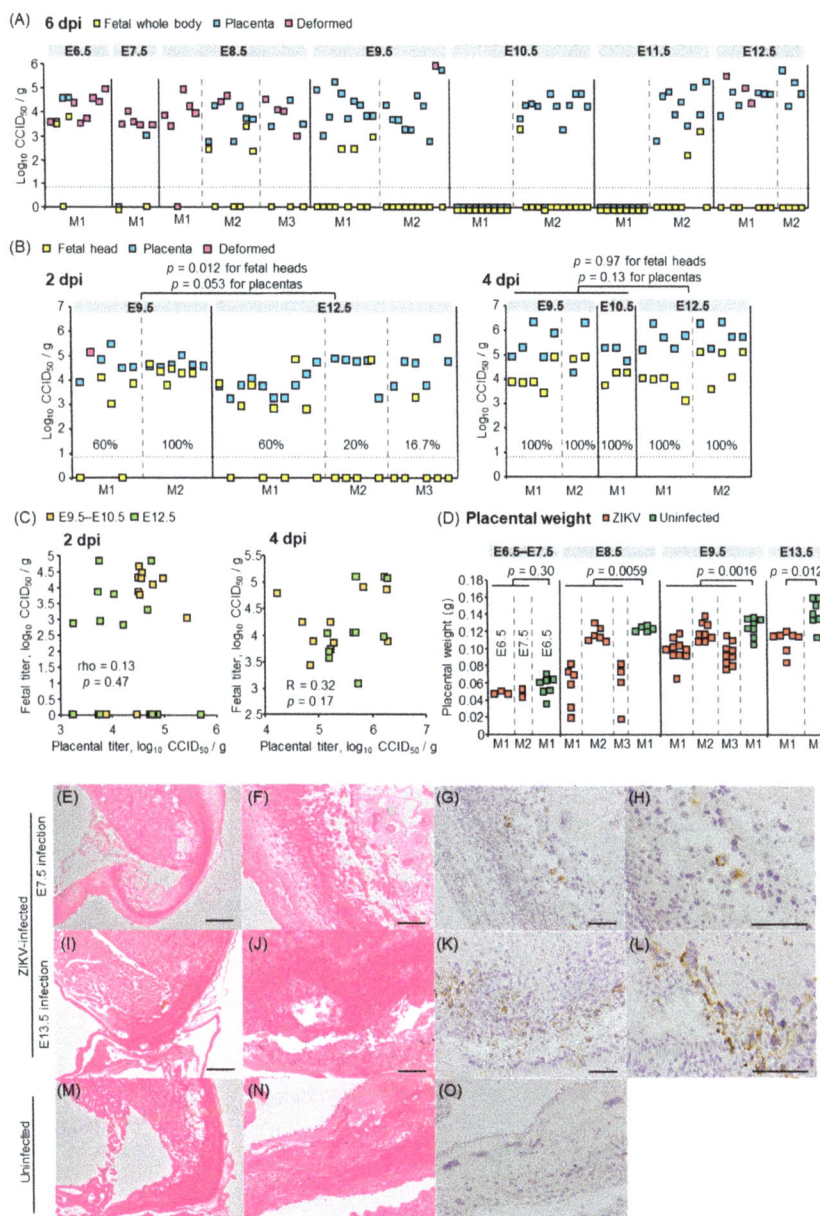

Figure 2. Viral titers and histological findings in fetal tissues or placentas. (**A**) Viral titers in fetal whole bodies, placentas, and deformed masses at 6 dpi. Dams were infected with ZIKV at the indicated embryonic days. Individual dams are indicated on the *x*-axis. Vertical dashed gray lines separate litters from each dam. Symbols represent individual fetus, placenta, or deformed mass. Limit of detection was 0.83 $\log_{10}CCID_{50}/g$ as indicated by the horizontal dashed line. (**B**) Viral titers in fetal heads, placentas, and deformed masses at 2 or 4 dpi, as described for panel A. Percentage of fetuses that were infected for each dam at 2 or 4 dpi is indicated. Kolmogorov–Smirnov test or *t*-test was used for statistical analysis. (**C**) Lack of correlation between virus titers in placentas and fetal heads at 2 dpi and 4 dpi as determined by Pearson or Spearman's correlation test. (**D**) Placental weights at 6 dpi. Dams were infected with ZIKV or inoculated with 2MEM (uninfected) at the

indicated embryonic days. Individual dams are indicated on the *x*-axis; each square represents one placenta. Significance was determined by *t*-test or Kolmogorov–Smirnov test. (**E**) H&E staining of placentas at 6 dpi; dams were infected at E7.5. Representative image of placentas from 2 dams. (**F**) As described for panel E at higher magnification. (**G**) IHC of placenta at 6 dpi at E7.5 using anti-ZIKV NS1 antibody. Positive staining (brown) was detected in decidual cells. Representative image of placentas from 2 dams. (**H**) As described for panel G at higher magnification. (**I–L**) H&E staining and IHC of placentas at 6 dpi; dams were infected at E13.5; otherwise as described for E–H. (**M**) H&E staining of placentas from uninfected dams. Representative image of placentas from 2 dams. (**N**) As described for panel M at higher magnification. (**O**) IHC of placenta from uninfected dams using anti-ZIKV NS1 antibody. Representative image of placentas from 2 dams. Scale bars; 500 µm (**E,I,M**), 100 µm (**F–H,J–L,N,O**).

3.3. Postnatal Outcomes

To assess postnatal outcomes, dams were infected with PRVABC59 at E8.5, E9.5, E10.5, E11.5, E12.5, E13.5, and E14.5, and their offspring were monitored from P1 to P14, including measuring body weight and head circumference from P3 to P11. All offspring born to dams infected at E8.5 or E9.5, died within one day after birth (Figure 3A). The survival of offspring born to dams infected at E10.5–E14.5 was significantly lower than that of uninfected offspring ($p = 0.0007$ for E10.5, $p < 0.0001$ for E11.5, $p = 0.0005$ for E12.5, $p = 0.042$ for E13.5, and $p < 0.0001$ for E14.5) (Figure 3A). Human infants with congenital ZIKV infection are typically small for gestational age (SGA) [1] and/or exhibit failure to thrive (FTT) [16]. SGA is defined as a birth weight at least two standard deviations (SDs) below the mean for gestational age [67]. FTT is defined as subnormal growth or subnormal weight gain in infants [68]. The weight of two litters (L1 and L2) infected at E12.5, and one offspring infected at E13.5, was less than 2SD of the mean weight of uninfected offspring at P3, which was the earliest time point of weight measurement (Figure 3B). The weights of offspring infected at E10.5 or E11.5 were comparable with those of uninfected offspring (Figure 3B). There was variability in offspring weights between litters (e.g., L1/L2 versus L3 after infection at E12.5). The absence of significance in offspring weights after infection at E10.5 or E11.5 when compared with uninfected offspring thus may be explained by the small sample size, which is a limitation of our study. The mean weight gain of L1 and L2 infected at E12.5 (Figure 3C) was lower than that of uninfected offspring ($p < 0.0001$ for L1, $p = 0.0005$ for L2), suggesting SGA and FTT. Microcephaly is defined postnatally as a small head circumference ≥ 2 SDs of the norm [69,70]. The head circumferences of L1 and one offspring from L2 infected at E12.5, were smaller than 2SD of the mean of uninfected offspring at P3 (Figure 3D). The mean head circumferences at P3–P11 of L1 infected at E12.5, at P3, P7, P8, P9, and P10 of L2 infected at E12.5, and at P5 and P6 of L1 infected at E13.5 were smaller than 2SD of the uninfected mean (Figure 3E), suggesting microcephaly. Thus, our mouse model recapitulates multiple postnatal outcomes including stillbirths (Figure 3A), neonatal death (Figure 3A), SGA (Figure 3B), FTT (Figure 3B,C), and microcephaly (Figure 3D,E), as observed in human cases [1,13,15,17,71].

To evaluate the outcomes in grown-up mice after congenital ZIKV infection, SHIRPA primary screening was performed on 4-week-old mice born to dams infected with PRBV-ABC59 at E12.5. Two mice born to dams infected at E12.5, were smaller than each littermate and died at P10 before SHIRPA was performed (Figure 3F). The SHIRPA scores of infected mice were compared with two age-matched control groups: (1) 2MEM inoculation at E12.5, or (2) no treatment during pregnancy and postnatal periods. The reduced body weight of infected mice (Figure 3G) was consistent with previous data (Figure 3B,C). Two mice remained small during adulthood (10-week-old) and reached the ethical endpoint for euthanasia at 10 weeks after birth (Supplemental Figure S2A), although the survival between the three groups did not reach statistical significance (Supplemental Figure S2B). Infected offspring had significantly deficient SHIRPA scores compared with 2MEM-inoculated and/or untreated offspring in 11 tests belonging to four SHIRPA functional categories (Figure 3G): neuropsychiatric state (touch escape, positional passivity, provoked biting, irritability, and aggression), motor behavior (limb grasping and negative geotaxis), autonomic function (salivation and body temperature), and reflex and sensory functions (visual placing and toe pinch). The abnormalities in the SHIRPA screen were also confirmed in IFNAR$^{-/-}$ offspring born to dams infected with the Natal RGN strain at E6.5. The mean body weight of one of the five litters infected with Natal RGN at E6.5 was lower than that of the uninfected litter at 3 weeks post-birth (Supplemental Figure S3A). The infected litter had abnormal scores in four tests: locomotor activity, tail elevation, gait, and grip strength (yellow boxes in Supplemental Figure S3A). Another infected litter showed an abnormality in a fifth test, namely, provoked biting (green box in Supplemental Figure S3A). The five tests belonged to three functional categories: neuropsychiatric state (provoked biting), motor behavior (locomotor activity, tail elevation, and gait), and muscle tone and strength (grip strength). ZIKV RNA was detected in the testis of one male offspring born to a Natal RGN-infected dam (Supplemental Figure S3B), confirming vertical transmission and offspring infection. Thus, our mouse model recapitulates a wide range of postnatal developmental sequelae [7,8,14,17,18].

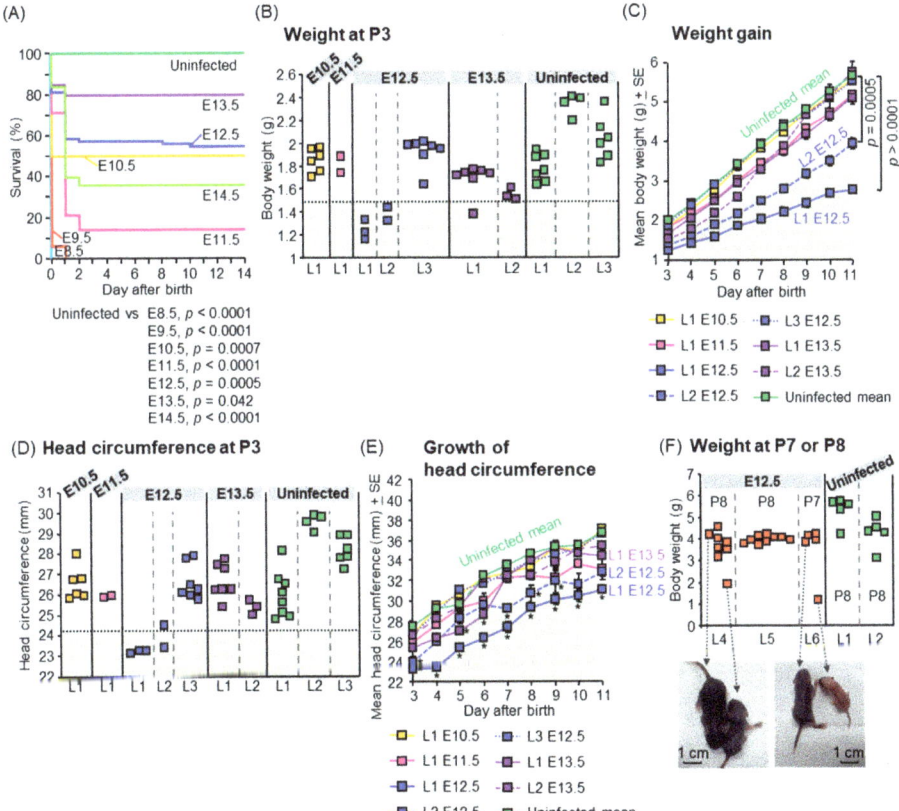

Figure 3. *Cont.*

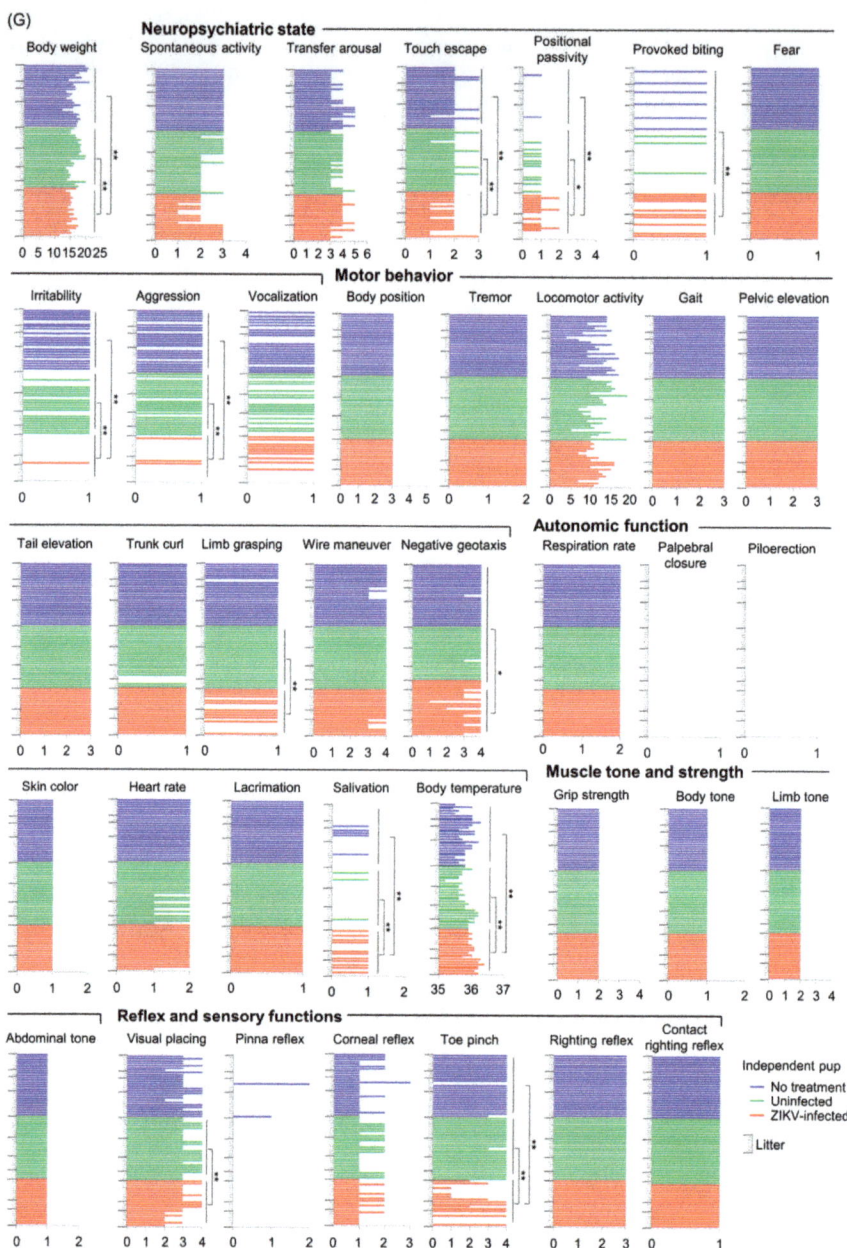

Figure 3. Postnatal outcomes. (**A**) Survival of offspring. Data are from 8 offspring from 1 dam infected at E8.5, 16 offspring from 3 dams infected at E9.5, 12 offspring from 2 dams infected at E10.5, 14 offspring from 2 dams infected at E11.5, 75 offspring from 9 dams infected at E12.5, 20 offspring from 3 dams infected at E13.5, 25 offspring from 4 dams infected at E14.5, and 19 offspring from 3 uninfected dams. Comparison of Kaplan–Meier survival curves between groups was performed by log-rank analysis. (**B**) Weight of offspring at P3. Individual litters are indicated on the *x*-axis; each square represents a single offspring. Vertical dashed gray lines separate each litter, which was infected at the indicated embryonic days. The pale green shaded area represents 2SD below the mean body weight of uninfected offspring. (**C**) Weight gain of

each litter. The pale green shaded area represents 2SD below the mean body weight of uninfected offspring. Data consist of 6 survived offspring out of 8 offspring (6/8) for litter 1 (L1) infected at E10.5, 2/7 for L1 infected at E11.5, 3/5 for L1 infected at E12.5, 2/4 for L2 infected at E12.5, 7/7 for L3 infected at E12.5, 7/7 for L1 infected at E13.5, and 3/5 for L2 infected at E13.5. The uninfected group consisted of 18 offspring from 3 litters. Statistical analyses were performed by repeated-measure ANOVA. (**D**) Head circumference of offspring at P3. Individual litters are indicated on the *x*-axis; each square represents a single offspring. Vertical dashed gray lines separate each litter, which was infected at the indicated embryonic days. The pale green shaded area represents 2SD below the mean head circumference of uninfected offspring. Head circumference was calculated by multiplying the head diameter by Pi (3.14). (**E**) Growth of head circumference of each litter. Data are from the same litters as described for panel C. The pale green shaded area represents 2SD below the mean head circumference of uninfected offspring. Asterisks show the value 2SD below that of the uninfected mean. (**F**) Weight of offspring born to ZIKV-infected or uninfected dams at P7 or P8. Individual litters are indicated on the *x*-axis; each square represents a single offspring. Vertical dashed gray lines separate each litter, which was infected at E12.5 or uninfected. Dorsal view of two small offspring infected at E12.5 compared with each littermate. (**G**) SHIRPA scores of 4-week-old mice born to ZIKV-infected dams at E12.5. The horizontal axis shows the score. Each bar represents one mouse. Statistical analyses were performed by Kolmogorov–Smirnov test or *t*-test: * $p < 0.05$; ** $p < 0.01$. Longer lines along the *y*-axis separate litters.

3.4. Maternal Neutralizing Antibodies Prevent Offspring Outcomes

To demonstrate the utility of our model, we performed a proof of principal experiment testing whether neonatal death could serve as criteria for screening of ZIKV vaccine candidates. There are no vaccines currently available for ZIKV infection, and female mice were infected with ZIKV prior to mating to induce neutralizing antibodies, which alone were sufficient to prevent vertical transmission of ZIKV in mice [72]. The dams were infected with ZIKV at E9.5, which caused neonatal death (Figure 3A), and the survival of their offspring was monitored. The experimental scheme is shown in Figure 4A. Briefly, female mice were infected with PRVABC59 40 days before mating (Groups A and B) or infected twice with a 57–60 days interval before mating (Groups C and D). Females in Group E were inoculated with 2MEM before mating. An increased neutralizing antibody titer was detected after plugging in Groups A, B, C, and D when compared with Group E or uninfected group (Figure 4B). Pregnant mice in Groups A, C, and E were infected s.c. with PRVABC59 at E9.5, whereas pregnant mice in Groups B and D were inoculated with 2MEM at E9.5. The survival of offspring in Groups A and C was significantly improved compared with Group E ($p < 0.0001$, Figure 4C). The 1-day-old offspring in Groups A and D were visually larger than those in Group E (Supplemental Figure S4). The survival of each litter infected at E9.5 (Groups A, C, and E) was correlated with the neutralizing antibody titer of each dam ($p = 0.0011$, Figure 4D). Taken together, the results demonstrated that maternal neutralizing antibodies (at least a PRNT titer of $1:10^{2.8}$, Figure 4B,D) prevent neonatal death in mice, and that neonatal death can serve as an in vivo phenotypic readout for screening the efficacy of candidate vaccines against ZIKV.

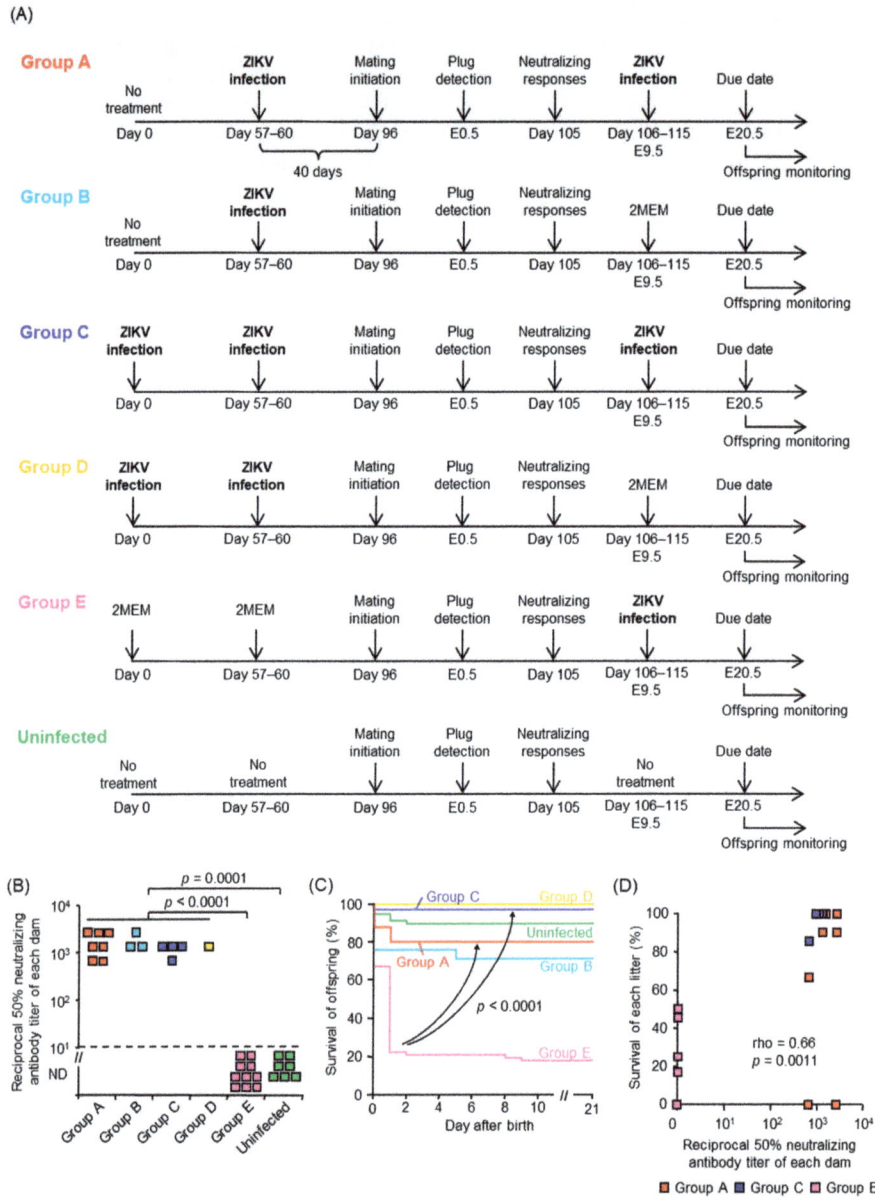

Figure 4. Neutralizing antibodies in dams protect the offspring from vertical ZIKV infection. (**A**) Experimental timeline of each group. (**B**) ZIKV-specific neutralizing antibody titers of each dam. Limit of detection was 1 in 10 dilutions as indicated by the horizontal dashed line. Titer was determined by $PRNT_{50}$ assays. Kolmogorov–Smirnov test was used for statistical analysis. (**C**) Survival of offspring. Comparisons for Group E versus either Group A or Group C, $p < 0.0001$. Comparisons of Kaplan–Meier survival curves between the different groups were performed by log-rank analyses. The data are from 51 offspring from 7 litters for Group A, 21 offspring from 3 litters for Group B, 35 offspring from 4 litters for Group C, 6 offspring from 1 litter for Group D, 67 offspring from 10 litters for Group E, and 60 offspring from 7 litters for the uninfected group. (**D**) Correlation between neutralizing antibody titers of each dam and the percent survival of each litter in Groups A, C, and E. Significance was determined by Spearman's correlation test.

4. Conclusions

Our mouse pregnancy model recapitulated multiple fetal and postnatal outcomes seen in humans after congenital ZIKV infection. The embryonic timing of ZIKV infection affected the outcomes; infection during early pregnancy caused fetal death and severe IUGR, and infection during mid to late pregnancy caused stillbirth, neonatal death, SGA, FTT, microcephaly, or developmental sequelae. Furthermore, neonatal death in our model may be useful as a readout phenotype to evaluate the efficacy of ZIKV vaccine candidates.

Supplementary Materials: The following are available online at https://www.mdpi.com/article/10.3390/v13091807/s1, Figure S1: Virus titers in maternal tissues, Figure S2: Offspring infected at E12.5 in adulthood, Figure S3: Offspring outcomes after ZIKV Natal RGN infection, Figure S4: Size of one-day-old offspring, Table S1: Mouse pregnancy models. References [73–77] are cited in supplemental materials.

Author Contributions: Conceptualization, E.N.; methodology, E.N., Y.K., J.E.H., B.T. and A.S.; formal analysis, E.N. and J.E.H.; investigation, E.N., Y.K., S.T. (Satoshi Taniguchi), J.E.H., K.-i.S., K.T., Y.S., B.T., K.Y., N.K., C.K.L. and T.S.; data curation, E.N., S.T. (Satoshi Taniguchi) and J.E.H.; writing—original draft preparation, E.N.; writing—review and editing, E.N., S.T. (Satoshi Taniguchi), K.T. and C.K.L.; supervision, A.S. and M.S.; funding acquisition, E.N., S.T. (Shigeru Tajima), C.K.L. and A.S. All authors have read and agreed to the published version of the manuscript.

Funding: This research was supported by the Research Program on Emerging and Re-emerging Infectious Diseases of the Japan Agency for Medical Research and Development (AMED; https://www.amed.go.jp/en/program/list/11/02/002.html; accessed on 26 August 2021), Grant numbers JP19fk0108035, JP20fk0108123 and JP21wm0225007, and JSPS KAKENHI (https://www.jsps.go.jp/english/index.html; accessed on 26 August 2021), Grant number JP20K07530. E.N. was supported in part by the Daiichi Sankyo Foundation of Life Science, Japan (http://www.ds-fdn.or.jp/support/studying_abroad.html; accessed on 26 August 2021). A.S. holds an investigator grant (APP1173880) from the National Health and Medical Research Council (NHMRC) of Australia (https://www.nhmrc.gov.au/; accessed on 26 August 2021). The project was also funded in part by an NHMRC project grant, grant number APP1144950. The funders had no role in the study design, data collection and analysis, decision to publish, or preparation of the manuscript.

Institutional Review Board Statement: All mouse experiments were conducted in accordance with the Guidelines for Animal Experiments performed at the National Institute of Infectious Diseases (NIID) or the Australian Code for Care and Use of Animals for Scientific Purposes, as outlined by the National Health and Medical Research Council of Australia. Animal experiments were approved by the Animal Welfare and Animal Care Committee of NIID (Ethics numbers: 116123 and 119155) or the QIMR Berghofer Medical Research Institute Animal Ethics Committee (Ethics number: A1604-611M). All mice were bred and housed under specific pathogen-free conditions.

Informed Consent Statement: Not applicable.

Data Availability Statement: The data presented in this study are available on request from the corresponding author.

Acknowledgments: The authors would like to thank Takahiro Maeki (NIID) for his suggestion, and Makiko Ikeda and Nor Azila Muhammad Azami (NIID) for their technical assistance.

Conflicts of Interest: The authors declare no conflict of interest. The funders had no role in the design of the study; in the collection, analyses, or interpretation of data; in the writing of the manuscript, or in the decision to publish the results.

References

1. Brasil, P.; Pereira, J.P., Jr.; Moreira, M.E.; Ribeiro Nogueira, R.M.; Damasceno, L.; Wakimoto, M.; Rabello, R.S.; Valderramos, S.G.; Halai, U.A.; Salles, T.S.; et al. Zika Virus Infection in Pregnant Women in Rio de Janeiro. *N. Engl. J. Med.* **2016**, *375*, 2321–2334. [CrossRef] [PubMed]
2. Franca, G.V.; Schuler-Faccini, L.; Oliveira, W.K.; Henriques, C.M.; Carmo, E.H.; Pedi, V.D.; Nunes, M.L.; Castro, M.C.; Serruya, S.; Silveira, M.F.; et al. Congenital Zika virus syndrome in Brazil: A case series of the first 1501 livebirths with complete investigation. *Lancet* **2016**, *388*, 891–897. [CrossRef]

3. van der Eijk, A.A.; van Genderen, P.J.; Verdijk, R.M.; Reusken, C.B.; Mogling, R.; van Kampen, J.J.; Widagdo, W.; Aron, G.I.; GeurtsvanKessel, C.H.; Pas, S.D.; et al. Miscarriage Associated with Zika Virus Infection. *N. Engl. J. Med.* **2016**, *375*, 1002–1004. [CrossRef] [PubMed]
4. Pereira, J.P., Jr.; Nielsen-Saines, K.; Sperling, J.; Maykin, M.M.; Damasceno, L.; Cardozo, R.F.; Valle, H.A.; Dutra, B.R.T.; Gama, H.D.; Adachi, K.; et al. Association of Prenatal Ultrasonographic Findings with Adverse Neonatal Outcomes Among Pregnant Women with Zika Virus Infection in Brazil. *JAMA Net. Open* **2018**, *1*, e186529. [CrossRef]
5. de Araújo, T.V.B.; de Alencar Ximenes, R.A.; de Barros Miranda-Filho, D.; Souza, W.V.; Montarroyos, U.R.; de Melo, A.P.L.; Valongueiro, S.; Braga, C.; Brandão Filho, S.P.; Cordeiro, M.T. Association between microcephaly, Zika virus infection, and other risk factors in Brazil: Final report of a case-control study. *Lancet Infect. Dis.* **2018**, *18*, 328–336. [CrossRef]
6. de Araújo, T.V.B.; Rodrigues, L.C.; de Alencar Ximenes, R.A.; de Barros Miranda-Filho, D.; Montarroyos, U.R.; de Melo, A.P.L.; Valongueiro, S.; Souza, W.V.; Braga, C.; Brandão Filho, S.P. Association between Zika virus infection and microcephaly in Brazil, January to May, 2016: Preliminary report of a case-control study. *Lancet Infect. Dis.* **2016**, *16*, 1356–1363. [CrossRef]
7. Pecanha, P.M.; Gomes Junior, S.C.; Pone, S.M.; Pone, M.; Vasconcelos, Z.; Zin, A.; Vilibor, R.H.H.; Costa, R.P.; Meio, M.; Nielsen-Saines, K.; et al. Neurodevelopment of children exposed intra-uterus by Zika virus: A case series. *PLoS ONE* **2020**, *15*, e0229434. [CrossRef] [PubMed]
8. Van der Linden, V.; Pessoa, A.; Dobyns, W.; Barkovich, A.J.; van der Linden Júnior, H.; Filho, E.L.R.; Ribeiro, E.M.; de Carvalho Leal, M.; de Araújo Coimbra, P.P.; de Fátima Viana Vasco Aragão, M. Description of 13 infants born during October 2015–January 2016 with congenital Zika virus infection without microcephaly at birth—Brazil. *Morb. Mortal. Wkly. Rep.* **2016**, *65*, 1343–1348. [CrossRef]
9. Frota, L.; Sampaio, R.F.; Miranda, J.L.; Brasil, R.M.C.; Gontijo, A.P.B.; Mambrini, J.V.M.; Brandao, M.B.; Mancini, M.C. Children with congenital Zika syndrome: Symptoms, comorbidities and gross motor development at 24 months of age. *Heliyon* **2020**, *6*, e04130. [CrossRef]
10. Ventura, P.A.; Lage, M.-L.C.; de Carvalho, A.L.; Fernandes, A.S.; Taguchi, T.B.; Nascimento-Carvalho, C.M. Early Gross Motor Development Among Brazilian Children with Microcephaly Born Right After Zika Virus Infection Outbreak. *J. Dev. Behav. Pediat.* **2020**, *41*, 134–140. [CrossRef]
11. Lage, M.-L.C.; Carvalho, A.L.; Ventura, P.A.; Taguchi, T.B.; Fernandes, A.S.; Pinho, S.F.; Santos-Junior, O.T.; Ramos, C.L.; Nascimento-Carvalho, C.M. Clinical, Neuroimaging, and Neurophysiological Findings in Children with Microcephaly Related to Congenital Zika Virus Infection. *Int. J. Env Res. Public Health* **2019**, *16*, 309. [CrossRef] [PubMed]
12. Nielsen-Saines, K.; Brasil, P.; Kerin, T.; Vasconcelos, Z.; Gabaglia, C.R.; Damasceno, L.; Pone, M.; Abreu de Carvalho, L.M.; Pone, S.M.; Zin, A.A.; et al. Delayed childhood neurodevelopment and neurosensory alterations in the second year of life in a prospective cohort of ZIKV-exposed children. *Nat. Med.* **2019**, *25*, 1213–1217. [CrossRef]
13. Franca, T.L.B.; Medeiros, W.R.; Souza, N.L.; Longo, E.; Pereira, S.A.; Franca, T.B.O.; Sousa, K.G. Growth and Development of Children with Microcephaly Associated with Congenital Zika Virus Syndrome in Brazil. *Int. J. Environ. Res. Public Health* **2018**, *15*, 1990. [CrossRef]
14. Aguilar Ticona, J.P.; Nery, N., Jr.; Ladines-Lim, J.B.; Gambrah, C.; Sacramento, G.; de Paula Freitas, B.; Bouzon, J.; Oliveira-Filho, J.; Borja, A.; Adhikarla, H. Developmental outcomes in children exposed to Zika virus in utero from a Brazilian urban slum cohort study. *PLoS Negl. Trop. Dis.* **2021**, *15*, e0009162. [CrossRef]
15. Wheeler, A.C. Development of infants with congenital Zika syndrome: What do we know and what can we expect? *Pediatrics* **2018**, *141*, S154–S160. [CrossRef] [PubMed]
16. Mulkey, S.B. Head Circumference as a Measure of In Utero Zika Virus Exposure and Outcomes. *JAMA Netw. Open* **2020**, *3*, e209461. [CrossRef] [PubMed]
17. Cranston, J.S.; Tiene, S.F.; Nielsen-Saines, K.; Vasconcelos, Z.; Pone, M.V.; Pone, S.; Zin, A.; Salles, T.S.; Pereira, J.P., Jr.; Orofino, D.; et al. Association Between Antenatal Exposure to Zika Virus and Anatomical and Neurodevelopmental Abnormalities in Children. *JAMA Netw. Open* **2020**, *3*, e209303. [CrossRef]
18. Cavalcante, T.B.; Ribeiro, M.R.C.; Sousa, P.D.S.; Costa, E.P.F.; Alves, M.; Simoes, V.M.F.; Batista, R.F.L.; Takahasi, E.H.M.; Amaral, G.A.; Khouri, R.; et al. Congenital Zika syndrome: Growth, clinical, and motor development outcomes up to 36 months of age and differences according to microcephaly at birth. *Int. J. Infect. Dis.* **2021**, *105*, 399–408. [CrossRef] [PubMed]
19. Soares de Souza, A.; Moraes Dias, C.; Braga, F.D.; Terzian, A.C.; Estofolete, C.F.; Oliani, A.H.; Oliveira, G.H.; Brandao de Mattos, C.C.; de Mattos, L.C.; Nogueira, M.L.; et al. Fetal Infection by Zika Virus in the Third Trimester: Report of 2 Cases. *Clin. Infect. Dis.* **2016**, *63*, 1622–1625. [CrossRef]
20. Wheeler, A.C.; Toth, D.; Ridenour, T.; Lima Nobrega, L.; Borba Firmino, R.; Marques da Silva, C.; Carvalho, P.; Marques, D.; Okoniewski, K.; Ventura, L.O.; et al. Developmental Outcomes among Young Children with Congenital Zika Syndrome in Brazil. *JAMA Netw. Open* **2020**, *3*, e204096. [CrossRef] [PubMed]
21. Cauchemez, S.; Besnard, M.; Bompard, P.; Dub, T.; Guillemette-Artur, P.; Eyrolle-Guignot, D.; Salje, H.; Van Kerkhove, M.D.; Abadie, V.; Garel, C.; et al. Association between Zika virus and microcephaly in French Polynesia, 2013–2015: A retrospective study. *Lancet* **2016**, *387*, 2125–2132. [CrossRef]

22. Kleber de Oliveira, W.; Cortez-Escalante, J.; De Oliveira, W.T.; do Carmo, G.M.; Henriques, C.M.; Coelho, G.E.; Araujo de Franca, G.V. Increase in Reported Prevalence of Microcephaly in Infants Born to Women Living in Areas with Confirmed Zika Virus Transmission During the First Trimester of Pregnancy-Brazil, 2015. *Mmwr. Morb. Mortal Wkly. Rep.* **2016**, *65*, 242–247. [CrossRef] [PubMed]
23. Shapiro-Mendoza, C.K.; Rice, M.E.; Galang, R.R.; Fulton, A.C.; VanMaldeghem, K.; Prado, M.V.; Ellis, E.; Anesi, M.S.; Simeone, R.M.; Petersen, E.E.; et al. Pregnancy Outcomes After Maternal Zika Virus Infection During Pregnancy-U.S.; Territories, January 1, 2016–April 25, 2017. *Mmwr. Morb. Mortal. Wkly. Rep.* **2017**, *66*, 615–621. [CrossRef]
24. Lin, H.Z.; Tambyah, P.A.; Yong, E.L.; Biswas, A.; Chan, S.Y. A review of Zika virus infections in pregnancy and implications for antenatal care in Singapore. *Singap. Med. J.* **2017**, *58*, 171–178. [CrossRef]
25. Pomar, L.; Malinger, G.; Benoist, G.; Carles, G.; Ville, Y.; Rousset, D.; Hcini, N.; Pomar, C.; Jolivet, A.; Lambert, V. Association between Zika virus and fetopathy: A prospective cohort study in French Guiana. *Ultrasound Obs. Gynecol.* **2017**, *49*, 729–736. [CrossRef] [PubMed]
26. Setoh, Y.X.; Prow, N.A.; Peng, N.; Hugo, L.E.; Devine, G.; Hazlewood, J.E.; Suhrbier, A.; Khromykh, A.A. De Novo Generation and Characterization of New Zika Virus Isolate Using Sequence Data from a Microcephaly Case. *mSphere* **2017**, *2*, e00190–17. [CrossRef]
27. Stanelle-Bertram, S.; Walendy-Gnirss, K.; Speiseder, T.; Thiele, S.; Asante, I.A.; Dreier, C.; Kouassi, N.M.; Preuss, A.; Pilnitz-Stolze, G.; Muller, U.; et al. Male offspring born to mildly ZIKV-infected mice are at risk of developing neurocognitive disorders in adulthood. *Nat. Microbiol.* **2018**, *3*, 1161–1174. [CrossRef]
28. Yockey, L.J.; Varela, L.; Rakib, T.; Khoury-Hanold, W.; Fink, S.L.; Stutz, B.; Szigeti-Buck, K.; Van den Pol, A.; Lindenbach, B.D.; Horvath, T.L.; et al. Vaginal Exposure to Zika Virus during Pregnancy Leads to Fetal Brain Infection. *Cell* **2016**, *166*, 1247–1256.e4. [CrossRef]
29. Miner, J.J.; Cao, B.; Govero, J.; Smith, A.M.; Fernandez, E.; Cabrera, O.H.; Garber, C.; Noll, M.; Klein, R.S.; Noguchi, K.K.; et al. Zika Virus Infection during Pregnancy in Mice Causes Placental Damage and Fetal Demise. *Cell* **2016**, *165*, 1081–1091. [CrossRef]
30. Valentine, G.C.; Seferovic, M.D.; Fowler, S.W.; Major, A.M.; Gorchakov, R.; Berry, R.; Swennes, A.G.; Murray, K.O.; Suter, M.A.; Aagaard, K.M. Timing of gestational exposure to Zika virus is associated with postnatal growth restriction in a murine model. *Am. J. Obs. Gynecol.* **2018**, *219*, 403.e1–403.e9. [CrossRef] [PubMed]
31. Shao, Q.; Herrlinger, S.; Yang, S.L.; Lai, F.; Moore, J.M.; Brindley, M.A.; Chen, J.F. Zika virus infection disrupts neurovascular development and results in postnatal microcephaly with brain damage. *Development* **2016**, *143*, 4127–4136. [CrossRef]
32. Shao, Q.; Herrlinger, S.; Zhu, Y.N.; Yang, M.; Goodfellow, F.; Stice, S.L.; Qi, X.P.; Brindley, M.A.; Chen, J.F. The African Zika virus MR-766 is more virulent and causes more severe brain damage than current Asian lineage and dengue virus. *Development* **2017**, *144*, 4114–4124. [CrossRef] [PubMed]
33. Li, C.; Xu, D.; Ye, Q.; Hong, S.; Jiang, Y.; Liu, X.; Zhang, N.; Shi, L.; Qin, C.F.; Xu, Z. Zika Virus Disrupts Neural Progenitor Development and Leads to Microcephaly in Mice. *Cell Stem Cell* **2016**, *19*, 672. [CrossRef] [PubMed]
34. Yuan, L.; Huang, X.Y.; Liu, Z.Y.; Zhang, F.; Zhu, X.L.; Yu, J.Y.; Ji, X.; Xu, Y.P.; Li, G.; Li, C.; et al. A single mutation in the prM protein of Zika virus contributes to fetal microcephaly. *Science* **2017**, *358*, 933–936. [CrossRef] [PubMed]
35. Cui, L.; Zou, P.; Chen, E.; Yao, H.; Zheng, H.; Wang, Q.; Zhu, J.N.; Jiang, S.; Lu, L.; Zhang, J. Visual and Motor Deficits in Grown-up Mice with Congenital Zika Virus Infection. *EBioMedicine* **2017**, *20*, 193–201. [CrossRef]
36. Wu, K.Y.; Zuo, G.L.; Li, X.F.; Ye, Q.; Deng, Y.Q.; Huang, X.Y.; Cao, W.C.; Qin, C.F.; Luo, Z.G. Vertical transmission of Zika virus targeting the radial glial cells affects cortex development of offspring mice. *Cell Res.* **2016**, *26*, 645–654. [CrossRef] [PubMed]
37. Jaeger, A.S.; Murrieta, R.A.; Goren, L.R.; Crooks, C.M.; Moriarty, R.V.; Weiler, A.M.; Rybarczyk, S.; Semler, M.R.; Huffman, C.; Mejia, A.; et al. Zika viruses of African and Asian lineages cause fetal harm in a mouse model of vertical transmission. *PLoS Negl. Trop. Dis.* **2019**, *13*, e0007343. [CrossRef]
38. Lanciotti, R.S.; Lambert, A.J.; Holodniy, M.; Saavedra, S.; Signor Ldel, C. Phylogeny of Zika Virus in Western Hemisphere, 2015. *Emerg. Infect. Dis.* **2016**, *22*, 933–935. [CrossRef]
39. Duggal, N.K.; McDonald, E.M.; Weger-Lucarelli, J.; Hawks, S.A.; Ritter, J.M.; Romo, H.; Ebel, G.D.; Brault, A.C. Mutations present in a low-passage Zika virus isolate result in attenuated pathogenesis in mice. *Virology* **2019**, *530*, 19–26. [CrossRef]
40. Nakayama, E.; Kato, F.; Tajima, S.; Ogawa, S.; Yan, K.; Takahashi, K.; Sato, Y.; Suzuki, T.; Kawai, Y.; Inagaki, T.; et al. Neuroinvasiveness of the MR766 strain of Zika virus in IFNAR-/- mice maps to prM residues conserved amongst African genotype viruses. *PLoS Pathog.* **2021**, *17*, e1009788. [CrossRef]
41. Setoh, Y.X.; Peng, N.Y.; Nakayama, E.; Amarilla, A.A.; Prow, N.A.; Suhrbier, A.; Khromykh, A.A. Fetal Brain Infection Is Not a Unique Characteristic of Brazilian Zika Viruses. *Viruses* **2018**, *10*, 541. [CrossRef]
42. Prow, N.A.; Liu, L.; Nakayama, E.; Cooper, T.H.; Yan, K.; Eldi, P.; Hazlewood, J.E.; Tang, B.; Le, T.T.; Setoh, Y.X.; et al. A vaccinia-based single vector construct multi-pathogen vaccine protects against both Zika and chikungunya viruses. *Nat. Commun.* **2018**, *9*, 1230. [CrossRef]
43. Kawai, Y.; Nakayama, E.; Takahashi, K.; Taniguchi, S.; Shibasaki, K.I.; Kato, F.; Maeki, T.; Suzuki, T.; Tajima, S.; Saijo, M.; et al. Increased growth ability and pathogenicity of American- and Pacific-subtype Zika virus (ZIKV) strains compared with a Southeast Asian-subtype ZIKV strain. *PLoS Negl. Trop. Dis.* **2019**, *13*, e0007387. [CrossRef] [PubMed]

44. Kato, F.; Tajima, S.; Nakayama, E.; Kawai, Y.; Taniguchi, S.; Shibasaki, K.; Taira, M.; Maeki, T.; Lim, C.K.; Takasaki, T.; et al. Characterization of large and small-plaque variants in the Zika virus clinical isolate ZIKV/Hu/S36/Chiba/2016. *Sci. Rep.* **2017**, *7*, 16160. [CrossRef] [PubMed]
45. Hobson-Peters, J.; Harrison, J.J.; Watterson, D.; Hazlewood, J.E.; Vet, L.J.; Newton, N.D.; Warrilow, D.; Colmant, A.M.G.; Taylor, C.; Huang, B.; et al. A recombinant platform for flavivirus vaccines and diagnostics using chimeras of a new insect-specific virus. *Sci. Transl. Med.* **2019**, *11*. [CrossRef]
46. Hazlewood, J.E.; Rawle, D.J.; Tang, B.; Yan, K.; Vet, L.J.; Nakayama, E.; Hobson-Peters, J.; Hall, R.A.; Suhrbier, A. A Zika Vaccine Generated Using the Chimeric Insect-Specific Binjari Virus Platform Protects against Fetal Brain Infection in Pregnant Mice. *Vaccines* **2020**, *8*, 496. [CrossRef] [PubMed]
47. Lanciotti, R.S.; Kosoy, O.L.; Laven, J.J.; Velez, J.O.; Lambert, A.J.; Johnson, A.J.; Stanfield, S.M.; Duffy, M.R. Genetic and serologic properties of Zika virus associated with an epidemic, Yap State, Micronesia, 2007. *Emerg. Infect. Dis.* **2008**, *14*, 1232–1239. [CrossRef] [PubMed]
48. Gardner, J.; Anraku, I.; Le, T.T.; Larcher, T.; Major, L.; Roques, P.; Schroder, W.A.; Higgs, S.; Suhrbier, A. Chikungunya virus arthritis in adult wild-type mice. *J. Virol.* **2010**, *84*, 8021–8032. [CrossRef] [PubMed]
49. Schroder, W.A.; Le, T.T.; Major, L.; Street, S.; Gardner, J.; Lambley, E.; Markey, K.; MacDonald, K.P.; Fish, R.J.; Thomas, R.; et al. A physiological function of inflammation-associated SerpinB2 is regulation of adaptive immunity. *J. Immunol.* **2010**, *184*, 2663–2670. [CrossRef]
50. Rogers, D.C.; Fisher, E.M.; Brown, S.D.; Peters, J.; Hunter, A.J.; Martin, J.E. Behavioral and functional analysis of mouse phenotype: SHIRPA, a proposed protocol for comprehensive phenotype assessment. *Mamm. Genome: Off. J. Int. Mamm. Genome Soc.* **1997**, *8*, 711–713. [CrossRef]
51. Martins, Y.C.; Werneck, G.L.; Carvalho, L.J.; Silva, B.P.; Andrade, B.G.; Souza, T.M.; Souza, D.O.; Daniel-Ribeiro, C.T. Algorithms to predict cerebral malaria in murine models using the SHIRPA protocol. *Malar. J.* **2010**, *9*, 1–13. [CrossRef]
52. Romeo, R.D.; Mueller, A.; Sisti, H.M.; Ogawa, S.; McEwen, B.S.; Brake, W.G. Anxiety and fear behaviors in adult male and female C57BL/6 mice are modulated by maternal separation. *Horm. Behav.* **2003**, *43*, 561–567. [CrossRef]
53. Parfitt, D.B.; Levin, J.K.; Saltstein, K.P.; Klayman, A.S.; Greer, L.M.; Helmreich, D.L. Differential early rearing environments can accentuate or attenuate the responses to stress in male C57BL/6 mice. *Brain Res.* **2004**, *1016*, 111–118. [CrossRef]
54. Lackner, P.; Beer, R.; Heussler, V.; Goebel, G.; Rudzki, D.; Helbok, R.; Tannich, E.; Schmutzhard, E. Behavioural and histopathological alterations in mice with cerebral malaria. *Neuropathol. Appl. Neurobiol.* **2006**, *32*, 177–188. [CrossRef]
55. Lacerda-Queiroz, N.; Rodrigues, D.H.; Vilela, M.C.; Miranda, A.S.; Amaral, D.C.; Camargos, E.R.; Carvalho, L.J.; Howe, C.L.; Teixeira, M.M.; Teixeira, A.L. Inflammatory changes in the central nervous system are associated with behavioral impairment in Plasmodium berghei (strain ANKA)-infected mice. *Exp. Parasitol.* **2010**, *125*, 271–278. [CrossRef] [PubMed]
56. Maeki, T.; Tajima, S.; Ikeda, M.; Kato, F.; Taniguchi, S.; Nakayama, E.; Takasaki, T.; Lim, C.K.; Saijo, M. Analysis of cross-reactivity between flaviviruses with sera of patients with Japanese encephalitis showed the importance of neutralization tests for the diagnosis of Japanese encephalitis. *J. Infect. Chemother. Off. J. Jpn. Soc. Chemother.* **2019**, *25*, 786–790. [CrossRef]
57. Tajima, S.; Yagasaki, K.; Kotaki, A.; Tomikawa, T.; Nakayama, E.; Moi, M.L.; Lim, C.K.; Saijo, M.; Kurane, I.; Takasaki, T. In vitro growth, pathogenicity and serological characteristics of the Japanese encephalitis virus genotype V Muar strain. *J. Gen. Virol.* **2015**, *96*, 2661–2669. [CrossRef] [PubMed]
58. Mu, J.; Slevin, J.C.; Qu, D.; McCormick, S.; Adamson, S.L. In vivo quantification of embryonic and placental growth during gestation in mice using micro-ultrasound. *Reprod. Biol. Endocrinol. RbE* **2008**, *6*, 34. [CrossRef]
59. de Paula Freitas, B.; de Oliveira Dias, J.R.; Prazeres, J.; Sacramento, G.A.; Ko, A.I.; Maia, M.; Belfort, R. Ocular findings in infants with microcephaly associated with presumed Zika virus congenital infection in Salvador, Brazil. *Jama Ophthalmol.* **2016**, *134*, 529–535. [CrossRef]
60. Guevara, J.G.; Agarwal-Sinha, S. Ocular abnormalities in congenital Zika syndrome: A case report, and review of the literature. *J. Med. Case Rep.* **2018**, *12*, 1–5. [CrossRef] [PubMed]
61. Sousa, A.Q.; Cavalcante, D.I.M.; Franco, L.M.; Araujo, F.M.C.; Sousa, E.T.; Valenca-Junior, J.T.; Rolim, D.B.; Melo, M.E.L.; Sindeaux, P.D.T.; Araujo, M.T.F.; et al. Postmortem Findings for 7 Neonates with Congenital Zika Virus Infection. *Emerg. Infect. Dis.* **2017**, *23*, 1164–1167. [CrossRef] [PubMed]
62. Ximenes, A.; Pires, P.; Werner, H.; Jungmann, P.M.; Rolim Filho, E.L.; Andrade, E.P.; Lemos, R.S.; Peixoto, A.B.; Zare Mehrjardi, M.; Tonni, G.; et al. Neuroimaging findings using transfontanellar ultrasound in newborns with microcephaly: A possible association with congenital Zika virus infection. *J. Matern. Fetal. Neonatal. Med.* **2019**, *32*, 493–501. [CrossRef] [PubMed]
63. Sones, J.L.; Davisson, R.L. Preeclampsia, of mice and women. *Physiol. Genom.* **2016**, *48*, 565–572. [CrossRef] [PubMed]
64. Szaba, F.M.; Tighe, M.; Kummer, L.W.; Lanzer, K.G.; Ward, J.M.; Lanthier, P.; Kim, I.J.; Kuki, A.; Blackman, M.A.; Thomas, S.J.; et al. Zika virus infection in immunocompetent pregnant mice causes fetal damage and placental pathology in the absence of fetal infection. *PLoS Pathog.* **2018**, *14*, e1006994. [CrossRef] [PubMed]
65. Ander, S.E.; Diamond, M.S.; Coyne, C.B. Immune responses at the maternal-fetal interface. *Sci. Immunol.* **2019**, *4*, eaat6114. [CrossRef] [PubMed]
66. Malassiné, A.; Frendo, J.L.; Evain-Brion, D. A comparison of placental development and endocrine functions between the human and mouse model. *Hum. Reprod. Update* **2003**, *9*, 531–539. [CrossRef] [PubMed]

67. Lee, P.A.; Chernausek, S.D.; Hokken-Koelega, A.C.; Czernichow, P. International Small for Gestational Age Advisory Board consensus development conference statement: Management of short children born small for gestational age, April 24–October 1, 2001. *Pediatrics* **2003**, *111*, 1253–1261. [CrossRef]
68. Shields, B.; Wacogne, I.; Wright, C.M. Weight faltering and failure to thrive in infancy and early childhood. *BMJ* **2012**, *345*, e5931. [CrossRef]
69. Ashwal, S.; Michelson, D.; Plawner, L.; Dobyns, W.B. Quality Standards Subcommittee of the American Academy of, N.; the Practice Committee of the Child Neurology, S. Practice parameter: Evaluation of the child with microcephaly (an evidence-based review): Report of the Quality Standards Subcommittee of the American Academy of Neurology and the Practice Committee of the Child Neurology Society. *Neurology* **2009**, *73*, 887–897. [CrossRef]
70. von der Hagen, M.; Pivarcsi, M.; Liebe, J.; von Bernuth, H.; Didonato, N.; Hennermann, J.B.; Buhrer, C.; Wieczorek, D.; Kaindl, A.M. Diagnostic approach to microcephaly in childhood: A two-center study and review of the literature. *Dev. Med. Child. Neurol.* **2014**, *56*, 732–741. [CrossRef]
71. Panchaud, A.; Stojanov, M.; Ammerdorffer, A.; Vouga, M.; Baud, D. Emerging Role of Zika Virus in Adverse Fetal and Neonatal Outcomes. *Clin. Microbiol. Rev.* **2016**, *29*, 659–694. [CrossRef]
72. Shan, C.; Xie, X.; Luo, H.; Muruato, A.E.; Liu, Y.; Wakamiya, M.; La, J.H.; Chung, J.M.; Weaver, S.C.; Wang, T.; et al. Maternal vaccination and protective immunity against Zika virus vertical transmission. *Nat. Commun.* **2019**, *10*, 5677. [CrossRef] [PubMed]
73. Aubry, F.; Jacobs, S.; Darmuzey, M.; Lequime, S.; Delang, L.; Fontaine, A.; Jupatanakul, N.; Miot, E.F.; Dabo, S.; Manet, C.; et al. Recent African strains of Zika virus display higher transmissibility and fetal pathogenicity than Asian strains. *Nat. Commun.* **2021**, *12*, 916. [CrossRef] [PubMed]
74. Cugola, F.R.; Fernandes, I.R.; Russo, F.B.; Freitas, B.C.; Dias, J.L.; Guimaraes, K.P.; Benazzato, C.; Almeida, N.; Pignatari, G.C.; Romero, S.; et al. The Brazilian Zika virus strain causes birth defects in experimental models. *Nature* **2016**, *534*, 267–271. [CrossRef]
75. Paul, A.M.; Acharya, D.; Neupane, B.; Thompson, E.A.; Gonzalez-Fernandez, G.; Copeland, K.M.; Garrett, M.; Liu, H.; Lopez, M.E.; de Cruz, M.; et al. Congenital Zika Virus Infection in Immunocompetent Mice Causes Postnatal Growth Impediment and Neurobehavioral Deficits. *Front. Microbiol.* **2018**, *9*, 2028. [CrossRef] [PubMed]
76. Julander, J.G.; Siddharthan, V.; Park, A.H.; Preston, E.; Mathur, P.; Bertolio, M.; Wang, H.; Zukor, K.; Van Wettere, A.J.; Sinex, D.G.; et al. Consequences of in utero exposure to Zika virus in offspring of AG129 mice. *Sci. Rep.* **2018**, *8*, 9384. [CrossRef]
77. Swann, J.B.; Hayakawa, Y.; Zerafa, N.; Sheehan, K.C.; Scott, B.; Schreiber, R.D.; Hertzog, P.; Smyth, M.J. Type I IFN contributes to NK cell homeostasis, activation, and antitumor function. *J. Immun.* **2007**, *178*, 7540–7549. [CrossRef] [PubMed]

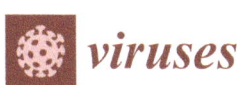

Review

The Current Evidence Regarding COVID-19 and Pregnancy: Where Are We Now and Where Should We Head to Next?

Theodoros Kalampokas [1,†], Anna Rapani [2,†], Maria Papageorgiou [1], Sokratis Grigoriadis [1,2], Evangelos Maziotis [1,2], George Anifandis [3], Olga Triantafyllidou [1], Despoina Tzanakaki [1], Spyridoula Neofytou [1], Panagiotis Bakas [1], Mara Simopoulou [1,2,*,‡] and Nikolaos Vlahos [1,‡]

1. Assisted Conception Unit, Second Department of Obstetrics and Gynecology, Aretaieion Hospital, Medical School, National and Kapodistrian University of Athens, 76, Vasilisis Sofias Avenue, 11528 Athens, Greece; kalamp@yahoo.com (T.K.); mariapap96@windowslive.com (M.P.); sokratis-grigoriadis@hotmail.com (S.G.); vagmaziotis@gmail.com (E.M.); triantafyllidouolga@gmail.com (O.T.); dtzanakaki@gmail.com (D.T.); spinik@yahoo.gr (S.N.); pbakas74@gmail.com (P.B.); nfvlahos@gmail.com (N.V.)
2. Laboratory of Physiology, Medical School, National and Kapodistrian University of Athens, 75, Mikras Asias, 11527 Athens, Greece; rapanianna@gmail.com
3. Department of Histology and Embryology, Faculty of Medicine, University of Thessaly, 41500 Larisa, Greece; ganif@uth.gr
* Correspondence: marasimopoulou@hotmail.com
† Joint first authors.
‡ Joint last authors.

Citation: Kalampokas, T.; Rapani, A.; Papageorgiou, M.; Grigoriadis, S.; Maziotis, E.; Anifandis, G.; Triantafyllidou, O.; Tzanakaki, D.; Neofytou, S.; Bakas, P.; et al. The Current Evidence Regarding COVID-19 and Pregnancy: Where Are We Head to Next? *Viruses* 2021, 13, 2000. https://doi.org/10.3390/v13102000

Academic Editors: David Baud and Leó Pomar

Received: 23 July 2021
Accepted: 28 September 2021
Published: 5 October 2021

Publisher's Note: MDPI stays neutral with regard to jurisdictional claims in published maps and institutional affiliations.

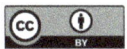

Copyright: © 2021 by the authors. Licensee MDPI, Basel, Switzerland. This article is an open access article distributed under the terms and conditions of the Creative Commons Attribution (CC BY) license (https://creativecommons.org/licenses/by/4.0/).

Abstract: Despite the volume of publications dedicated to unraveling the biological characteristics and clinical manifestations of SARS-CoV-2, available data on pregnant patients are limited. In the current review of literature, we present an overview on the developmental course, complications, and adverse effects of COVID-19 on pregnancy. A comprehensive review of the literature was performed in PubMed/Medline, Embase, and Cochrane Central databases up to June 2021. This article collectively presents what has been so far reported on the identified critical aspects, namely complications during pregnancy, delivery challenges, neonatal health care, potential routes of viral transmission, including vertical transmission or breastfeeding, along with the risks involved in the vaccination strategy during pregnancy. Despite the fact that we are still largely navigating uncharted territory, the observed publication explosion in the field is unprecedented. The overwhelming need for data is undoubtable, and this serves as the driver for the plethora of publications witnessed. Nonetheless, the quality of data sourced is variable. In the midst of the frenzy for reporting on SARS-CoV-2 data, monitoring this informational overload is where we should head to next, considering that poor quality research may in fact hamper our attempts to prevail against this unparalleled pandemic outbreak.

Keywords: pregnancy; COVID-19; complications; delivery; neonatal health; transmission; breast-feeding; vaccination

1. Introduction

A global effort to investigate the pathophysiological mechanisms of SARS-CoV-2 has been noted since the beginning of the current pandemic. The noted explosion of interest in investigating COVID-19 to provide data, map the virus' biological identity, and guide clinicians towards prevention and management strategies [1] is unparalleled. Fertility and reproduction have been in the spotlight of recent publications, since SARS-CoV-2 targets female reproductive organs that express its main receptor ACE2 [2,3]. Hitherto, studies have described the symptomatology, the developmental course and the complications characterizing the COVID-19 disease, while identifying certain patient characteristics that constitute risk factors for manifesting poor outcomes. Nonetheless, the effect of COVID-19 on pregnancy, leading to a unique state of different human physiology, has yet to be fully elucidated [4].

The limited and contradicting data on pregnant patients have resulted in a lack of established guidelines. Coupled by the fact that the vast discrepancies in management may be a strong indication of poor standards and fast track publication policies, these circumstances cause uncertainty both for the patients and clinicians. The current review of literature provides an all-inclusive overview of the published studies concerning the impact of COVID-19 on several aspects of pregnancy. The complications and adverse effects on maternal health status are presented, along with data on the optimal delivery method for pregnant patients who have tested positive for COVID-19. The subsequent neonatal health and potential risk of vertical transmission or a potential viral transmission during breastfeeding are further discussed. The debated matter of vaccination policy during pregnancy is presented, as well as the latest available data in this field of interest. The aim of this review is to collectively present evidence on the impact of COVID-19 on several aspects of pregnancy and discuss how data contribute to the scientific progress during this pandemic. The wealth of information is overwhelming, yet fails to provide definitive conclusions. What becomes apparent is the challenge in navigating this maze of publications, while the variable quality of data sourced adds another level of complexity.

2. Materials and Methods

A comprehensive review of the literature was performed in PubMed/Medline, Embase, and Cochrane Central databases up to June 2021. Literature screening was performed employing a combination of Medical Subject Headings (MeSH) terms and keywords, including: "2019 novel coronavirus pandemic"'; "COVID-19"; "severe acute respiratory syndrome coronavirus 2"; "SARS-CoV-2"; "coronavirinae"; "coronavirus infection"; "pregnancy"; "pregnancy outcome"; "pregnancy complications"; "neonatal outcomes"; "perinatal outcomes"; "delivery"; "labor"; "vertical transmission"; "mother to fetus transmission"; "breastfeeding"; "vaccination"; "vaccines"; "vaccination safety". The search was limited to full-length manuscripts published in English in international peer-reviewed journals. Original research articles describing studies performed in humans as well as review papers were sourced. In order to provide an all-inclusive analysis of the current evidence, no specific inclusion and exclusion criteria regarding study selection process were employed. Regarding type of study, different types of studies were considered eligible to be included in this review, namely prospective and retrospective observational and interventional studies, randomized controlled trials, case reports and case series, as well as systematic reviews and meta-analysis. From the articles retrieved in the first round of search, additional references were identified by manual citation mining. Following literature assessment, authors categorized the sourced studies according to the specific topic of research investigated in five categories, namely: 1. studies investigating complications of COVID-19 reported during pregnancy; 2. studies investigating labor-related challenges in pregnant women infected by SARS-CoV-2; 3. studies investigating neonatal and perinatal outcomes in neonates born from COVID-19 positive mothers; 4. studies aiming to address the possible mechanisms of SARS-CoV-2 vertical transmission; 5. studies examining breastfeeding-related concerns; and 6. studies debating vaccination efficacy and safety during pregnancy and lactation. A critical analysis of these aspects was performed in order to provide an all-inclusive overview of the current evidence.

3. Complications of COVID-19 Reported in Pregnancy

Prior to discussing the complications of COVID-19 during pregnancy, a primary factor that seems to exert a substantial impact on the manifestation of the disease is the timing of viral exposure. The association between the risk of viral transmission and certain stages of pregnancy remains vague. The cases of two pregnant women who were found to be positive for SARS-CoV-2 during the first weeks of pregnancy have been reported [5]. In the second trimester of their pregnancy, both underwent amniocentesis for the evaluation of the existence of SARS-CoV-2 RNA, as well as for an assessment of antibodies in amniotic fluid samples. Despite the negative results, the concern of a potential in utero transmission during the first trimester merits further investigation. Concerning cases of COVID-19 infection during the second trimester of pregnancy, interesting conclusions are proposed. Tang et al. revealed two second trimester pregnancies that tested positive for COVID-19 [6]. At the time of delivery, both women had a negative SARS-CoV-2 RNA test in throat swab samples, but elevated titles of antibodies. Both babies were healthy and throat swabs tested negative. IgG antibodies levels were elevated in both cases, due to transmission from the mother, despite lacking any sign indicative of acute infection. One case of a COVID-19 positive pregnant woman who delivered in the second trimester has been also reported [7], with no evidence supporting the potential transmission of the virus.

Regarding the complications and their severity attributed to the diagnosis of COVID-19, a special interest has been noted in unveiling the factors contributing to adverse health outcomes and to the deterioration of health status. The range of clinical manifestations described in cases of pregnant patients diagnosed with COVID-19 includes mild flu-like symptoms to the onset of severe pneumonia. Fever and cough constitute the most frequent symptoms described in pregnant women, while myalgia, shortness of breath, sore throat, nasal congestion, diarrhea, headache, and chills are further contributing to the symptomatology (Table 1). The clinical course of the disease in pregnant and non-pregnant women has been investigated by Wang et al. Interestingly, a milder clinical course was described in pregnant women, along with a higher rate of asymptomatic cases and a reduced duration of hospitalization [8]. Based on the observations of 43 pregnant women who tested positive for SARS-CoV-2, 29 of them presented to the hospital suffering from COVID-19 symptoms, while the remaining 14 were asymptomatic. In two cases, severe complications involving respiratory distress syndrome were developed [9].

Table 1. An overview of the reported symptomatology in pregnant patients diagnosed with COVID-19, as described in the included studies.

Study	No of Pregnant Women	Trimester/ Gestation	No of Asymptomatic Women	Fever	Cough	Dyspnea	Myalgia	Headache	Diarrhea	Other
[10]	1	33 w	-	0	1	1	1	0	0	Nausea, vomiting, acute pancreatitis
[11]	1	21 w	-	1	1	0	0	0	0	Anosmia, ageusia
[12]	1	32 w	-	1	1	0	1	0	0	Anorexia, nausea
[13]	1	20 w	-	0	1	0	0	0	0	Acroparaesthesia, bilateral lower extremity weakness, dysphonia, dysphagia, Guillain-Barré syndrome
[14]	1219	37.7 w (median)	579	214	414	230	232	188	63	Nasal stiffness, chills, anosmia, fatigue, sore throat, nausea
[15]	427	29–38 w	-	>250	>200	>150	>50	>50	>20	Vomiting, rhinorrhea, lethargy, sore throat
[16]	118	3rd (75)	6	84	81	8	-	7	8	Chest tightness, fatigue
[17]	13	1st (5) 2nd (3) 3rd (5)	-	8	5	1	1	-	1	-
[18]	51	3rd	26	27	31	-	14	-	-	Fatigue
[19]	16	3rd	-	12	0	0	-	-	-	-
[20]	1	22 w	-	1	1	-	1	-	1	Vaginal bleeding, abdominal pain
[21]	78	27–41 w	20	24	29	8	11	7	5	Anosmia, rhinorrhea

Table 1. Cont.

Study	No of Pregnant Women	Trimester/ Gestation	No of Asymptomatic Women	Fever	Cough	Dyspnea	Myalgia	Headache	Diarrhea	Other
[22]	594 (including 6 w postpartum Women)	1st (77) 2nd (241) 3rd (196) Postpartum (76)	-	71	119	-	71	-	-	Sore throat
[23]	1	38 w	-	-	1	-	-	-	-	Chest tightness
[6]	2	24 w, 27 w	-	2	0	1	-	0	-	-
[7]	15	37 w	-	10	6	-	-	-	1	-
[24]	1	34 w	-	-	-	1	1	-	-	-
[25]	1	38 w	-	1	1	-	-	1	1	Rhinorrhea, sore throat
[26]	1	22 w	-	1	-	-	-	-	-	Rhinitis
[27]	1	34 w	-	1	-	-	-	-	1	-
[28]	2	34 w, 37 w	-	1	1	1	-	-	1	-
[8]	30	30–40.9 w	8	11	5	-	-	-	-	Abdominal pain, haemoptysis, fatigue, poor appetite
[29]	1	33 w	-	-	-	-	-	-	-	-
[30]	1	32 w	-	1	-	-	-	-	-	Flu-like symptoms
[31]	1	38 w	-	1	-	-	-	-	-	-
[32]	64	29.9 ± 5.8 w	-	-	-	-	-	-	-	-
[33]	1	19 w	-	1	1	-	1	-	1	Sore throat, fatigue
[34]	38	29.3 ± 8.5	-	10	25	13	-	-	7	Sore throat, fatigue, anosmia
[35]	100	31.3 w (median)	-	62	80	30	26	-	10	Anosmia, sore throat
[36]	9	36–39 w	-	7	4	1	3	-	1	Sore throat, malaise
[37]	7	37–41 w	-	6	1	1	-	-	1	-
[38]	1	35 w	-	-	1	-	-	-	-	-
[39]	19	35–41 w	-	11	5	5	-	-	2	-
[40]	17	35–41 w	-	3	6	2	-	-	3	Nasal congestion, sputum production
[36]	1	35 w	-	1	-	1	-	-	-	Fatigue
[41]	3	34–38 w	-	2	3	1	-	-	-	-
[42]	1	35 w	-	-	1	-	-	-	-	-
[43]	1	39 w	-	-	1	-	-	-	-	-
[44]	1	29 w	-	1	-	1	-	-	-	Rhinitis
[45]	1	34 w	-	1	-	1	-	-	-	Nasal congestion
[46]	7	>36 w	-	7/7	6/7	-	-	-	6/7	-
[47]	4	3rd	-	3/4	2/4	2/4	2/4	-	-	Fatigue
[48]	1	30 w	-	1/1	-	-	-	-	-	-
[49]	9	-	-	9/9	9/9	-	-	-	1	-
[50]	7	28–37 w	2/7	2/7	3/7	-	3/7	2/7	-	Chest pain
[51]	1	35 w	-	1/1	1/1	-	-	-	-	-
[52]	1	38 w	1	-	-	-	-	-	-	-
[53]	1	33 w	-	1/1	-	1/1	-	-	-	-
[54]	9	24–36 w	-	9/9	9/9	5/9	4/9	-	-	-

Another study including symptomatic pregnant women showcased the need for closer and meticulous monitoring of these patients when they are older than thirty-five years, and while characterized by at least one comorbidity, namely obesity, gestational diabetes, or hypertension [34]. Eight out of the seventy pregnant women with a severe or critical diagnosis of COVID-19 that were included in the study by Blitz et al. required intubation, with subsequent documentation of two deaths [55]. To emphasize the significance of obesity, a 10% ICU hospitalization rate has been reported in pregnant women with increased body mass index, attributed as the sole statistically significant factor contributing to this outcome [35]. Moreover, in a UK cohort study involving four hundred twenty-seven pregnant women with COVID-19, one in ten women were hospitalized and required respiratory support in ICU, while 70% of the patients were reported with increased BMI, 40% were >35 years old, and a third had comorbidities [15]. A case report of a 41-year-old obese and diabetic pregnant patient who manifested respiratory failure and required mechanical ventilation [53], as well as the case of two asymptomatic patients who developed symptoms of an upper respiratory tract infection following labor have been documented. In the last report, it should be emphasized that both of these two patients were obese and diabetic, while one of them had a history of chronic hypertension and asthma [50].

Besides the investigation of obesity as a factor contributing to the manifestation of severe complications, the role of the week of gestation during the time of diagnosis has been assessed and concluded as a potential parameter affecting severity of the disease. According to a case-control study evaluating ICU admissions and the requirement of respiratory support among pregnant and non-pregnant women diagnosed with COVID-19, pregnant women diagnosed when they were over the 20th week mark of gestation were at a higher risk of severe adverse outcomes, in comparison to the non-pregnant group. Amongst the two groups of patients, other comorbidities or obesity were not found to be remarkably differentiated [56]. A study including 64 women with severe or critical manifestations of COVID-19 demonstrated that all of the patients who experienced critical symptoms were >24th week of gestation at the time of the initial symptoms. Contrary to the abovementioned study, in this report comorbidities were documented, including pulmonary conditions and cardiac diseases in 25% and 17%, respectively [32].

Little is known in regard to the cardiovascular complications of coronavirus disease 2019 in pregnancy. Differentiating between postpartum cardiomyopathy and COVID-19-related cardiomyopathy in infected pregnant women is challenging. The case of a young pregnant woman who exhibited signs of heart failure with pulmonary edema following cesarean section has been presented in the literature [57]. Coagulopathy is considered to be associated with COVID-19, which in turn may result in the onset of further complications, including deep vein thrombosis [58]. The case of an obese, young, pregnant woman who developed ovarian vein thrombosis while being diagnosed with COVID-19 has been documented in the literature [59]. Another report on an obese, young, pregnant woman showcased an event of pulmonary embolism despite her being administered with prophylactic anticoagulation protocol [44]. The case of a pregnant woman who tested positive for COVID-19 has been published, showcasing the onset of venous sinus thrombosis following symptoms of headache and hemiparesis. As concluded in that case report, in the presence of suspected hypercoagulability and atypical features, venous sinus thrombosis should be considered in the differential diagnosis for patients with COVID-19 [60]. Acute pancreatitis constitutes a rare complication of primary COVID-19 infection, as presented in a case report describing a patient who was diagnosed while being hospitalized due to COVID-19-related pneumonia. The patient exhibited signs of improvement postpartum and was further discharged home [10]. Moreover, the impact of SARS-CoV-2 on the neurological system has been emphasized, as the virus's neurotropism potential has been in the spotlight of research. Some cases of Guillain–Barre Syndrome associated with COVID-19 have been recently revealed [13,61].

Considering the impact of SARS-CoV-2 infection during pregnancy on maternal and neonatal morbidity and mortality, recent published data from large epidemiological studies warrant great interest and thus should be highlighted. One of the largest cohorts that have been published so far is the INTERCOVID study [62]. This is a multicenter multinational cohort study, including 2130 women from 43 institutions and 18 countries, from March to

October 2020. The authors of this study investigated to what extent SARS-CoV-2 infection during pregnancy could increase the risk of adverse maternal and neonatal outcomes in comparison to pregnant women without COVID-19. In total, 706 pregnant women positive for SARS-CoV-2 were included in the study. To minimize the respective bias, for each of the study participants, the authors included two matched not-infected women, serving as controls. In total, 1424 not-infected women were allocated to the control group. The study and the control groups were matched according to the stage of pregnancy, the type and stage of delivery, as well as the level of patient care received. The primary outcome measures were the incidence of adverse pregnancy, neonatal, and perinatal outcomes, including morbidity and mortality. Statistical analysis was performed, employing models to adjust the findings according to country, month entering study, maternal age, and medical history. Provided data indicated that SARS-CoV-2 infection during pregnancy is strongly associated with adverse pregnancy outcomes, including pre-eclampsia/eclampsia, severe infections, intensive care unit admission, and medically induced preterm labor. The risk of adverse neonatal and perinatal outcomes, such as severe neonatal morbidity and severe perinatal morbidity and mortality, also presented to be statistically significantly increased. In addition, COVID-19-related symptoms, such as fever and shortness of breath were associated with increased risk of severe maternal and neonatal complications. Interestingly, even the asymptomatic women presented with an increased risk of pregnancy complications, including pre-eclampsia and higher maternal morbidity. Infant positivity for SARS-CoV-2 was calculated to be 13%. Delivery via cesarean section but not breast feeding was associated with an increased risk of neonatal transmission [62]. Similar results are also provided from other smaller cohort studies performed in different populations worldwide, including cohorts in Spain, Turkey, India, and Iran [63–66]. These recently published data demonstrate that in comparison to the general pregnant population, COVID-19 infected pregnant women present with increased risk of adverse maternal, neonatal, and perinatal outcomes, highlighting the need for careful monitoring of pregnancies implicating COVID-19.

On the antipode of this influx of evidence demonstrating that pregnant women may experience a more severe clinical manifestation of COVID-19, one study reported that pregnant women with comorbidities were not characterized by a higher risk of hospitalization. Moreover, in this study, non-pregnant patients more frequently reported fever, contrary to pregnant patients who frequently reported symptoms of myalgia, fatigue, and headaches [22]. On the same note, pregnant women exhibit a lower risk of developing a severe symptomatology if diagnosed with COVID-19 in comparison to the general population [16]. However, the cases describing and raising awareness on the phenomenon of maternal deaths call for cautious conclusions regarding the actual risk that pregnant women may experience. Amongst published studies referring to maternal deaths, Hantoushzadeh et al. presented the cases of nine severely affected pregnant women. Seven out of nine died due to cardiopulmonary complications, one remained intubated in the ICU, and one recovered, while it should be noted that the majority of the patients had no comorbidities [54].

Clinical manifestations of pregnant women that tested positive for COVID-19 should be further examined and considered when managing this cohort of patients. In an effort to evaluate the common laboratory test findings in pregnant women with COVID-19, interesting observations have been published. In the majority of these patients, a normal count of white blood cells has been reported, while lymphopenia constitutes the most common finding. In cases of women with severe symptomatology who require admission to the ICU, the lymphocyte count was found to be lower [35]. Thrombocytopenia has been described in three mild cases of pregnant patients [67]. Such a finding should be highlighted and acknowledged prior to initiating any invasive pregnancy-related procedure, such as the placement of an epidural catheter. Increased levels of alanine aminotransferase (ALT) and aspartate aminotransferase (AST), as well as elevated C-reactive protein (CRP) is present in many cases of pregnant patients. Inflammation marker levels are remarkably higher in pregnant patients who have tested positive for the SARS-CoV-2 in comparison to the non-pregnant group [8]. Regarding the computed tomography (CT) findings, pregnant women were subjected to chest CT, representing the modality of choice for early detection. The typical findings of viral pneumonia were detected similarly to the cases of non-pregnant patients [68]. These findings include decreased diffuse and ground glass opacities, patchy lung consolidation, blurred borders, and lesions merged into strips in some cases [49]. As evident in literature, severe pneumonia, tracheal intubation and artificial ventilation, as well as an emergency cesarean section were performed under general anesthesia in a 39-year-old woman diagnosed with COVID-19 at 25 weeks of gestation. This suggests the need to explore the risk of increased coronavirus disease severity during pregnancy, the impact on perinatal prognosis, as well as the management that pregnancy requires under such circumstances [69].

4. Challenges during Delivery of Pregnant Patients with COVID-19

Since SARS-CoV-2 transmission and COVID-19 pathophysiology remain vague, the timing and mode of delivery constitute a challenging issue. Based on current evidence, the guidelines suggest that the delivery mode should be individualized and personalized, based on the obstetric indications and the maternal–fetal status [70]. The indications for performing a C-section include prematurity, breech presentation, fetal intrauterine distress, premature rapture of membrane, arrest of descent, arrest of dilation, failed induction, decrease in the fetal heart rate, severe pre-eclampsia, history of another C-section, abnormal amniotic fluid, umbilical cord or placenta (placenta previa), and no fetal movement or no variability of fetal heart monitoring. As evident in several studies, due to the lack of data on determining the risk of intrapartum mother-to-child transmission, vaginal delivery was avoided.

A higher risk of adverse outcomes related to delivery have been attributed to cases of pregnant women with COVID-19. More specifically, iatrogenic preterm births and C-sections are more often expected in comparison to pregnant women who tested negative for COVID-19 [71]. To add to this observation, Knight et al. reported that among the preterm births that were observed, 80% were required due to the deterioration of the maternal health status [15]. Furthermore, the rate of preterm births and C-sections among critically ill pregnant patients was notably elevated. Interestingly, as it has been voiced, 75% of critically ill pregnant women gave birth prematurely, while the 94% delivered by C-section due to the deterioration of their health status [32]. Amongst patients hospitalized in the ICU, 80% delivered via C-section [35]. Several studies report the performance of C-sections on the grounds of severely compromised maternal status, such as respiratory insufficiency and pulmonary embolism that required urgent attention and intervention [44,53,54]. Contrary to the above, there is a case of a COVID-19 positive pregnant woman in the 33rd week of gestation, for whom delivery was required in order to improve the maternal respiratory status. Following labor induction, vaginal delivery was performed while the patient was under ventilation with an impressive outcome. Therefore, the need for strict patient selection when contemplating delivery method should be prioritized, since despite the worsening respiratory status of some pregnant patients indicating the need for performing a C-section, they may still undergo an induced vaginal labor [29].

Whether delivery itself could ameliorate the severe effects of COVID-19 and restore maternal health status is a valid question. A study demonstrated that an improvement of the respiratory status may be observed following delivery. Nonetheless, whether the delivery mode is implicated to affect maternal status post-partum remains to be validated [72]. When concrete data concerning the risks involved in delivery method is published, clinicians should be able to establish a common strategy that will ascertain optimal obstetric and perinatal results, safeguarding both the women's and the newborn's safety.

5. Neonates' Health Status

No significant differences have been observed regarding the clinical course and the laboratory findings in neonates born to mothers diagnosed as positive, compared to those who have tested negative for COVID-19. The only finding of significance concerns the significantly decreased birthweight in neonates born by mothers positive for COVID-19 [7]. Moreover, Hantoushzadeh et al. have reported three cases of fetal deaths in cases of critically ill mothers [54]. The case of a newborn that tested positive for SARS-CoV-2 immediately following birth via C-section has been published. The baby manifested a severe course of the disease with tachypnea, cyanosis, and dyspnea subsequently requiring respiratory support. Both the baby and mother, who were intubated for twenty-four hours, were safely discharged home [25]. Sisman et al. described the case of a premature neonate born by a COVID-19 positive mother who developed fever, hypoxia, and neonatal respiratory distress syndrome in the second day of life, and tested positive in the throat swab test for COVID-19. It was assumed that this case constitutes a congenital infection based on the placenta findings [27]. Two severely ill premature neonates born by COVID-19 positive mothers were intubated in the neonatal intensive care unit and underwent a prolonged hospitalization [73]. In this study, an interesting point is raised with regard to the potential association between premature neonates and a more severe course of COVID-19. However, in such cases, prematurity stands as a confounder, allowing for no further extrapolations to be drawn concerning the severity of the disease in these babies.

Regarding the reported complications observed in neonates, neonatal pneumonia, mild grunting following birth due to mild Newborn Respiratory Distress Syndrome (NRDS), tachypnea, and moaning are reported. All these cases were successfully treated, employing continuous positive airway pressure ventilation [40,46,74]. Zhu et al. described one neonate, delivered at a gestational age of 34 + 5 weeks, who developed shortness of breath, moaning, and thrombocytopenia along with abnormal liver function. Due to multiple organ failure and disseminated intravascular coagulation, its death was reported on the ninth day of admission. However, another case presenting with a common symptomatology was successfully treated by employing respiratory support, and recovered fifteen days later [49]. In a study by Vivanti et al., a neonate, whose mother tested positive for SARS-CoV-2, developed neurological symptoms. Three days following birth, it exhibited irritability, poor feeding, axial hypertonia, and opisthotonos, whereas a sample of cerebrospinal fluid was collected and further tested negative for the virus. The neonate gradually recovered and was finally discharged eighteen days later [51]. An overview of neonates' health status born by mothers that were positive for COVID-19 is depicted in Table 2.

Table 2. An overview of the reported neonatal outcomes in pregnant patients diagnosed with COVID-19 as described in the included studies.

Study	No of Pregnant Women	Completed Pregnancy	Vaginal Birth	C-Section	Preterm Delivery	Neonatal Adverse Outcomes	NICU Admission	Neonatal Death	Stillbirth	Miscarriage
[10]	1	1	1	0	1	0	1	0	0	0
[11]	1	1	0	1	1	SGA	1	1	0	0
[12]	1	1	0	1	1	Respiratory distress	1	0	0	0
[14]	1219	1196	-	450	204	-	254	5	-	-
[15]	427	266	106	156	66	Neonatal encephalopathy	67	2	3	4
[16]	118	68	5	63	14	-	-	0	0	-
[17]	1	1	-	1	-	-	-	-	-	-
[18]	13	6	1	4	2	Neonatal pneumonia	0	0	0	1
[19]	51	51	26	25	10	-	-	0	0	0
[20]	16	16	2	14	3	-	-	0	0	0
[21]	1	0	0	0	0	-	-	-	-	1
[75]	31	31	25	6	1	2 infected neonates	2	0	0	0

Table 2. Cont.

Study	No of Pregnant Women	Completed Pregnancy	Vaginal Birth	C-Section	Preterm Delivery	Neonatal Adverse Outcomes	NICU Admission	Neonatal Death	Stillbirth	Miscarriage
[22]	116	106	63	43	14	Prolonged QT syndrome, mild respiratory distress, short bowel syndrome, tachycardia	12	0	0	0
[6]	1	1	1	-	-	-	1: quarantine	-	-	-
[71]	65	65	13	52	9	Asphyxia, fever, diarrhea	-	-	-	-
[7]	2	2	1	1	0	Jaundice	0	0	0	0
[24]	15	15	1	14	1	NRDS	15: quarantine	0	0	0
[25]	1	1	-	1	1	-	1	0	0	0
[26]	1	1	-	1	-	Severe COVID-19	1	0	0	0
[27]	1	1	1	-	2	-	-	-	-	2 (twins)
[28]	1	1	1	-	1	Jaundice, fever, respiratory distress hypoxia	1	0	0	0
[8]	2	2	-	2	1	-	-	-	-	-
[29]	30	30	7	23	5	-	-	-	-	-
[30]	1	1	1	-	1	Intubation	1	-	-	-
[31]	1	1 (triplets)	-	3	3	1: NCPAP	3	0	0	0
[32]	1	1	1	-	-	Abdominal distension, respiratory acidosis, intubation	1	0	0	0
[33]	64	32	8	24	29	2: IUGR	21	0	0	0
[34]	1	1	1	-	-	-	-	-	-	1
[35]	38	17	10	7	10	3: intubated	3	0	0	1
[36]	100	33	17	16	20	6: intubated	10	1	0	0
[36]	9	9	0	9	4	-	0	0	0	0
[37]	7	7	0	7	0	1: mild pulmonary infection	0	0	0	0
[38]	1	1	-	1	1	-	0	0	0	0
[39]	19	19	1	18	0	-	19: isolation	0	0	0
[40]	17	17	0	17	3	5: neonatal pneumonia	-	0	0	0
[36]	1	1	-	1	1	Tachypnea, moaning, periodic breath	1	0	0	0
[41]	3	3	3	0	1	-	0	0	0	0
[42]	1	1	0	1	1	-	0	0	0	0
[43]	1	1	0	1	0	-	0	0	0	0
[44]	1	1	0	1	1	-	1	0	0	0
[45]	1	1	0	1	0	-	1: quarantine	0	0	0
[46]	7	7	0	7	4	Respiratory distress	5	0	0	0
[47]	4	4	1	3	0	TTN, rash	2	0	0	0
[48]	1	1	0	1	1	-	1: isolation	0	0	0
[49]	9	9	2	7	6	Dyspnea, fever, vomit, NRDS, pneumothorax, thrombopenia	-	1	0	0
[51]	1	1	0	1	1	Intubation, neurological symptoms	1	0	0	0
[52]	1	1	0	1	0	-	0	0	0	0
[53]	1	1	0	1	1	Intubation	1	0	0	0
[54]	9	9	1	8	-	Intubation, pneumonia	-	2	4	-

6. Delineating the Phenomenon of Vertical Transmission

A crucial concern that challenges obstetricians is whether a transplacental transmission could occur in cases of pregnant patients diagnosed with COVID-19. The placenta constitutes a specialized organ, vital for the development of the fetus as well as for the protection of the fetus. However, as depicted in the literature, many bacteria or viruses, such as cytomegalovirus, human immunodeficiency virus, and rubella virus, could cross the placenta barrier and infect the fetus [76]. Despite the fact that many placenta pathologies have been described [77], transplacental transmission and its frequency still remain a controversial topic of scientific interest.

In a study performed by Yu et al., the nucleic acid test for the throat swab of one neonate was positive for SARS-CoV-2 thirty-six hours following birth [37]. However, in the abovementioned case, intrauterine tissue samples, including placenta and cord blood, were detected as negative, rendering the hypothesis of a potential intrauterine vertical transmission vague. Another report describes a case of vertical transmission from the asymptomatic mother to the baby. The molecular detection of SARS-CoV-2 in mother's blood at delivery and in the neonatal nasopharyngeal confirmed the infection [78]. Alwardi et al. reported a case of preterm triplets born by a coronavirus positive pregnant woman. All of them tested positive from the nasopharyngeal swab drawn twenty hours following birth, while one of the triplets required nasal ventilation for eight hours [30]. In a study by Khan et al., seventeen swab samples were tested for SARS-CoV-2, out of which two were positive. However, the viral nucleic acid test of placenta, cord blood, or amniotic fluid were not tested to confirm whether intrauterine vertical transmission has occurred [40]. Along the same lines, Alzamora et al. confirmed infection on a neonate's nasopharyngeal swab sixteen hours following birth. Nonetheless, amniotic fluid, cord blood, or placental tissue samples were not tested in order to investigate the presence of the virus [53]. Interestingly, Marzollo et al. revealed the case of a possible congenital COVID-19 infection. A full-term neonate who was delivered vaginally by a positive tested mother demonstrated respiratory and gastrointestinal symptoms soon after birth [31].

A proven case of transplacental transmission of SARS-CoV-2 from a pregnant woman affected by COVID-19 during the third trimester of pregnancy has been published [51]. The nasopharyngeal and rectal swabs, as well as placenta samples were collected and further tested positive for SARS-CoV-2 by employing RT-PCR. It should be noted that the viral load was significantly higher in the placental tissue than in amniotic fluid or in maternal or neonatal blood. Moreover, the first study to report persistent placental infection of SARS-CoV-2 and its congenital transmission has been recently published. As mentioned, the transmission is associated with hydrops fetalis and intrauterine fetal demise during the stages of early pregnancy. In this study, the case of a pregnant asymptomatic woman in the first trimester who tested positive for COVID-19 at the 8th week of gestation is presented. At 13 weeks of gestation, the patient tested negative, however viral RNA was detected in the placenta, suggesting that the SARS-CoV-2 had crossed the placental barrier, and viral RNA was then detected in the amniotic fluid [79].

The risk of infection during vaginal delivery further perplexes any attempts to delineate the vertical viral transmission process. The increased risk of mother to infant transmission by intrapartum exposure to amniotic fluid, sac, or membranes has been demonstrated by a study examining eleven placental and membranal swabs for the detection of the virus [80]. Fenizia's et al. findings also support the in utero transmission of SARS-CoV-2. The virus's genome was isolated in cord plasma, which is exclusively fetal [75]. The second case that was described supports an in utero transmission, due to the state of an infected placenta and the presence of antibodies in cord blood. While the first case refers to a patient with a severe course of COVID-19 disease, the second one refers to a patient with mild symptoms. Therefore, establishing a connection between the risk of transmission and the severity of the disease cannot be concluded.

Delineating whether a vertical viral transmission may occur is a crucial and urgent matter. Not only due to the fact that it could compromise the fetal health status, but further—as demonstrated by the following studies—a vertical transmission could be indicative of severe adverse effects during pregnancy that will require a clinician's special attention and management strategy. The case of a patient at 22nd week of gestation, whose pregnancy was complicated by severe pre-eclampsia resulting in termination has also been described. The placenta findings demonstrated the presence of SARS-CoV-2, localized predominantly at the maternal–fetal interface of the placenta. This viral invasion of the placenta should be emphasized, as it may constitute a crucial factor of severe morbidity in pregnant patients [20]. Moreover, another report presented the case of a pregnancy with normal development, which following the mother's COVID-19 infection exhibited severe complications including critical blood flow in the fetal umbilical artery, fetal growth restriction (first percentile), hydropericardium, right ventricular hypertrophy, and intraventricular hemorrhage. As a result, the baby was prematurely delivered in the 26th week, resulting in its death due to asystole. Test results indicated that a vertical transmission of SARS-CoV-2 had occurred from mother to the fetus [11]. A preterm infant born to a mother with severe COVID-19 pneumonia has been reported in the literature. The amniotic fluid tested positive for SARS-CoV-2, while the newborn exhibited signs of an early-onset infection with SARS-CoV-2, suggesting the possibility of vertical transmission [12]. On the other hand, a patient with monochorionic–diamniotic twins being diagnosed with COVID-19 at 15 weeks of gestation has been described. Following severe complications, namely stage II twin–twin transfusion syndrome, subchorionic hematoma, *Escherichia coli* bacteremia, and septic shock, a preterm delivery was initiated at 21 weeks of gestation. Amniotic fluid and placenta were negative for SARS-CoV-2, arguing the case against transplacental transmission following a second-trimester infection [81]. Another issue of great importance that remains unknown is whether the intervillositis that was described in the abovementioned study was provoked by COVID-19 infection, since this finding is known to be associated with miscarriage, fetal growth restriction, or pre-eclampsia. Similarly, in another study, miscarriage of preterm twins born by a mother who experienced COVID-19 symptoms two weeks prior to delivery has been reported. SARS-CoV-2 was detected in placenta samples and amniotic fluid, nonetheless it was absent in the amniotic sac. Moreover, the placenta histology showed signs of chronic intervillositis. All these findings are consistent with the hypothesis of vertical transmission and further reinforce the potential link between miscarriages and COVID-19 infection [26]. Despite the fact that placental COVID-19 infection has been reported in some cases during the second and third trimester, no documentation of such phenomenon has been published considering the first trimester of pregnancy. However, it has been recently indicated that in the placenta and fetal organs examined from an early pregnancy miscarriage in a COVID-19 positive mother, SARS-CoV-2 nucleocapsid protein, viral RNA, and particles consistent with coronavirus have been detected. These findings validated for the first time that congenital SARS-CoV-2 infection could be feasible during the first trimester of pregnancy. This constitutes an alarming observation that should be considered when clinicians assess and manage pregnant patients, since the risk of adverse perinatal outcomes in cases of infection during the early pregnancy stage could be detrimental [82]. A report investigating the impact of SARS-CoV-2 on a twin pregnancy diagnosed with infection at the third trimester of gestation, identified a pattern of cytokines including IL1-Ra, IL-9 G-CSF, IL-12, and IL-8 that were differently expressed in both twins, suggesting that the SARS-CoV-2-induced cytokine storm is not impaired during the placental passage [83]. On the other hand, in an analysis of nineteen placentas of COVID-19 positive women, a variety of pathologies were described, albeit the absence of chronic intervillositis was validated [84]. Smithgall et al. compared fifty-one third trimester placentas of women positive for COVID-19, with twenty-five placentas of pregnant women testing negative. Although the first group exhibited signs of maternal–fetal vascular malperfusion, no definite association of SARS-CoV-2 could be concluded [18]. Therefore, it has become evident that the absence of a typical placental pathology indicates the need for further studies, in order to investigate the possibility of placenta infection.

Since IgG and IgM antibody testing for SARS-CoV-2 became widely available, new criteria were established in order to determine a potential intrauterine viral transmission. Maternal IgG is passively transferred across the placenta from mother to fetus, while this transmission primarily occurs during the last trimester of gestation. On the other hand, IgM cannot be transferred through the placenta due to its larger size [85]. Therefore, elevated levels of IgM antibodies could probably indicate in utero infection, assuming that the virus was transmitted through the placenta and IgM antibodies were then produced by the infant. Dong et al. studied an infant delivered by a mother with COVID-19 via C-section [45]. Although the viral nucleic acid tests of the neonate's nasopharyngeal swab and the breastmilk sample were both negative, IgM and IgG antibody levels were elevated in the infant's blood sample collected two hours post birth. In another study, two neonates had elevated IgM antibodies and five neonates exhibited elevated IgG antibodies [1]. Gao et al. proposed the case of a potential intrauterine transmission of coronavirus, based on the elevated IgM antibodies in neonate's serum, attributed to the mother's exposure to the virus six weeks prior to delivery [86]. The case of a pregnant patient with COVID-19, whose pregnancy was complicated with RhD alloimmunization, makes for an interesting observation [87]. Due to fetal anemia, three intrauterine transfusions were performed by the 30th week of gestation. Following the procedure, IgM and IgG antibodies measured in the fetal blood sample were negative, indicating no signs of virus transmission from the mother to the fetus. In the 32nd week of gestation, due to maternal complications including progressive shortness of breath, a cesarean section was performed. Amniotic fluid, cord blood, and the neonate's throat swab tested negative for SARS-CoV-2, while the mother's nasopharyngeal swab was positive for COVID-19. Consequently, data regarding antibodies against severe acute respiratory syndrome coronavirus 2 are therefore limited. More serologic data should be accumulated in controlled, meticulously designed studies with control groups, in order to investigate the neonatal exposure to the virus.

The dynamic changes of antibodies against coronavirus in neonates born by COVID-19 positive mothers have been described [88]. Fifteen out of twenty-four neonates had increased levels of IgG antibodies and six had increased IgM levels, while none developed respiratory symptoms and all tested negative for the presence of the virus. The levels of the IgG antibodies which may reflect the passive immunity [76] in neonates decreased slower in neonates who exhibited elevated IgM antibodies. As the literature suggests, maternal IgG antibodies remain in neonate's serum for approximately six months, providing them with essential protection from infections [89]. The findings of Dong et al. are extremely interesting, since they emphasize a rapid decrease in the levels of IgG antibodies against SARS-CoV-2 in neonates' blood in a time frame of less than one and a half months. This indicates the potential increased risk of COVID-19 infection for the neonates [23]. Table 3 and Figure 1 portray the current evidence on the potential routes of vertical transmission, as presented in the included studies herein.

Table 3. An overview of the reported evidence on vertical transmission in pregnant patients diagnosed with COVID-19 as described in the included studies.

Study	Neonatal Throat Swab (+)	Amniotic Fluid (+)	Vaginal Secretions (+)	Placenta (+)	Breastmilk Viral RNA (+)	IgM (+)	IgG (+)	Cord Blood Viral RNA (+)	IgM (+)	IgG (+)	Neonatal Serum IgM (+)	IgG (+)	Other (+)
[83]	0/1	-	-	-	-	-	-	-	-	-	-	1/1	-
[11]	-	-	-	1/1	-	-	-	-	-	-	-	-	Umbilical cord
[12]	1/1	1/1	-	-	-	-	-	-	-	-	-	-	-
[81]	-	0/1	-	0/1	-	-	-	-	-	-	-	-	-
[78]	1/1	-	-	-	-	-	-	-	-	-	1/1	1/1	-
[79]	-	1/1	-	1/1	-	-	-	-	-	-	-	-	Fetal membranes
[82]	-	-	-	2/2	-	-	-	-	-	-	-	-	Fetal lungs and kidneys
[15]	12/240	-	-	-	-	-	-	-	-	-	-	-	-

Table 3. Cont.

Study	Neonatal Throat Swab (+)	Amniotic Fluid (+)	Vaginal Secretions (+)	Placenta (+)	Breastmilk Viral RNA (+)	IgM (+)	IgG (+)	Cord Blood Viral RNA (+)	IgM (+)	IgG (+)	Neonatal Serum IgM (+)	IgG (+)	Other (+)
[16]	0/8	-	-	-	0/3	-	-	-	-	-	-	-	
[17]	-	0/1	-	0/1	0/1	1/1	1/1	0/1	1/1	1/1	-	-	
[18]	0/5	0/9	0/13	0/9	1/3	-	-	-	-	-	1/5	1/5	
[20]	0/3	-	-	-	-	-	-	-	-	-	-	-	
[21]	-	-	-	1/1	-	-	-	-	-	-	-	-	Umbilical cord
[75]	2/31	0/3	1/30	2/31	1/11	1/10	0/10	1/30	1/30	12/30	-	-	
[22]	0/120	-	-	-	-	-	-	-	-	-	-	-	
[6]	0/1	-	0/1	-	0/1	0/1	1/1	-	-	-	0/1	1/1	
[71]	0/38	-	-	-	-	-	-	-	-	-	-	-	
[7]	0/2	-	-	-	-	-	-	-	-	-	0/2	2/2	
[24]	0/15	0/15	-	0/15	-	-	-	-	-	-	-	-	
[25]	1/1	-	-	-	-	-	-	-	-	-	-	-	
[26]	1/1	-	-	-	1/1	-	-	-	-	-	-	-	Infant's and mother's stool sample
[27]	-	2/2	-	2/2	-	-	-	-	-	-	-	-	Maternal Blood sample
[28]	1/1	-	-	-	-	-	-	-	-	-	-	-	
[8]	0/2	0/2	-	1/2	1/2	-	-	1/2	-	-	-	-	
[29]	0/30	-	-	-	-	-	-	-	-	-	-	-	
[30]	0/1	0/1	-	0/1	0/1	-	-	-	-	-	-	-	
[31]	3/3	-	-	-	-	-	-	-	-	-	-	-	
[32]	1/1	-	-	-	-	-	-	-	-	-	-	-	Tracheal aspiration, anal swab
[33]	1/33	-	-	-	-	-	-	-	-	-	-	-	
[34]	-	0/1	0/1	1/1	-	-	-	-	-	-	-	-	
[36]	1/36	-	-	-	-	-	-	-	-	-	-	-	
[36]	0/6	0/6	-	-	0/6	-	-	0/6	-	-	-	-	
[37]	1/3	-	-	0/1	-	-	-	0/1	-	-	-	-	
[38]	0/1	0/1	-	0/1	0/1	-	-	0/1	-	-	-	-	
[39]	0/19	0/19	-	-	0/10	-	-	0/19	-	-	-	-	
[40]	2/17	-	-	-	-	-	-	-	-	-	-	-	
[36]	0/1	0/1	0/1	0/1	0/1	-	-	0/1	-	-	-	-	
[41]	0/3	-	-	-	-	-	-	-	-	-	-	-	
[42]	0/1	0/1	-	0/1	0/1	-	-	0/1	-	-	-	-	
[43]	0/1	-	-	-	-	-	-	-	-	-	-	-	
[45]	0/1	-	0/1	-	0/1	-	-	-	-	-	1/1	1/1	
[46]	0/6	0/5	-	-	-	-	-	0/5	-	-	-	-	
[47]	0/3	-	-	-	-	-	-	-	-	-	-	-	
[48]	0/1	0/1	-	0/1	-	-	-	0/1	-	-	-	-	
[49]	0/9	-	-	-	-	-	-	-	-	-	-	-	
[51]	1/1	1/1	1/1	1/1	-	-	-	-	-	-	-	-	Rectal swab, neonatal blood
[52]	0/1	-	-	1/1	-	-	-	-	-	-	0/1	0/1	
[53]	1/1	-	-	-	-	-	-	-	-	-	0/1	0/1	

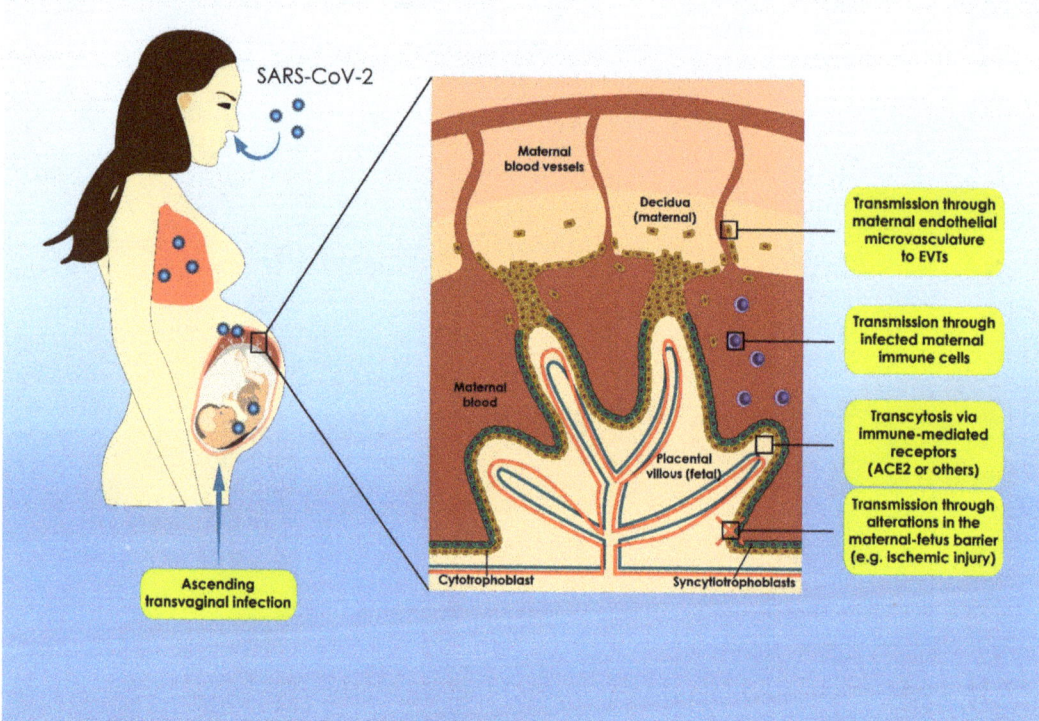

Figure 1. Suggested pathways for SARS-CoV-2 transmission from infected mothers to fetuses during pregnancy. Limited data are available regarding the role of placenta in SARS-CoV-2 infection, and thus the mechanisms of possible vertical transmission are still poorly understood. Considering the current knowledge, five possible infection routes have been proposed. Following infection of the mother, SARS-CoV-2 virions spread throughout the body via maternal circulation, finally reaching the maternal–fetal interface. According to the first suggested mechanism, transmission of SARS-CoV-2 could be achieved through maternal endothelial microvasculature to extravillous trophoblasts (EVTs) and other placenta cells expressing angiotensin converting enzyme 2 (ACE2) receptors. According to the second mechanism, SARS-CoV-2 virions could stimulate immune response in the maternal–fetal interface, inducing accumulation of maternal immune cells in the infected area, such as macrophages. Maternal immune cells could then be infected, as these cells express ACE2 receptors. Following this, the infected maternal immune cells could infiltrate the placenta and transmit the virus to the fetal cells (cell-to-cell transmission). The third proposed mechanism involves possible alterations in the maternal–fetal barrier, including ischemic injury and increased release of inflammatory regulators. These alterations lead to increased SARS-CoV-2 virions' permeability throughout the placenta, leading finally to virions spreading in the fetal environment. According to the fourth proposed mechanism, both syncytiotrophoblasts and their rupture could directly be infected by virion transcytosis, mediated via immune receptors, including ACE2 and Fc (FcR). Finally, fetal infection originating from ascending vaginal infection has also been proposed.

7. Risks Entailed in Breastfeeding

Apart from intrauterine vertical transmission and infection during delivery, the issue of breastfeeding along with the viral transmission risks entailed raise concerns for obstetricians. In order to evaluate this hypothesis, breastmilk samples have been assessed for RNA presence, while in some cases IgM and IgG antibodies against SARS-CoV-2 were further measured. The cases of two mothers positive to SARS-CoV-2 who were lactating have been described [90]. Breastmilk samples of one mother, who experienced mild symptoms of COVID-19, were positive for four continuous days. The newborn exhibited symptoms relevant to the respiratory system and tested positive for SARS-CoV-2, while the transmission route could not be assessed.

In the study by Lang et al., several breastmilk samples were repeatedly tested following delivery in order to measure viral RNA. In total, all results were negative and mothers were encouraged to breastfeed following a fourteen day isolation period [42]. In another study, the case of direct breastfeeding by a mother who tested positive for SARS-CoV-2 has been described. Breastmilk samples were continuously tested for viral presence, while antibodies against SARS-CoV-2 were measured. SARS-CoV-2 nucleic acid was not detected in the breast milk, whereas antibodies were detected in both the mother's serum and milk. Therefore, this case provided a confirmation that the viral transmission via breastmilk alone might be extremely rare, rendering breastfeeding a safe feeding method for an infant [91]. On the same note, the study by Salvatore et al. reports a cohort of neonates born by mothers positive to SARS-CoV-2, and follows the results of rooming in and breastfeeding up to one month following birth [21]. All the neonates tested negative for SARS-CoV-2, either immediately following birth or fourteen days later. This indicates that rooming in and breastfeeding may be safe when the necessary precautions are taken into consideration, including hand hygiene and use of surgical masks.

It is widely known that breastfeeding provides infants with protection against infections, mainly via secretory IgA antibodies [92]. Dong et al. report the presence of IgG and IgA antibodies in breast milk, which seem to trigger the immune protection in the neonate [23]. Another study reports the case of a premature neonate born by a healthy asymptomatic mother, who developed symptoms and tested positive for coronavirus three days following birth. Although the newborn was breastfed, and milk was later tested positive for COVID-19, but the newborn did not develop any symptomatology [93]. The potential protective role of maternal antibodies against COVID-19 should be taken into consideration, in order to assess the risk-benefit of breastfeeding [75]. More recently, a study including 55 newborns of SARS-CoV-2-positive mothers reported that no viral infection was detected in the neonates who received unpasteurized breast milk following birth. All infants were breastfed at home and remained SARS-CoV-2 negative. These findings may provide an insight regarding the safety of breastfeeding [94].

8. Vaccination Debate

It is well established in clinical practice that the majority of vaccines are permitted during pregnancy, as their benefit often outweighs the potential risk entailed [95]. Therefore, a few observations have been reported concerning women included in vaccine clinical trials who experienced an unanticipated pregnancy. Pharmaceutical companies developing COVID-19 vaccines exclude pregnant individuals from their clinical trials. Moreover, due to the limited available information on the safety and efficacy of vaccines during pregnancy, it has been proposed to avoid conceiving for weeks to months following vaccination [96]. Furthermore, since mRNA vaccines do not utilize an adjuvant nor do they constitute live vaccines, the American College of Obstetricians and Gynecologists (ACOG) along with the Society for Maternal-Fetal Medicine (SMFM) have stated that "these vaccines should not be withheld from pregnant and breastfeeding women". Nonetheless, the FDA has yet to issue any guidelines delineating employment of COVID-19 vaccines during pregnancy, while the emergency authorization use (EAU) letters that mRNA vaccines have received label pregnant women as "a population of interest" [97].

Interestingly, the main point of concern is that vaccination may initiate a cascade of symptoms, namely headache, fatigue, chills, and most importantly fever. Maternal fever during the third trimester of pregnancy has been linked to an increased risk of developing neonatal birth defects [98]. The transplacental transfer of SARS-CoV-2 antibodies following maternal vaccination in the third trimester may pose as a strong indicator that when a mother receives a COVID-19 vaccine, the neonate is protected to an extent. The role of the timing of vaccination when considering the level of protection that the transferred autoantibodies may offer has yet to be decoded. As proposed, additional longitudinal follow-up studies of a larger scale that will strictly monitor vaccinated patients are required to correlate pregnancy and neonatal outcomes with maternal vaccination. In the meantime, patients' own preference along with their healthcare provider's suggestion should determine whether vaccination should be considered [99]. As a prerequisite, the evaluation of individualized risk factors should be undertaken [100].

9. Discussion

Management of pregnant patients during these unprecedented times encompasses numerous aspects of investigation. It is prudent to thoroughly consider the risks and concerns entailed in all phases and stages of pregnancy to identify the COVID-19-related parameters that may jeopardize the end goal of a healthy "take-home baby". Crucial aspects are still under investigation, including the concerns raised on the route of transmission from the mother to the fetus, along with the developmental course and severity of complications of COVID-19 during pregnancy [101]. Could the physiological changes that occur during pregnancy involving the cardiovascular, respiratory, and coagulation system, coupled by a COVID-19 diagnosis establish an increased morbidity risk? Thus far, data suggest that pregnant patients with severe SARS-CoV-2 infection are at an increased risk of perinatal complications compared to asymptomatic pregnant patients [14]. Most studies reporting on the consequences of COVID-19 infection concern the third trimester of pregnancy. Moreover, the role of certain risk factors, such as obesity, should be evaluated. Management and monitoring of pregnant patients of different profiles may differ, hence we are called to thoroughly profile pregnant patients to ascertain appropriate management.

Our intention was to provide an all-inclusive overview on what is thus far known and reported on COVID-19 and pregnancy, highlighting current concerns and areas of special interest. Undoubtably, this has been an extraordinary year for medicine that has shaped and transformed scientific research. An accelerating pace in COVID-19-related research has been noted, as there are thousands of publications dedicated to COVID-19 and pregnancy. Nonetheless, this wealth of published data presents with amplified weaknesses in research methodology, and current publication policies that could prognosticate the challenges researchers may face in the future [102]. The high heterogeneity observed among the studies led the authors to refrain from performing a systematic review on this topic. It is well documented that systematic reviews provide an objective analysis of the relevant evidence, in contrast to the narrative reviews which are characterized by subjectivity. Nonetheless, the quality of evidence provided by a systematic review is strongly associated with the quality of the included studies. Considering the lack of robust data on COVID-19 aspects, a systematic review could potentially, at present, fail to serve its own purpose, which is reaching a robust conclusion and may further present the risk of confusing the readership. However, the authors acknowledge that the quality of a narrative review may be improved by following a systematic approach for literature evaluation, and have herein adopted an effective search strategy, using specific key-words and data assessment strategy [103].

The critical analysis of the current data—constituting the aim of this comprehensive review—results in certain aspects becoming clear. It becomes evident that a risk assessment is vital for pregnant women who are diagnosed as positive for COVID-19. Especially when comorbidities are present, the complications may be severe, demanding close monitoring similar to a high-risk pregnancy. Up until now, studies' findings in the literature are collectively pointing to the direction that certain identified risk factors in pregnant patients indicate a higher risk of complications. Studying the inevitable heterogeneity of pregnant patients diagnosed with COVID-19 who are included in current and future studies will further unravel additional risk factors that play a crucial role in the developmental course of the disease. Regarding the delivery mode, a vast number of studies were characterized by missing outcome data and selection report bias, therefore, assessing the short-term and long-term repercussions of opting for vaginal delivery or c-section is still under investigation. For the time being, the lack of sufficient data and high-quality methodology leads clinicians to assess the risks and benefits based on the individual's health status alone. Interestingly, regardless of delivery mode, most of the cases of newborns in the literature seem to respond well and achieve health status restoration. However, 2019-nCoV infection may exert severe adverse effects on newborns, such as neonatal pneumonia, prematurity, neonatal respiratory distress syndrome, and even neonatal death. The deafening heterogeneity amongst studies along with the preliminary nature of the published data dictate that interpretation of results sourced hitherto should be performed with caution. Despite the increasing number of publications dedicated to this topic, unbiased conclusions cannot be drawn due to the inadequacy of good quality evidence.

Moving on to the matter of viral transmission, delineating the routes of transmission is of paramount significance, that will enable us to optimize the management of COVID-19 pregnant patients and their delivery options. Clinical research should soon be qualified to provide definitive evidence on the mechanisms and the physiology entailed when considering the possibility of COVID-19 vertical transmission. Thus far, no safe conclusions can be drawn with respect to the routes of transmission, due to the lack of consistency in the evidence reporting on mother to newborn transmission. In regard to breastfeeding, larger cohort studies are essential to confirm the rarity of perinatal transmission when strict safety measures are applied. What is more, the physiology mechanisms entailed in the protection that breastfeeding appears to offer should be further evaluated. Current publications investigating the matter of breastfeeding in COVID-19 patients raise the concern stemming from the heterogeneity of patients examined. Following the recommendations from World Health Organization, there is no indication to stop breastfeeding as advocated by the vast majority of concordant published data, as evident in literature thus far. The concerns for the safety of breastfeeding should be validated by larger studies, since isolating the newborn and the mother as a precautionary protection measure while lacking conclusive evidence may affect the newborn's emotional attachment. In an effort to draw conclusions on the heated topic of vaccination, data thus far suggest that considering the risks associated with COVID-19 in pregnant patients, vaccination should be encouraged. Contemplating the wide application of vaccination in this group of patients, follow-up and assessment in both the mother and the fetus from cases that have already received the vaccine will allow us to draw a safer conclusion in the future [104].

The responsibility of the scientific community should be highlighted. Research topics unrelated to COVID-19 may come second best while as estimated 80% of clinical trials have been interrupted during the past few months in an effort to dedicate available resources to this crusade against SARS-CoV-2 [102]. Thus, where do we go from here? The pandemic is new and old at the same time. Due to the rapid emergence of new data, several studies are now outdated—despite the recent dates of publication—and novel ones appear to present the minor updated findings. Perhaps the eagerness to share, report, and publish on "everything COVID-19 related" may not in fact be as beneficial. The question raised is, what is the true impact of this overwhelming volume of publications? Does it assist physicians to achieve their goal in optimizing their clinical practice during this pandemic? Or could it be that this vast influx of data stands as a backpedal, hindering scientific progress? This is a time to ponder on whether "any data is good data" and the answer may be no. Instead of being fast-tracked and prioritized, it should be recommended for value and standards to be rigorously assessed in COVID-19 data, in the context of "what it offers". It is of paramount significance to ensure that publications of research on COVID-19 are more regulated. Until this informational overload that bombards the scientific community is effectively managed, clinicians should abide by an ethical, moral, and legal duty towards their patients regarding shared decision making, while prioritizing patients' safety [105].

10. Conclusions

There is an urgency to define the optimal strategy to manage pregnant patients diagnosed with SARS-CoV-2. It becomes evident that the huge volume of articles published since the beginning of the pandemic is impressive. However, this is coupled by a lack of conclusive theses, due to discrepancies and heterogeneity which is almost alarming, albeit anticipated. Extrapolated hypotheses emerge daily, perhaps lacking filtering mechanisms to exclude data that may be of poor quality. What becomes clear is that this overload of data fails to lead to robust conclusions, but rather paradoxically reflects the current unknown situation we are still facing nearing two years into the pandemic. The research field as a whole may be affected by the inevitable urgency to address COVID-19, albeit failing to lead to robust data and clear conclusions. Based on the current contradicting findings referring to the role of COVID-19 on the various phases of pregnancy, and the lack of robust original studies, no safe conclusions can be drawn. To prevail against this unparalleled pandemic outbreak, high quality information is needed. Perhaps it is time for the scientific community to suggest a strategy to monitor and control COVID-19-related data flow in every discipline, to ascertain a successful and timely response to this ongoing crisis.

Author Contributions: Conceptualization, T.K. and A.R.; methodology, M.P., S.G. and G.A.; investigation, M.P., S.G., E.M., G.A., O.T., D.T., S.N. and P.B.; writing—original draft preparation, A.R., M.P., S.G. and E.M.; writing—review and editing, T.K., A.R., S.G. and M.S.; supervision, M.S. and N.V.; project administration, M.S. and N.V. All authors have read and agreed to the published version of the manuscript.

Funding: This research received no external funding.

Institutional Review Board Statement: Not applicable.

Informed Consent Statement: Not applicable.

Data Availability Statement: Not applicable.

Conflicts of Interest: The authors declare no conflict of interest.

References

1. Zeng, H.; Xu, C.; Fan, J.; Tang, Y.; Deng, Q.; Zhang, W.; Long, X. Antibodies in Infants Born to Mothers with COVID-19 Pneumonia. *JAMA* **2020**, *323*, 1848–1849. [CrossRef] [PubMed]
2. Anifandis, G.; Tempest, H.G.; Oliva, R.; Swanson, G.M.; Simopoulou, M.; Easley, C.A.; Primig, M.; Messini, C.I.; Turek, P.J.; Sutovsky, P.; et al. COVID-19 and human reproduction: A pandemic that packs a serious punch. *Syst. Biol. Reprod. Med.* **2021**, *67*, 3–23. [CrossRef]
3. Anifandis, G.; Messini, C.I.; Simopoulou, M.; Sveronis, G.; Garas, A.; Daponte, A.; Messinis, I.E. SARS-CoV-2 vs. human gametes, embryos and cryopreservation. *Syst. Biol. Reprod. Med.* **2021**, *67*, 260–269. [CrossRef] [PubMed]
4. Narang, K.; Enninga, E.A.L.; Gunaratne, M.D.S.K.; Ibirogba, E.R.; Trad, A.T.A.; Elrefaei, A.; Theiler, R.N.; Ruano, R.; Szymanski, L.M.; Chakraborty, R.; et al. SARS-CoV-2 Infection and COVID-19 during Pregnancy: A Multidisciplinary Review. *Mayo Clin. Proc.* **2020**, *95*, 1750–1765. [CrossRef] [PubMed]
5. Yu, N.; Li, W.; Kang, Q.; Zeng, W.; Feng, L.; Wu, J. No SARS-CoV-2 detected in amniotic fluid in mid-pregnancy. *Lancet Infect. Dis.* **2020**, *20*, 1364. [CrossRef]
6. Tang, J.-Y.; Song, W.-Q.; Xu, H.; Wang, N. No evidence for vertical transmission of SARS-CoV-2 in two neonates with mothers infected in the second trimester. *Infect. Dis. Lond. Engl.* **2020**, *52*, 913–916. [CrossRef] [PubMed]
7. Liu, W.; Cheng, H.; Wang, J.; Ding, L.; Zhou, Z.; Liu, S.; Chang, L.; Rong, Z. Clinical Analysis of Neonates Born to Mothers with or without COVID-19: A Retrospective Analysis of 48 Cases from Two Neonatal Intensive Care Units in Hubei Province. *Am. J. Perinatol.* **2020**, *37*, 1317–1323. [CrossRef]
8. Wang, Z.; Wang, Z.; Xiong, G. Clinical characteristics and laboratory results of pregnant women with COVID-19 in Wuhan, China. *Int. J. Gynaecol. Obstet. Off. Organ Int. Fed. Gynaecol. Obstet.* **2020**, *150*, 312–317. [CrossRef]
9. Breslin, N.; Baptiste, C.; Gyamfi-Bannerman, C.; Miller, R.; Martinez, R.; Bernstein, K.; Ring, L.; Landau, R.; Purisch, S.; Friedman, A.M.; et al. Coronavirus disease 2019 infection among asymptomatic and symptomatic pregnant women: Two weeks of confirmed presentations to an affiliated pair of New York City hospitals. *Am. J. Obstet. Gynecol. MFM* **2020**, *2*, 100118. [CrossRef]
10. Narang, K.; Szymanski, L.M.; Kane, S.V.; Rose, C.H. Acute Pancreatitis in a Pregnant Patient with Coronavirus Disease 2019 (COVID-19). *Obstet. Gynecol.* **2021**, *137*, 431–433. [CrossRef]

11. Sukhikh, G.; Petrova, U.; Prikhodko, A.; Starodubtseva, N.; Chingin, K.; Chen, H.; Bugrova, A.; Kononikhin, A.; Bourmenskaya, O.; Brzhozovskiy, A.; et al. Vertical Transmission of SARS-CoV-2 in Second Trimester Associated with Severe Neonatal Pathology. *Viruses* **2021**, *13*, 447. [CrossRef] [PubMed]
12. Farhadi, R.; Mehrpisheh, S.; Ghaffari, V.; Haghshenas, M.; Ebadi, A. Clinical course, radiological findings and late outcome in preterm infant with suspected vertical transmission born to a mother with severe COVID-19 pneumonia: A case report. *J. Med. Case Rep.* **2021**, *15*, 213. [CrossRef]
13. Garcia, J.J.; Turalde, C.W.; Bagnas, M.A.; Anlacan, V.M. Intravenous immunoglobulin in COVID-19 associated Guillain-Barré syndrome in pregnancy. *BMJ Case Rep.* **2021**, *14*, e242365. [CrossRef] [PubMed]
14. Metz, T.D.; Clifton, R.G.; Hughes, B.L.; Sandoval, G.; Saade, G.R.; Grobman, W.A.; Manuck, T.A.; Miodovnik, M.; Sowles, A.; Clark, K.; et al. Disease Severity and Perinatal Outcomes of Pregnant Patients with Coronavirus Disease 2019 (COVID-19). *Obstet. Gynecol.* **2021**, *137*, 571–580. [CrossRef]
15. Knight, M.; Bunch, K.; Vousden, N.; Morris, E.; Simpson, N.; Gale, C.; O'Brien, P.; Quigley, M.; Brocklehurst, P.; Kurinczuk, J.J.; et al. Characteristics and outcomes of pregnant women admitted to hospital with confirmed SARS-CoV-2 infection in UK: National population based cohort study. *BMJ* **2020**, *369*, m2107. [CrossRef] [PubMed]
16. Chen, L.; Li, Q.; Zheng, D.; Jiang, H.; Wei, Y.; Zou, L.; Feng, L.; Xiong, G.; Sun, G.; Wang, H.; et al. Clinical Characteristics of Pregnant Women with COVID-19 in Wuhan, China. *N. Engl. J. Med.* **2020**, *382*, e100. [CrossRef] [PubMed]
17. Wu, Y.; Liu, C.; Dong, L.; Zhang, C.; Chen, Y.; Liu, J.; Zhang, C.; Duan, C.; Zhang, H.; Mol, B.W.; et al. Coronavirus disease 2019 among pregnant Chinese women: Case series data on the safety of vaginal birth and breastfeeding. *BJOG Int. J. Obstet. Gynaecol.* **2020**, *127*, 1109–1115. [CrossRef]
18. Smithgall, M.C.; Liu-Jarin, X.; Hamele-Bena, D.; Cimic, A.; Mourad, M.; Debelenko, L.; Chen, X. Third-trimester placentas of severe acute respiratory syndrome coronavirus 2 (SARS-CoV-2)-positive women: Histomorphology, including viral immunohistochemistry and in-situ hybridization. *Histopathology* **2020**, *77*, 994–999. [CrossRef] [PubMed]
19. Li, N.; Han, L.; Peng, M.; Lv, Y.; Ouyang, Y.; Liu, K.; Yue, L.; Li, Q.; Sun, G.; Chen, L.; et al. Maternal and Neonatal Outcomes of Pregnant Women with Coronavirus Disease 2019 (COVID-19) Pneumonia: A Case-Control Study. *Clin. Infect. Dis. Off. Publ. Infect. Dis. Soc. Am.* **2020**, *71*, 2035–2041. [CrossRef]
20. Hosier, H.; Farhadian, S.F.; Morotti, R.A.; Deshmukh, U.; Lu-Culligan, A.; Campbell, K.H.; Yasumoto, Y.; Vogels, C.B.; Casanovas-Massana, A.; Vijayakumar, P.; et al. SARS-CoV-2 infection of the placenta. *J. Clin. Investig.* **2020**, *130*, 4947–4953. [CrossRef]
21. Salvatore, C.M.; Han, J.-Y.; Acker, K.P.; Tiwari, P.; Jin, J.; Brandler, M.; Cangemi, C.; Gordon, L.; Parow, A.; DiPace, J.; et al. Neonatal management and outcomes during the COVID-19 pandemic: An observation cohort study. *Lancet Child Adolesc. Health* **2020**, *4*, 721–727. [CrossRef]
22. Afshar, Y.; Gaw, S.L.; Flaherman, V.J.; Chambers, B.D.; Krakow, D.; Berghella, V.; Shamshirsaz, A.A.; Boatin, A.A.; Aldrovandi, G.; Greiner, A.; et al. Clinical Presentation of Coronavirus Disease 2019 (COVID-19) in Pregnant and Recently Pregnant People. *Obstet. Gynecol.* **2020**, *136*, 1117–1125. [CrossRef]
23. Dong, Y.; Chi, X.; Hai, H.; Sun, L.; Zhang, M.; Xie, W.-F.; Chen, W. Antibodies in the breast milk of a maternal woman with COVID-19. *Emerg. Microbes Infect.* **2020**, *9*, 1467–1469. [CrossRef]
24. Majachani, N.; Francois, J.L.M.; Fernando, A.K.; Zuberi, J. A Case of a Newborn Baby Girl Infected with SARS-CoV-2 Due to Transplacental Viral Transmission. *Am. J. Case Rep.* **2020**, *21*, e925766. [CrossRef]
25. Hinojosa-Velasco, A.; de Oca, P.V.B.-M.; García-Sosa, L.E.; Mendoza-Durán, J.G.; Pérez-Méndez, M.J.; Dávila-González, E.; Ramírez-Hernández, D.G.; García-Mena, J.; Zárate-Segura, P.; Reyes-Ruiz, J.M.; et al. A case report of newborn infant with severe COVID-19 in Mexico: Detection of SARS-CoV-2 in human breast milk and stool. *Int. J. Infect. Dis. IJID Off. Publ. Int. Soc. Infect. Dis.* **2020**, *100*, 21–24. [CrossRef] [PubMed]
26. Pulinx, B.; Kieffer, D.; Michiels, I.; Petermans, S.; Strybol, D.; Delvaux, S.; Baldewijns, M.; Raymaekers, M., Cartuyvels, R.; Maurissen, W. Vertical transmission of SARS-CoV-2 infection and preterm birth. *Eur. J. Clin. Microbiol. Infect. Dis.* **2020**, *39*, 2441–2445. [CrossRef] [PubMed]
27. Sisman, J.; Jaleel, M.A.; Moreno, W.; Rajaram, V.; Collins, R.R.J.; Savani, R.C.; Rakheja, D.; Evans, A.S. Intrauterine Transmission of SARS-CoV-2 Infection in a Preterm Infant. *Pediatr. Infect. Dis. J.* **2020**, *39*, e265–e267. [CrossRef] [PubMed]
28. Costa, S.; Posteraro, B.; Marchetti, S.; Tamburrini, E.; Carducci, B.; Lanzone, A.; Valentini, P.; Buonsenso, D.; Sanguinetti, M.; Vento, G.; et al. Excretion of SARS-CoV-2 in human breast milk. *Clin. Microbiol. Infect.* **2020**, *26*, 1430–1432. [CrossRef] [PubMed]
29. Slayton-Milam, S.; Sheffels, S.; Chan, D.; Alkinj, B. Induction of Labor in an Intubated Patient with Coronavirus Disease 2019 (COVID-19). *Obstet. Gynecol.* **2020**, *136*, 962–964. [CrossRef]
30. Alwardi, T.H.; Ramdas, V.; Al Yahmadi, M.; Al Aisari, S.; Bhandari, S.; Saif Al Hashami, H.; Al Jabri, A.; Manikoth, P.; Malviya, M. Is Vertical Transmission of SARS-CoV-2 Infection Possible in Preterm Triplet Pregnancy? A Case Series. *Pediatr. Infect. Dis. J.* **2020**, *39*, e456–e458. [CrossRef]
31. Marzollo, R.; Aversa, S.; Prefumo, F.; Saccani, B.; Perez, C.R.; Sartori, E.; Motta, M. Possible Coronavirus Disease 2019 Pandemic and Pregnancy: Vertical Transmission Is Not Excluded. *Pediatr. Infect. Dis. J.* **2020**, *39*, e261–e262. [CrossRef]
32. Pierce-Williams, R.A.M.; Burd, J.; Felder, L.; Khoury, R.; Bernstein, P.S.; Avila, K.; Penfield, C.A.; Roman, A.S.; DeBolt, C.A.; Stone, J.L.; et al. Clinical course of severe and critical coronavirus disease 2019 in hospitalized pregnancies: A United States cohort study. *Am. J. Obstet. Gynecol. MFM* **2020**, *2*, 100134. [CrossRef] [PubMed]

33. Baud, D.; Greub, G.; Favre, G.; Gengler, C.; Jaton, K.; Dubruc, E.; Pomar, L. Second-Trimester Miscarriage in a Pregnant Woman with SARS-CoV-2 Infection. *JAMA* **2020**, *323*, 2198–2200. [CrossRef]
34. Sentilhes, L.; De Marcillac, F.; Jouffrieau, C.; Kuhn, P.; Thuet, V.; Hansmann, Y.; Ruch, Y.; Fafi-Kremer, S.; Deruelle, P. Coronavirus disease 2019 in pregnancy was associated with maternal morbidity and preterm birth. *Am. J. Obstet. Gynecol.* **2020**, *223*, 914.e1–914.e15. [CrossRef]
35. Vivanti, A.J.; Mattern, J.; Vauloup-Fellous, C.; Jani, J.; Rigonnot, L.; El Hachem, L.; Le Gouez, A.; Desconclois, C.; Ben M'Barek, I.; Sibiude, J.; et al. Retrospective Description of Pregnant Women Infected with Severe Acute Respiratory Syndrome Coronavirus 2, France. *Emerg. Infect. Dis.* **2020**, *26*, 2069–2076. [CrossRef]
36. Chen, H.; Guo, J.; Wang, C.; Luo, F.; Yu, X.; Zhang, W.; Li, J.; Zhao, D.; Xu, D.; Gong, Q.; et al. Clinical characteristics and intrauterine vertical transmission potential of COVID-19 infection in nine pregnant women: A retrospective review of medical records. *Lancet* **2020**, *395*, 809–815. [CrossRef]
37. Yu, N.; Li, W.; Kang, Q.; Xiong, Z.; Wang, S.; Lin, X.; Liu, Y.; Xiao, J.; Liu, H.; Deng, D.; et al. Clinical features and obstetric and neonatal outcomes of pregnant patients with COVID-19 in Wuhan, China: A retrospective, single-centre, descriptive study. *Lancet Infect. Dis.* **2020**, *20*, 559–564. [CrossRef]
38. Li, Y.; Zhao, R.; Zheng, S.; Chen, X.; Wang, J.; Sheng, X.; Zhou, J.; Cai, H.; Fang, Q.; Yu, F.; et al. Lack of Vertical Transmission of Severe Acute Respiratory Syndrome Coronavirus 2, China. *Emerg. Infect. Dis.* **2020**, *26*, 1335–1336. [CrossRef] [PubMed]
39. Liu, W.; Wang, J.; Li, W.; Zhou, Z.; Liu, S.; Rong, Z. Clinical characteristics of 19 neonates born to mothers with COVID-19. *Front. Med.* **2020**, 193–198. [CrossRef]
40. Khan, S.; Jun, L.; Siddique, R.; Li, Y.; Han, G.; Xue, M.; Nabi, G.; Liu, J. Association of COVID-19 with pregnancy outcomes in health-care workers and general women. *Clin. Microbiol. Infect. Off. Publ. Eur. Soc. Clin. Microbiol. Infect. Dis.* **2020**, *26*, 788–790. [CrossRef] [PubMed]
41. Khan, S.; Peng, L.; Siddique, R.; Nabi, G.; Xue, M.; Liu, J.; Han, G. Impact of COVID-19 infection on pregnancy outcomes and the risk of maternal-to-neonatal intrapartum transmission of COVID-19 during natural birth. *Infect. Control Hosp. Epidemiol.* **2020**, 748–750. [CrossRef]
42. Lang, G.; Zhao, H. Can SARS-CoV-2-infected women breastfeed after viral clearance? *J. Zhejiang Univ. Sci. B* **2020**, 405–407. [CrossRef]
43. Lyra, J.; Valente, R.; Rosário, M.; Guimarães, M. Cesarean Section in a Pregnant Woman with COVID-19: First Case in Portugal. *Acta Med. Port.* **2020**, *33*, 429–431. [CrossRef]
44. Martinelli, I.; Ferrazzi, E.; Ciavarella, A.; Erra, R.; Iurlaro, E.; Ossola, M.; Lombardi, A.; Blasi, F.; Mosca, F.; Peyvandi, F. Pulmonary embolism in a young pregnant woman with COVID-19. *Thromb. Res.* **2020**, *191*, 36–37. [CrossRef]
45. Dong, L.; Tian, J.; He, S.; Zhu, C.; Wang, J.; Liu, C.; Yang, J. Possible Vertical Transmission of SARS-CoV-2 from an Infected Mother to Her Newborn. *JAMA* **2020**, *323*, 1846–1848. [CrossRef]
46. Yang, P.; Wang, X.; Liu, P.; Wei, C.; He, B.; Zheng, J.; Zhao, D. Clinical characteristics and risk assessment of newborns born to mothers with COVID-19. *J. Clin. Virol. Off. Publ. Pan Am. Soc. Clin. Virol.* **2020**, *127*, 104356. [CrossRef]
47. Chen, Y.; Peng, H.; Wang, L.; Zhao, Y.; Zeng, L.; Gao, H.; Liu, Y. Infants Born to Mothers with a New Coronavirus (COVID-19). *Front. Pediatr.* **2020**, *8*, 104. [CrossRef] [PubMed]
48. Wang, X.; Zhou, Z.; Zhang, J.; Zhu, F.; Tang, Y.; Shen, X. A Case of 2019 Novel Coronavirus in a Pregnant Woman With Preterm Delivery. *Clin. Infect. Dis. Off. Publ. Infect. Dis. Soc. Am.* **2020**, *71*, 844–846. [CrossRef] [PubMed]
49. Zhu, H.; Wang, L.; Fang, C.; Peng, S.; Zhang, L.; Chang, G.; Xia, S.; Zhou, W. Clinical analysis of 10 neonates born to mothers with 2019-nCoV pneumonia. *Transl. Pediatr.* **2020**, *9*, 51–60. [CrossRef]
50. Breslin, N.; Baptiste, C.; Miller, R.; Fuchs, K.; Goffman, D.; Gyamfi-Bannerman, C.; D'Alton, M. Coronavirus disease 2019 in pregnancy: Early lessons. *Am. J. Obstet. Gynecol. MFM* **2020**, *2*, 100111. [CrossRef] [PubMed]
51. Vivanti, A.J.; Vauloup-Fellous, C.; Prevot, S.; Zupan, V.; Suffee, C.; Do Cao, J.; Benachi, A.; De Luca, D. Transplacental transmission of SARS-CoV-2 infection. *Nat. Commun.* **2020**, *11*, 3572. [CrossRef]
52. Ferraiolo, A.; Barra, F.; Kratochwila, C.; Paudice, M.; Vellone, V.G.; Godano, E.; Varesano, S.; Noberasco, G.; Ferrero, S.; Arioni, C. Report of Positive Placental Swabs for SARS-CoV-2 in an Asymptomatic Pregnant Woman with COVID-19. *Medicina* **2020**, *56*, 306. [CrossRef]
53. Alzamora, M.C.; Paredes, T.; Caceres, D.; Webb, C.M.; Valdez, L.M.; La Rosa, M. Severe COVID-19 during Pregnancy and Possible Vertical Transmission. *Am. J. Perinatol.* **2020**, *37*, 861–865. [CrossRef]
54. Hantoushzadeh, S.; Shamshirsaz, A.A.; Aleyasin, A.; Seferovic, M.D.; Aski, S.K.; Arian, S.E.; Pooransari, P.; Ghotbizadeh, F.; Aalipour, S.; Soleimani, Z.; et al. Maternal death due to COVID-19. *Am. J. Obstet. Gynecol.* **2020**, *223*, 109.e1–109.e16. [CrossRef] [PubMed]
55. Blitz, M.J.; Rochelson, B.; Minkoff, H.; Meirowitz, N.; Prasannan, L.; London, V.; Rafael, T.J.; Chakravarthy, S.; Bracero, L.A.; Wasden, S.W.; et al. Maternal mortality among women with coronavirus disease 2019 admitted to the intensive care unit. *Am. J. Obstet. Gynecol.* **2020**, *223*, 595–599.e5. [CrossRef] [PubMed]
56. Badr, D.A.; Mattern, J.; Carlin, A.; Cordier, A.-G.; Maillart, E.; El Hachem, L.; El Kenz, H.; Andronikof, M.; De Bels, D.; Damoisel, C.; et al. Are clinical outcomes worse for pregnant women at ≥20 weeks' gestation infected with coronavirus disease 2019? A multicenter case-control study with propensity score matching. *Am. J. Obstet. Gynecol.* **2020**, *223*, 764–768. [CrossRef] [PubMed]

57. Nejadrahim, R.; Khademolhosseini, S.; Kavandi, H.; Hajizadeh, R. Severe acute respiratory syndrome coronavirus-2- or pregnancy-related cardiomyopathy, a differential to be considered in the current pandemic: A case report. *J. Med. Case Rep.* **2021**, *15*, 143. [CrossRef] [PubMed]
58. Goswami, J.; MacArthur, T.A.; Sridharan, M.; Pruthi, R.K.; McBane, R.D.; Witzig, T.E.; Park, M.S. A Review of Pathophysiology, Clinical Features, and Management Options of COVID-19 Associated Coagulopathy. *Shock* **2020**, *55*, 700. [CrossRef] [PubMed]
59. Mohammadi, S.; Abouzaripour, M.; Hesam Shariati, N.; Hesam Shariati, M.B. Ovarian vein thrombosis after coronavirus disease (COVID-19) infection in a pregnant woman: Case report. *J. Thromb. Thrombolysis* **2020**, *50*, 604–607. [CrossRef]
60. Gunduz, Z.B. Venous sinus thrombosis during COVID-19 infection in pregnancy: A case report. *Sao Paulo Med. J. Rev. Paul. Med.* **2021**, *139*, 190–195. [CrossRef] [PubMed]
61. Tekin, A.B.; Zanapalioglu, U.; Gulmez, S.; Akarsu, I.; Yassa, M.; Tug, N. Guillain Barre Syndrome following delivery in a pregnant woman infected with SARS-CoV-2. *J. Clin. Neurosci.* **2021**, *86*, 190–192. [CrossRef]
62. Villar, J.; Ariff, S.; Gunier, R.B.; Thiruvengadam, R.; Rauch, S.; Kholin, A.; Roggero, P.; Prefumo, F.; do Vale, M.S.; Cardona-Perez, J.A.; et al. Maternal and Neonatal Morbidity and Mortality Among Pregnant Women with and without COVID-19 Infection: The INTERCOVID Multinational Cohort Study. *JAMA Pediatr.* **2021**, *175*, 817–826. [CrossRef]
63. Carrasco, I.; Muñoz-Chapuli, M.; Vigil-Vázquez, S.; Aguilera-Alonso, D.; Hernández, C.; Sánchez-Sánchez, C.; Oliver, C.; Riaza, M.; Pareja, M.; Sanz, O.; et al. SARS-CoV-2 infection in pregnant women and newborns in a Spanish cohort (GESNEO-COVID) during the first wave. *BMC Pregnancy Childbirth* **2021**, *21*, 326. [CrossRef] [PubMed]
64. Oncel, M.Y.; Akın, I.M.; Kanburoglu, M.K.; Tayman, C.; Coskun, S.; Narter, F.; Er, I.; Oncan, T.G.; Memisoglu, A.; Cetinkaya, M.; et al. A multicenter study on epidemiological and clinical characteristics of 125 newborns born to women infected with COVID-19 by Turkish Neonatal Society. *Eur. J. Pediatr.* **2021**, *180*, 733–742. [CrossRef] [PubMed]
65. Taghavi, S.-A.; Heidari, S.; Jahanfar, S.; Amirjani, S.; Aji-Ramkani, A.; Azizi-Kutenaee, M.; Bazarganipour, F. Obstetric, maternal, and neonatal outcomes in COVID-19 compared to healthy pregnant women in Iran: A retrospective, case-control study. *Middle East Fertil. Soc. J.* **2021**, *26*, 17. [CrossRef] [PubMed]
66. Singh, V.; Choudhary, A.; Datta, M.R.; Ray, A. Maternal and Neonatal Outcomes of COVID-19 in Pregnancy: A Single-Centre Observational Study. *Cureus* **2021**, *13*, e13184. [CrossRef]
67. Le Gouez, A.; Vivanti, A.J.; Benhamou, D.; Desconclois, C.; Mercier, F.J. Thrombocytopenia in pregnant patients with mild COVID-19. *Int. J. Obstet. Anesth.* **2020**, *44*, 13–15. [CrossRef] [PubMed]
68. Omar, S.; Motawea, A.M.; Yasin, R. High-resolution CT features of COVID-19 pneumonia in confirmed cases. *Egypt. J. Radiol. Nucl. Med.* **2020**, *51*, 121. [CrossRef]
69. Waratani, M.; Ito, F.; Tanaka, Y.; Mabuchi, A.; Mori, T.; Kitawaki, J. Severe coronavirus disease pneumonia in a pregnant woman at 25 weeks' gestation: A case report. *J. Obstet. Gynaecol. Res.* **2021**, *47*, 1583–1588. [CrossRef]
70. Coronavirus Disease (COVID-19): Pregnancy and Childbirth. Available online: https://www.who.int/news-room/q-a-detail/coronavirus-disease-COVID-19-pregnancy-and-childbirth (accessed on 24 January 2021).
71. Yang, R.; Mei, H.; Zheng, T.; Fu, Q.; Zhang, Y.; Buka, S.; Yao, X.; Tang, Z.; Zhang, X.; Qiu, L.; et al. Pregnant women with COVID-19 and risk of adverse birth outcomes and maternal-fetal vertical transmission: A population-based cohort study in Wuhan, China. *BMC Med.* **2020**, *18*, 330. [CrossRef]
72. McLaren, R.A.; London, V.; Atallah, F.; McCalla, S.; Haberman, S.; Fisher, N.; Stein, J.L.; Minkoff, H.L. Delivery for respiratory compromise among pregnant women with coronavirus disease 2019. *Am. J. Obstet. Gynecol.* **2020**, *223*, 451–453. [CrossRef]
73. Sagheb, S.; Lamsehchi, A.; Jafary, M.; Atef-Yekta, R.; Sadeghi, K. Two seriously ill neonates born to mothers with COVID-19 pneumonia- a case report. *Ital. J. Pediatr.* **2020**, *46*, 137. [CrossRef]
74. Peng, Z.; Wang, J.; Mo, Y.; Duan, W.; Xiang, G.; Yi, M.; Bao, L.; Shi, Y. Unlikely SARS-CoV-2 vertical transmission from mother to child: A case report. *J. Infect. Public Health* **2020**, *13*, 818–820. [CrossRef] [PubMed]
75. Fenizia, C.; Biasin, M.; Cetin, I.; Vergani, P.; Mileto, D.; Spinillo, A.; Gismondo, M.R.; Perotti, F.; Callegari, C.; Mancon, A.; et al. Analysis of SARS-CoV-2 vertical transmission during pregnancy. *Nat. Commun.* **2020**, *11*, 5128. [CrossRef]
76. Gude, N.M.; Roberts, C.T.; Kalionis, B.; King, R.G. Growth and function of the normal human placenta. *Thromb. Res.* **2004**, *114*, 397–407. [CrossRef] [PubMed]
77. Komine-Aizawa, S.; Takada, K.; Hayakawa, S. Placental barrier against COVID-19. *Placenta* **2020**, *99*, 45–49. [CrossRef]
78. Carbayo-Jiménez, T.; Carrasco-Colom, J.; Epalza, C.; Folgueira, D.; Pérez-Rivilla, A.; Barbero-Casado, P.; Blázquez-Gamero, D.; Galindo-Izquierdo, A.; Pallás-Alonso, C.; Moral-Pumarega, M.T. Severe Acute Respiratory Syndrome Coronavirus 2 Vertical Transmission from an Asymptomatic Mother. *Pediatr. Infect. Dis. J.* **2021**, *40*, e115–e117. [CrossRef]
79. Shende, P.; Gaikwad, P.; Gandhewar, M.; Ukey, P.; Bhide, A.; Patel, V.; Bhagat, S.; Bhor, V.; Mahale, S.; Gajbhiye, R.; et al. Persistence of SARS-CoV-2 in the first trimester placenta leading to transplacental transmission and fetal demise from an asymptomatic mother. *Hum. Reprod.* **2021**, *36*, 899–906. [CrossRef]
80. Penfield, C.A.; Brubaker, S.G.; Limaye, M.A.; Lighter, J.; Ratner, A.J.; Thomas, K.M.; Meyer, J.A.; Roman, A.S. Detection of severe acute respiratory syndrome coronavirus 2 in placental and fetal membrane samples. *Am. J. Obstet. Gynecol. MFM* **2020**, *2*, 100133. [CrossRef] [PubMed]
81. Mok, T.; Contreras, D.; Chmait, R.H.; Goldstein, J.; Pluym, I.D.; Tabsh, K.; Aldrovandi, G.; Afshar, Y. Complicated Monochorionic–Diamniotic Twins in a Pregnant Woman with COVID-19 in the Second Trimester. *Am. J. Perinatol.* **2021**, *38*, 747–752. [CrossRef]

82. Valdespino-Vázquez, M.Y.; Helguera-Repetto, C.A.; León-Juárez, M.; Villavicencio-Carrisoza, O.; Flores-Pliego, A.; Moreno-Verduzco, E.R.; Díaz-Pérez, D.L.; Villegas-Mota, I.; Carrasco-Ramírez, E.; López-Martínez, I.E.; et al. Fetal and placental infection with SARS-CoV-2 in early pregnancy. *J. Med. Virol.* **2021**, *93*, 4480–4487. [CrossRef] [PubMed]
83. Trombetta, A.; Comar, M.; Tommasini, A.; Canton, R.; Campisciano, G.; Zanotta, N.; Cason, C.; Maso, G.; Risso, F.M. SARS-CoV-2 Infection and Inflammatory Response in a Twin Pregnancy. *Int. J. Environ. Res. Public. Health* **2021**, *18*, 3075. [CrossRef]
84. Hecht, J.L.; Quade, B.; Deshpande, V.; Mino-Kenudson, M.; Ting, D.T.; Desai, N.; Dygulska, B.; Heyman, T.; Salafia, C.; Shen, D.; et al. SARS-CoV-2 can infect the placenta and is not associated with specific placental histopathology: A series of 19 placentas from COVID-19-positive mothers. *Mod. Pathol.* **2020**, *33*, 2092–2103. [CrossRef]
85. Fouda, G.G.; Martinez, D.R.; Swamy, G.K.; Permar, S.R. The Impact of IgG transplacental transfer on early life immunity. *ImmunoHorizons* **2018**, *2*, 14–25. [CrossRef]
86. Gao, J.; Hu, X.; Sun, X.; Luo, X.; Chen, L. Possible intrauterine SARS-CoV-2 infection: Positive nucleic acid testing results and consecutive positive SARS-CoV-2-specific antibody levels within 50 days after birth. *Int. J. Infect. Dis.* **2020**, *99*, 272–275. [CrossRef] [PubMed]
87. Filimonovic, D.; Lackovic, M.; Filipovic, I.; Orlic, N.K.; Markovic, V.M.; Djukic, V.; Stevanovic, I.P.; Mihajlovic, S. Intrauterine transfusion in COVID-19 positive mother vertical transmission risk assessment. *Eur. J. Obstet. Gynecol. Reprod. Biol.* **2020**, *252*, 617–618. [CrossRef] [PubMed]
88. Gao, J.; Li, W.; Hu, X.; Wei, Y.; Wu, J.; Luo, X.; Chen, S.; Chen, L. Disappearance of SARS-CoV-2 Antibodies in Infants Born to Women with COVID-19, Wuhan, China. *Emerg. Infect. Dis.* **2020**, *26*, 2491–2494. [CrossRef]
89. Niewiesk, S. Maternal Antibodies: Clinical Significance, Mechanism of Interference with Immune Responses, and Possible Vaccination Strategies. *Front. Immunol.* **2014**, *5*, 446. [CrossRef]
90. Groß, R.; Conzelmann, C.; Müller, J.A.; Stenger, S.; Steinhart, K.; Kirchhoff, F.; Münch, J. Detection of SARS-CoV-2 in human breastmilk. *Lancet* **2020**, *395*, 1757–1758. [CrossRef]
91. Yu, Y.; Li, Y.; Hu, Y.; Li, B.; Xu, J. Breastfed 13 month-old infant of a mother with COVID-19 pneumonia: A case report. *Int. Breastfeed. J.* **2020**, *15*, 68. [CrossRef]
92. Hanson, L.A. Breastfeeding provides passive and likely long-lasting active immunity. *Ann. Allergy Asthma Immunol. Off. Publ. Am. Coll. Allergy Asthma Immunol.* **1998**, *81*, 523–533. [CrossRef]
93. Lugli, L.; Bedetti, L.; Lucaccioni, L.; Gennari, W.; Leone, C.; Ancora, G.; Berardi, A. An Uninfected Preterm Newborn Inadvertently Fed SARS-CoV-2-Positive Breast Milk. *Pediatrics* **2020**, *146*, e2020004960. [CrossRef]
94. Shlomai, N.O.; Kasirer, Y.; Strauss, T.; Smolkin, T.; Marom, R.; Shinwell, E.S.; Simmonds, A.; Golan, A.; Morag, I.; Waisman, D.; et al. Neonatal SARS-CoV-2 Infections in Breastfeeding Mothers. *Pediatrics* **2021**, *147*. [CrossRef]
95. Rasmussen, S.A.; Watson, A.K.; Kennedy, E.D.; Broder, K.R.; Jamieson, D.J. Vaccines and pregnancy: Past, present, and future. *Semin. Fetal. Neonatal Med.* **2014**, *19*, 161–169. [CrossRef]
96. Rasmussen, S.A.; Kelley, C.F.; Horton, J.P.; Jamieson, D.J. Coronavirus Disease 2019 (COVID-19) Vaccines and Pregnancy. *Obstet. Gynecol.* **2021**, *137*, 408–414. [CrossRef] [PubMed]
97. Anand, P.; Stahel, V.P. Review the safety of COVID-19 mRNA vaccines: A review. *Patient Saf. Surg.* **2021**, *15*, 20. [CrossRef]
98. Graham, J.M. Update on the gestational effects of maternal hyperthermia. *Birth Defects Res.* **2020**, *112*, 943–952. [CrossRef]
99. Shimabukuro, T.T.; Kim, S.Y.; Myers, T.R.; Moro, P.L.; Oduyebo, T.; Panagiotakopoulos, L.; Marquez, P.L.; Olson, C.K.; Liu, R.; Chang, K.T.; et al. Preliminary Findings of mRNA COVID-19 Vaccine Safety in Pregnant Persons. *N. Engl. J. Med.* **2021**, *384*, 2273–2282. [CrossRef] [PubMed]
100. Levy, A.T.; Singh, S.; Riley, L.E.; Prabhu, M. Acceptance of COVID-19 vaccination in pregnancy: A survey study. *Am. J. Obstet. Gynecol. MFM* **2021**, *3*, 100399. [CrossRef] [PubMed]
101. Panahi, L.; Amiri, M.; Pouy, S. Risks of Novel Coronavirus Disease (COVID-19) in Pregnancy; a Narrative Review. *Arch. Acad. Emerg. Med.* **2020**, *8*, e34.
102. Lancet, T. Science during COVID-19: Where do we go from here? *Lancet* **2020**, *396*, 1941. [CrossRef]
103. Ferrari, R. Writing narrative style literature reviews. *Med. Writ.* **2015**, *24*, 230–235. [CrossRef]
104. Male, V. Are COVID-19 vaccines safe in pregnancy? *Nat. Rev. Immunol.* **2021**, *21*, 200–201. [CrossRef] [PubMed]
105. Simopoulou, M.; Sfakianoudis, K.; Giannelou, P.; Rapani, A.; Siristatidis, C.; Bakas, P.; Vlahos, N.; Pantos, K. Navigating assisted reproduction treatment in the time of COVID-19: Concerns and considerations. *J. Assist. Reprod. Genet.* **2020**, *37*, 2663–2668. [CrossRef] [PubMed]

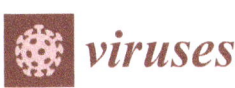

Article

Maternal and Neonatal Outcomes of SARS-CoV-2 Infection in a Cohort of Pregnant Women with Comorbid Disorders

Maria de Lourdes Benamor Teixeira [1,2], Orlando da Costa Ferreira Júnior [3], Esaú João [1,*], Trevon Fuller [1,2], Juliana Silva Esteves [4], Wallace Mendes-Silva [4,5], Carolina Carvalho Mocarzel [4], Richard Araújo Maia [3], Lídia Theodoro Boullosa [3], Cássia Cristina Alves Gonçalves [3], Patrícia Pontes Frankel [4] and Maria Isabel Fragoso da Silveira Gouvêa [1,2]

1. Infectious Diseases Department, Hospital Federal dos Servidores do Estado, Rua Sacadura Cabral, 178, Anexo IV 4° Andar, Rio de Janeiro 20221-161, RJ, Brazil; mlbenamor@hotmail.com (M.d.L.B.T.); trevon@diphse.com.br (T.F.); bebelsgouvea@uol.com.br (M.I.F.d.S.G.)
2. Instituto Nacional de Infectologia Evandro Chagas, Fundação Oswaldo Cruz, Av. Brasil, 4365—Manguinhos, Rio de Janeiro 21040-360, RJ, Brazil
3. Laboratório de Biologia Molecular, Departamento de Genética, Instituto de Biologia, Universidade Federal do Rio de Janeiro, Av. Carlos Chagas Filho, 373—Sala A1-050—Cidade Universitária da Universidade Federal do Rio de Janeiro, Rio de Janeiro 21941-902, RJ, Brazil; orlandocfj@gmail.com (O.d.C.F.J.); richardmaia.a@hotmail.com (R.A.M.); ldthboullosa@hotmail.com (L.T.B.); cassia.alves@gmail.com (C.C.A.G.)
4. Maternal Fetal Department and Infectious Diseases Department, Hospital Federal dos Servidores do Estado, Rua Sacadura Cabral, 178, Rio de Janeiro 20221-161, RJ, Brazil; drajulianaesteves@gmail.com (J.S.E.); drwallacemendes@yahoo.com.br (W.M.-S.); carolinac.mocarzel@gmail.com (C.C.M.); patricia_frankel@hotmail.com (P.P.F.)
5. Perinatal Health Program, Maternidade Escola, Universidade Federal do Rio de Janeiro, Av. Carlos Chagas Filho, 373—Sala A1-050—Cidade Universitária da Universidade Federal do Rio de Janeiro, Rio de Janeiro 21941-902, RJ, Brazil
* Correspondence: esaujoao@gmail.com; Tel.: +55-21-2233-0018

Abstract: There are some reports and case series addressing Coronavirus Disease 2019 (COVID-19) infections during pregnancy in upper income countries, but there are few data on pregnant women with comorbid conditions in low and middle income Countries. This study evaluated the proportion and the maternal and neonatal outcomes associated with SARS-CoV-2 infection among pregnant women with comorbidities. Participants were recruited consecutively in order of admission to a maternity for pregnant women with comorbidities. Sociodemographic, clinical, and laboratory data were prospectively collected during hospitalization. Pregnant women were screened at entry: nasopharyngeal swabs were tested by RT-PCR; serum samples were tested for IgG antibodies against spike protein by ELISA. From April to June 2020, 115 eligible women were included in the study. The proportion of SARS-CoV-2 infection was 28.7%. The rate of obesity was 60.9%, vascular hypertension 40.0%, and HIV 21.7%. The most common clinical presentations were ageusia (21.2%), anosmia (18.2%), and fever (18.2%). Prematurity was higher among mothers who had a SARS-CoV-2 infection based on RT-PCR. There were two cases of fetal demise. We found a high proportion of COVID-19 among pregnant women with comorbidities. This underscores the importance of antenatal care during the pandemic to implement universal SARS-CoV-2 screening, precautionary measures, and the rollout of vaccination programs for pregnant women.

Keywords: SARS-CoV-2; HIV; obesity; obstetrics; pregnancy

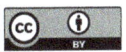

1. Introduction

In 2019, cases of a new respiratory disease caused by a novel Coronavirus emerged in Wuhan, China. The disease, now named Coronavirus disease 19 (COVID-19) is caused by the SARS-CoV-2 virus and rapidly spread worldwide. Since 26 February 2020, when the first case was reported in Brazil, COVID-19 has caused a huge number of infections [1]. On

11 March 2020, COVID-19 was declared a pandemic by the World Health Organization, and is continuing to spread globally. As of June 2021, 180 million cases with more than 3.89 million deaths have been confirmed worldwide. In much of South America, the pandemic is currently spreading out of control. A total of 18.2 million SARS-CoV-2 cases have been reported in Brazil through June 2021, resulting in 507,109,000 deaths [1]. Among these confirmed COVID-19 cases in Brazil, 14,484 have been in pregnant women, 1461 (10.1%) of whom have died [2].

A study of COVID-19 cases reported electronically to the US National Notifiable Diseases Surveillance System analyzed lab-confirmed cases among women of child-bearing age, of whom 8207 were pregnant [3]. Compared to non-pregnant women, non-white pregnant women with underlying medical conditions were 5.4 time more likely to be hospitalized, 1.5 times more likely to be admitted to an intensive care unit (ICU), and 1.7 times more likely to receive mechanical ventilation [3].

COVID-19 screening tests, vaccination, social distancing, mask-wearing, hand hygiene, and avoidance of crowds are among the policies recommended by the WHO and CDC to control the pandemic. According to a systematic review, COVID-19 during pregnancy is associated with increased rates of adverse maternal and neonatal outcomes, particularly in low and middle income countries (LMIC) countries [4]. Universal screening of pregnant women upon admission is already recommended in the United Kingdom, and suggested in other countries such as the United States [5,6]. Allotey et al. in a systematic review reported that 7–12% of pregnant women hospitalized for any reason tested positive for SARS-CoV-2, 62–82% of whom were asymptomatic [7].

The aim of this study was to evaluate the proportion and the maternal and neonatal outcomes associated with SARS-CoV-2 infection in pregnant women with comorbid conditions admitted to a maternal referral center for high-risk prenatal care in Rio de Janeiro.

2. Materials and Methods

This was a pilot study motivated by the need to assess possible pregnancy complications during the COVID-19 epidemic. Participants were offered enrollment consecutively in order of admission to the maternity.

This study was conducted at a referral maternity unit for pregnant women with comorbid disorders at Hospital Federal dos Servidores do Estado (HFSE), Rio de Janeiro, a public federal institution funded by the Brazilian Ministry of Health. From 13 April to 17 June 2020, all pregnant women admitted to the maternity unit were invited to participate in this study. The inclusion criteria were: admission to the maternity unit during gestation, ≥ 18 years of age, willingness to have nasopharyngeal swabs and blood samples collected for diagnosis of SARS-CoV-2 infection, and provided signed informed consent. The exclusion criteria were women not willing to participate and subsequent admissions in the same pregnancy during the study period. Sampling was not longitudinal as most patients received prenatal care at other health institutions, delivered at our hospital, and post-natal follow-up occurred elsewhere.

Sociodemographic, clinical, and laboratory data were prospectively collected during hospitalization using a structured standardized form designed for the study.

We used the Brazilian Diabetes Society criteria for gestational diabetes according to which it is defined as fasting glycemia of 92–125 mg/dL during the first trimester, or 1-h plasma glucose >180 mg/dL or 2-h plasma glucose of 153–199 following a 75 g glucose load during the second and third trimesters [8,9]. This study defined HIV using the following testing algorithm [10]: 1. A plasma sample was tested for HIV-1 by either a chemiluminescence immunoassay (CLIA) (Abbott ARCHITECT HIV Ag/Ab Combo, Abbott Diagnostics, Abbott Park, IL, USA) or an Abbott real time HIV-1 viral load test (Abbott Real-time HIV-1 Abbott Laboratories, Abbott Park, IL, USA). Next, a second sample from the same participant was tested by CLIA or an Abbott. If both samples were positive for HIV-1, the participant was classified as living with HIV.

Nasopharyngeal swabs were systematically collected according to established protocols [11] within 24 h of admission to the maternity. Swabs were refrigerated upon collection and were transported within 2 h to the Molecular Virology Reference Laboratory at Universidade Federal do Rio de Janeiro. Briefly, SARS-CoV-2 RNA from swab media were extracted in the Maxwell MDX Promega automated machine using the Maxwell16 Viral Total Nucleic Acid Purification Kit (Promega, Madison, WI, USA). RT-PCR was standardized in the laboratory using RT-PCR 7500 Thermal Cycler (Applied Biosystems, Foster City, CA, USA) and the Gotaq one-step Probe RT-qPCR System (Pomega). We have strictly followed the CDC protocol [12] which uses the SARS-CoV-2 nucleocapsid targets—N1 and N2—and human RNase P (RP) as control target. After 45 amplification cycles, RT-PCR positive were defined for samples with cycle threshold (ct) below or equal to 38, negative above 40 ct and inconclusive between these ct values. To define the assay limit of detection (LoD) value, we first defined the number of RNA copies of a SARS-CoV-2 isolate by digital PCR. We then made 12 dilutions (a Log2 series) of this viral isolate specimen and eight replicates of each dilution to calculate the LoD by Probit analysis. We figure that the assay has a LoD of 10 copies of viral RNA per 200 µL of swab media. Serum samples were collected within 24 h of admission to the maternity for serology diagnosis of SARS-CoV-2 infection (IgG serology) and processed at Virology Molecular Reference Laboratory (LVM) at Universidade Federal do Rio de Janeiro. The ELISA assay for detection of IgG was developed and validated at the LVM, using the spike protein as antigen, according to protocol described by Perera et al. [13].

Mann–Whitney tests were used for median comparisons, and interquartile range (IQR) intervals were also calculated. Chi-squared or Fisher's exact tests were used to compare proportions. In parallel, subgroup analysis of only the RT-PCR data was conducted. Associations between SARS-CoV-2 infection and sociodemographic, clinical, and laboratory variables were evaluated. The level of significance was set at 0.05 for all tests. Statistical analysis was performed using SPSS version 20.0. Imbalanced variables (diabetes and ethnicity) were adjusted between the SARS-CoV-2 positive and negative groups using propensity score matching with SAS 9.4.

The study was approved by the institutional review board of the Hospital Federal dos Servidores do Estado (CAAE# 13139720.5.0000.5252, April 2020).

3. Results

From 13 April to 17 June 2020, 128 women were admitted to the HFSE maternity center. Of these 128 women, 13 were excluded: 8 did not agree to participate and 5 women did not have swabs collected. The 115 eligible women were included in the study and had nasopharyngeal swabs for SARS-CoV-2 and plasma collected for serology. See the flowchart for the inclusion and exclusion characteristics of the study population (Figure 1).

Among the 115 women investigated, 28.7% were diagnosed with SARS-CoV-2 infection (33/115). Of the 33 positives, 16 were positive by IgG only, 7 were positive both by IgG and RT-PCR, 6 were positive only by RT-PCR, and 4 were positive by IgG and inconclusive by RT-PCR (Figure 1). In total, 80 tested negative both by RT-PCR and serology, and 2 had inconclusive RT-PCR and negative serology. Those with RT-PCR inconclusive and negative serology or indeterminate serology and negative RT-PCR were classified as negative.

The sociodemographic (Table 1), clinical characteristics and laboratory findings (Table 2), and the maternal and obstetric outcomes (Table 3) are presented below. Both COVID-19 positive and negative pregnant women had similar demographic characteristics (Table 1). The only imbalanced variables were the number of household contacts and diabetes. SARS-CoV-2 positive mothers had an average of 4 household contacts while negative mothers had 3.5 (standardized difference: 0.29). Diabetes was more or less frequent in the SARS-CoV-2 positive women (13.4%) than the SARS-CoV-2 negative ones (25%) (standardized difference: 0.28).

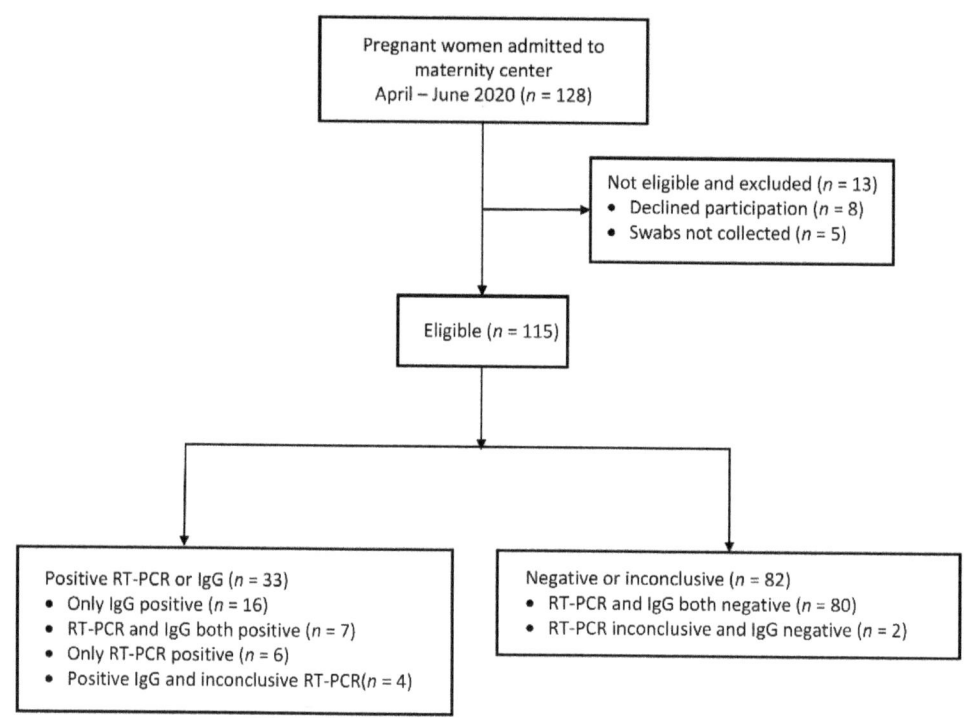

Figure 1. Flowchart of the inclusion and exclusion characteristics of the study population.

Table 1. Baseline demographic and clinical characteristics in a cohort of pregnant women screened for SARS-CoV-2 infection at a prenatal care reference center in Rio de Janeiro, March–June 2020.

		COVID-19		
Variables	All Pregnant Women	Positive	Negative	Standardized Difference
Demographics				
Ethnicity (n = 114) (number,%)				
White	33 (28.9%)	11 (34.4%)	22 (26.8%)	0.165
Non-white	81 (71.1%)	21 (65.6%)	60 (73.2%)	
Age at entry (y) (n = 114) (median, IQR)	29 (25–35.2)	28 (24–35)	30 (25–36)	0.005
Number of household contacts (n = 108) (median, IQR)	4 (3–5)	4 (3–6)	3.5 (3–5)	0.26
Diabetes (gestational or type II) (n = 105) (number,%)				
Yes	23 (21.9%)	4 (13.8%)	19 (25.0%)	−0.286
No	82 (78.1%)	24 (86.2%)	57 (75.0%)	
Vascular Hypertension (n = 115) (number,%)				
Yes	46 (40%)	13 (39.4%)	33 (40.2%)	−0.016
No	69 (60%)	20 (60.6%)	50 (59.8%)	
Obesity (n = 115) (number,%)				
Yes	70 (60.9%)	21 (63.6%)	49 (59.8%)	0.078
No	45 (39.1%)	12 (36.4%)	33 (40.2%)	

Table 1. Cont.

Variables	All Pregnant Women	COVID-19 Positive	COVID-19 Negative	Standardized Difference
Living with HIV (n = 115) (number,%)				
Yes	25 (21.7%)	8 (24.2%)	17 (20.7%)	0.084
No	90 (78.3%)	25 (75.8%)	65 (79.3%)	
Tobacco Use during gestation (n = 112) (number,%)				
Yes	6 (5.4%)	1 (3.1%)	5 (6.3%)	−0.15
No	106 (94.6%)	31 (96.9%)	75 (93.8%)	
Illicit Drug Use during gestation (n = 112) (number,%)				
Yes	2 (1.8%)	1 (3.1%)	1 (1.2%)	
No	110 (98.2%)	31 (96.9%)	79 (98.8%)	0.13
Alcohol use during gestation (n = 111) (number,%)				
Yes	5 (4.5%)	1 (3.1%)	4 (5.1%)	−0.1
No	106 (95.5%)	31 (96.9%)	75 (94.9%)	

Table 2. Maternal signs and symptoms.

Variables	All Pregnant Women	COVID-19 Positive	COVID-19 Negative	Statistical Test	p-Value
Signs and Symptoms	All pregnant women (n = 115)	Positive (n = 33)	Negative (n = 82)	p-Value Fisher's Exact Test	
Fever	9 (7.8%)	6 (18.2%)	3 (3.7%)		0.016
Chills	2 (1.7%)	1 (3.0%)	1 (1.2%)		0.493
Headache	16 (13.9%)	5 (15.2%)	11 (13.4%)		0.774
Dry cough	8 (7.0%)	4 (12.1%)	4 (4.9%)		0.163
Sore throat	5 (4.3%)	3 (9.1%)	2 (2.4%)		0.141
Runny nose	6 (5.2%)	2 (6.1%)	4 (4.9%)		1
Anosmia	7 (6.1%)	6 (18.2%)	1 (1.2%)		<0.01
Ageusia	7 (6.1%)	7 (21.2%)	0 (0%)		<0.01
Persistent pain in the chest	2 (1.7%)	2 (6.1%)	0 (0%)		0.081
Dyspnea	7 (6.1%)	5 (15.2%)	2 (2.4%)		0.020
Myalgia	5 (4.3%)	4 (12.1%)	1 (1.2%)		0.023
Fatigue	3 (2.6%)	3 (9.1%)	0 (0%)		0.022
Vomiting/ nausea	6 (5.2%)	3 (9.1%)	3 (3.7%)		0.352
Diarrhea	4 (3.5%)	2 (6.1%)	2 (2.4%)		0.577

There were 14 participants who were positive by RT-PCR or serology and presented with at least one symptom. The most common clinical presentation was ageusia (7/14), anosmia (6/14), fever (6/14), headache (5/14), dyspnea (5/14), and myalgia (4/14) (Table 2).

The principal maternal comorbid conditions among the participants of the study were obesity 60.9% (70/115), vascular hypertension 40.0% (46/115), HIV 21.7% (25/115), diabetes (gestational diabetes 14.3% (15/105) and type II diabetes 7.0% (8/115)), smoking/tobacco use 5.4% (6/112), alcohol use 4.5% (5/111), use of illicit drugs 1.8% (2/112), rheumatological 0.9% (1/115), and hematological diseases 5.2% (6/115).

We also conducted a separate analysis comparing obstetric outcomes of SARS-CoV-2 RT-PCR positive women to those who were RT-PCR negative, without considering the IgG antibodies. Of 13 women who tested positive for SARS-CoV-2 by RT-PCR, four were asymptomatic when sampled. In a univariate model, gestational age at birth was lower for infants born to mothers who had a SARS-CoV-2 infection based on RT-PCR ($p = 0.005$). In particular, the average gestational age at delivery was 36 weeks for COVID-positive mothers and 38 weeks in negative mothers. All of the 26% of pregnant women with SARS-CoV-2 had preterm deliveries (Table 3). After we performed propensity matching, gestational age at delivery was significantly higher in the group of PCR-positive mothers ($p = 0.027$).

Table 3. Obstetrical and neonatal outcomes.

Variables	COVID-19			Statistical Test	p-Value
	All Pregnant Women	Positive	Negative		
Obstetrical characteristics and outcomes					
Preeclampsia ($n = 105$) (number,%)				Fisher's Exact Test	0.227
Yes	15 (14.3%)	2 (6.9%)	13 (17.1%)		
No	90 (85.7%)	27 (93.1%)	63 (82.9%)		
Gestational age at delivery (weeks) ($n = 99$) (median, IQR)	38 (37–39)	38 (35.7–39)	38 (37–39)	Mann-Whitney	0.249
Mode of Delivery ($n = 102$) (number,%)				Pearson Chi-Square	0.956
Vaginal	66 (64.7%)	18 (64.3%)	48 (64.9%)		
C-section	36 (35.3%)	10 (35.7%)	26 (35.1%)		
Neonatal Outcomes ($n = 102$)					
Birth weight (g) ($n = 100$) (number,%)				Fisher's Exact Test	0.505
<2500	12 (12.0%)	2 (7.4%)	10 (13.7%)		
≥2500	88 (88.0%)	25 (92.6%)	63 (86.3%)		
Preterm delivery ($n = 99$) (number,%)	17 (17.2%)	7 (26.9%)	10 (13.7%)	Fisher's Exact Test	0.139

Of the reasons for admission to the maternity center 103 (89.6%) were for delivery, 12 (10.4%) were due to clinical conditions and obstetrical complaints. Among those who delivered during the study, there were 66 vaginal and 36 cesarean births. The principal maternal complications are shown in Table 1, and three pregnant women required admission to the intensive care unit due to oxygen desaturation. There were no maternal deaths.

There was only one case of a malformation, holoprosencephaly, in a mother who was seropositive for SARS-CoV-2. All the pregnant women living with HIV participating in the study were using combined antiretroviral therapy (cART). Among these women, the median CD4+ T cell count was 619 cells/mm^3. All of them (71% (17/24)) had an undetectable HIV-1 viral load. Concerning neonatal outcomes, there were two cases of fetal demise. One was to an obese woman with SARS-CoV-2 positive serology and negative RT-PCR. The other was to a mother living with HIV, who was RT-PCR inconclusive and had positive serology for SARS-CoV-2. Only the placenta of the woman who was living with HIV was tested and was determined to be RT-PCR-positive for SARS-CoV-2.

4. Discussion

The proportion of SARS-CoV-2 in this study population of pregnant women with co-morbid conditions at a reference center for high risk gestation was 28.7%. This is higher than the proportion reported in previous studies of pregnant women, which have ranged from 0.56% to 15.4%, and a recent meta-analysis reported a similar range of 7% to 13% [7,14–20]. This proportion may depend on a variety of factors including the local attack rate, the risk profile of the population investigated and the type of screening assay [21–24].

The clinical manifestations of COVID-19 in pregnant women in this cohort were largely similar to those of non-pregnant adults in settings with high incidence of SARS-CoV-2 infection, as has been noted in a number of other studies and international guidelines [5,21]. In symptomatic pregnant women, the frequency of fever was similar to that of a multicentric study [25], but lower than in a large CDC registry [26]. This may be explained by the fact that the population of this study were being admitted to our hospital for obstetric and clinical reasons. Three pregnant women were admitted due to signs and symptoms related to COVID-19, all of whom were RT-PCR positive.

Among the principal comorbid conditions in this population were obesity, vascular hypertension, and living with HIV. Obesity has been recognized as one the most important risk factors for severe COVID-19 [27,28]. While in this cohort, obesity was the most frequent comorbid condition, it was not a significant risk factor for SARS-CoV-2 infection.

With respect to neonatal outcomes, in this study the rate of preterm birth among pregnant women with SARS-CoV-2 infection based on PCR tests was 26%, which is higher than the overall rate of preterm birth in Brazil of 11.5% [29]. Concerning malformations, as holoprosencephaly is far more common among diabetic mothers and arises early in gestation, we do not consider it likely that the malformation was associated with maternal SARS-CoV-2 infection. As the sample size of our study was limited, the extent to which these findings can be generalized is unknown. Furthermore, as the site is a reference center for high-risk pregnancies, it is not surprising that preterm births and malformations occurred during the study. It should be noted that a robust review study found no evidence of teratogenicity of SARS-CoV-2 [30].

Coagulation disorders are a concern during pregnancy and can be exacerbated by COVID-19 infection and obesity. However, none of the patients in the cohort experienced complications related to coagulation, perhaps because in this unit, they received antithrombotic prophylaxis as the standard of care for this subpopulation.

There have been few studies of the effects of co-infection of HIV and SARS-CoV-2 in pregnant women. One such study was conducted in South Africa and found that of six pregnant women who were positive for COVID-19 and died, three were living with HIV [31]. In our study, fully 25 (22%) of the study participants were women living with HIV. As the study site is a reference center for HIV in pregnancy, one of the principal comorbidities was HIV. This institution is also a center for prevention of perinatal HIV transmission where testing for HIV is universal during prenatal care and at delivery and cART is the standard of care. Another study in South Africa reported that living with HIV worsened the severity of COVID-19; however, like our study, a number of others have found no evidence of worse clinical outcomes [32–35]. This population has a higher prevalence of HIV than other populations of pregnant women in which COVID-19 has been investigated, have taken cART as the standard of care with good adherence, had suppressed viral load and high CD4 cell counts. This could partially explain why the severity of COVID-19 among the participants was minimal in our setting.

Universal screening of pregnant women for COVID-19 has been extensively implemented in high income countries experiencing the pandemic. It is widely accepted that in these settings such screening is worthwhile as it can detect asymptomatic cases of COVID-19 [14,36,37]. While in LMICs affected by the COVID-19 pandemic with limited resources, putting universal screening of pregnant women in place will be more difficult. In our view, effort should be made to implement such programs as they can have a positive impact on public health.

Among the strengths of this study is that it was conducted in a maternity for patients with comorbidities and substantial prevalence of HIV, and underscores the importance of establishing governmental policies for pregnant women in LMICs, as has already been implemented in high income countries. These include universal screening, precautionary measures and the rollout of a vaccine program for pregnant women.

Among the limitations of the study was that the follow-up after discharge was limited. In addition, serologic tests for SARS-CoV-2 have a number of limitations, such as false-negative results due to improper timing for collecting a sample for testing or cross-reaction with other Coronaviruses. Additionally, the study did not screen for IgM antibodies.

In conclusion, this study showed high proportion of SARS-CoV-2 infection among pregnant women. This underscores the importance of antenatal care during the pandemic to implement universal SARS-CoV-2 screening, precautionary measures and the rollout of vaccination programs [5,11,38] for pregnant women.

Author Contributions: Conceptualization, M.d.L.B.T., E.J. and M.I.F.d.S.G.; investigation, O.d.C.F.J., R.A.M., L.T.B., C.C.A.G., J.S.E., W.M.-S., C.C.M. and P.P.F.; writing—original draft preparation, M.d.L.B.T., E.J. and M.I.F.d.S.G.; writing—review and editing, M.d.L.B.T., E.J., M.I.F.d.S.G. and T.F.; supervision, E.J. All authors have read and agreed to the published version of the manuscript.

Funding: This research received no external funding.

Institutional Review Board Statement: The study was conducted according to the guidelines of the Declaration of Helsinki, and approved by the Institutional Review Board of the Hospital Federal dos Servidores do Estado.

Informed Consent Statement: Informed consent was obtained from all subjects involved in the study.

Data Availability Statement: The data presented in this study are available on request from the corresponding author. The data are not publicly available due to privacy restrictions.

Acknowledgments: We thank the Laboratório de Biologia Molecular, Departamento de Genética, Instituto de Biologia, Universidade Federal do Rio de Janeiro, the pregnant women who participated in the study, all the staff of the Infectious Diseases Department, the Neonatology Department, and the Maternal Fetal Department at the Hospital Federal dos Servidores do Estado, and the Brazilian Ministry of Health.

Conflicts of Interest: The authors declare no conflict of interest.

References

1. Ministry of Health. *Coronavirus COVID-19 Cases Portal*; Ministry of Health: Brasília, Brazil, 2021.
2. Rodrigues, A.; Lacerda, L.; Rossana Pulcineli Vieira Francisco. Brazilian Obstetric Observatory. *arXiv* **2021**, arXiv:2105.06534.
3. Ellington, S.; Strid, P.; Tong, V.T.; Woodworth, K.; Galang, R.R.; Zambrano, L.D.; Nahabedian, J.; Anderson, K.; Gilboa, S.M. Characteristics of women of reproductive age with laboratory-confirmed SARS-CoV-2 infection by pregnancy status—United States, 22 January–7 June 2020. *MMWR Morb. Mortal. Wkly. Rep.* **2020**, *69*, 769–775. [CrossRef] [PubMed]
4. Chmielewska, B.; Barratt, I.; Townsend, R.; Kalafat, E.; van der Meulen, J.; Gurol-Urganci, I.; O'Brien, P.; Morris, E.; Draycott, T.; Thangaratinam, S.; et al. Effects of the COVID-19 pandemic on maternal and perinatal outcomes: A systematic review and meta-analysis. *Lancet Glob. Health* **2021**, *9*, e759–e772. [CrossRef]
5. Royal College of Obstetricians & Gynaecologists. *Coronavirus (COVID-19) Infection in Pregnacy. Version 13. Friday 19 February 2021*; Royal College of Obstetricians & Gynaecologists: London, UK, 2021; p. 98.
6. American College of Obstetricians and Gynecologists. *Novel Coronavirus 2019 (COVID-19). Updated December 2020*; American College of Obstetricians and Gynecologists: Washington, DC, USA, 2020.
7. Allotey, J.; Stallings, E.; Bonet, M.; Yap, M.; Chatterjee, S.; Kew, T.; Debenham, L.; Llavall, A.C.; Dixit, A.; Zhou, D.; et al. Clinical manifestations, risk factors, and maternal and perinatal outcomes of coronavirus disease 2019 in pregnancy: Living systematic review and meta-analysis. *BMJ* **2020**, *370*, m3320. [CrossRef] [PubMed]
8. Volanski, W.; do Prado, A.L.; Al-Lahham, Y.; Teleginski, A.; Pereira, F.S.; Alberton, D.; Rego, F.G.D.; Valdameri, G.; Picheth, G. d-GDM: A mobile diagnostic decision support system for gestational diabetes. *Arch. Endocrinol. Metab.* **2019**, *63*, 524–530. [CrossRef] [PubMed]
9. Ministério da Saúde. *Diagnóstico da Infecção pelo HIV em Adultos e Crianças*; Minstério da Saúde: Brasília, Brazil, 2018.
10. International Maternal Pediatric Adolescent AIDS Clinical Trials (IMPAACT) Network. *Pharmacokinetic Properties of Antiretroviral and Anti-Tuberculosis Drugs during Pregnancy and Postpartum (IMPAACT Protocol 2026) Manual of Procedures*; IMPAACT: Washington, DC, USA, 2021.
11. CDC. *Interim Guidelines for Collecting, Handling, and Testing Clinical Specimens from Persons for Coronavirus Disease 2019 (COVID-19)*; CDC: Atlanta, GA, USA, 2020.

12. CDC. *2019-Novel Coronavirus (2019-nCoV) Real-Time RT-PCR Diagnostic Panel—CDC-006-00019, Revision: 06*; CDC/DDID/NCIRD/Division of Viral Diseases: Centers for Disease Control and Prevention: Atlanta, Georgia, 2020.
13. Perera, R.A.; Mok, C.K.; Tsang, O.T.; Lv, H.; Ko, R.L.; Wu, N.C.; Yuan, M.; Leung, W.S.; Chan, J.M.; Chik, T.S.; et al. Serological assays for severe acute respiratory syndrome coronavirus 2 (SARS-CoV-2), 1 April 2020. *Eur. Commun. Dis. Bull.* **2020**, *25*, 2000421.
14. Breslin, N.; Baptiste, C.; Gyamfi-Bannerman, C.; Miller, R.; Martinez, R.; Bernstein, K.; Ring, L.; Landau, R.; Purisch, S.; Friedman, A.M.; et al. Coronavirus disease 2019 infection among asymptomatic and symptomatic pregnant women: Two weeks of confirmed presentations to an affiliated pair of New York City hospitals. *Am. J. Obstet. Gynecol. MFM* **2020**, *2*, 100118. [CrossRef]
15. LaCourse, S.M.; Kachikis, A.; Blain, M.; Simmons, L.E.; Mays, J.A.; Pattison, A.D.; Salerno, C.C.; McCartney, S.A.; Kretzer, N.M.; Resnick, R.; et al. Low prevalence of SARS-CoV-2 among pregnant and postpartum patients with universal screening in Seattle, Washington. *Clin. Infect. Dis.* **2020**, *72*, 869–872. [CrossRef] [PubMed]
16. Ochiai, D.; Kasuga, Y.; Iida, M.; Ikenoue, S.; Tanaka, M. Universal screening for SARS-CoV-2 in asymptomatic obstetric patients in Tokyo, Japan. *Int. J. Gynecol. Obstet.* **2020**, *150*, 268–269. [CrossRef]
17. Savasi, V.M.; Parisi, F.; Patanè, L.; Ferrazzi, E.; Frigerio, L.; Pellegrino, A.; Spinillo, A.; Tateo, S.; Ottoboni, M.; Veronese, P.; et al. Clinical findings and disease severity in hospitalized pregnant women with Coronavirus Disease 2019 (COVID-19). *Obstet. Gynecol.* **2020**, *136*. [CrossRef] [PubMed]
18. Miller, E.S.; Grobman, W.A.; Sakowicz, A.; Rosati, J.; Peaceman, A.M. Clinical implications of universal Severe Acute Respiratory Syndrome Coronavirus 2 (SARS-CoV-2) testing in pregnancy. *Obstet. Gynecol.* **2020**, *136*, 232–234. [CrossRef]
19. Sutton, D.; Fuchs, K.; D'Alton, M.; Goffman, D. Universal screening for SARS-CoV-2 in women admitted for delivery. *N. Engl. J. Med.* **2020**, *382*, 2163–2164. [CrossRef] [PubMed]
20. Salvatore, C.M.; Han, J.-Y.; Acker, K.P.; Tiwari, P.; Jin, J.; Brandler, M.; Cangemi, C.; Gordon, L.; Parow, A.; DiPace, J.; et al. Neonatal management and outcomes during the COVID-19 pandemic: An observation cohort study. *Lancet Child Adolesc. Health* **2020**, *4*, 721–727. [CrossRef]
21. Li, N.; Han, L.; Peng, M.; Lv, Y.; Ouyang, Y.; Liu, K.; Yue, L.; Li, Q.; Sun, G.; Chen, L.; et al. Maternal and neonatal outcomes of pregnant women with COVID-19 pneumonia: A case-control study. *Clin. Infect Dis.* **2020**, *17*, 2035–2041. [CrossRef] [PubMed]
22. Campbell, K.H.; Tornatore, J.M.; Lawrence, K.E.; Illuzzi, J.L.; Sussman, L.S.; Lipkind, H.S.; Pettker, C.M. Prevalence of SARS-CoV-2 among patients admitted for childbirth in southern Connecticut. *JAMA* **2020**, *323*, 2520–2522. [CrossRef]
23. Khalil, A.; Hill, R.; Ladhani, S.; Pattisson, K.; O'Brien, P. Severe acute respiratory syndrome coronavirus 2 in pregnancy: Symptomatic pregnant women are only the tip of the iceberg. *Am. J. Obstet. Gynecol.* **2020**, *223*, 296–297. [CrossRef]
24. Buitrago-Garcia, D.; Egli-Gany, D.; Counotte, M.J.; Hossmann, S.; Imeri, H.; Ipekci, A.M.; Salanti, G.; Low, N. Occurrence and transmission potential of asymptomatic and presymptomatic SARS-CoV-2 infections: A living systematic review and meta-analysis. *PLoS Med.* **2020**, *17*, e1003346. [CrossRef]
25. Afshar, Y.; Gaw, S.L.; Flaherman, V.J.; Chambers, B.D.; Krakow, D.; Berghella, V.; Shamshirsaz, A.A.; Boatin, A.A.; Aldrovandi, G.; Greiner, A.; et al. Clinical Presentation of Coronavirus Disease 2019 (COVID-19) in Pregnant and Recently Pregnant People. *Obstet. Gynecol.* **2020**, *136*, 1117–1125. [CrossRef] [PubMed]
26. Zambrano, L.D.; Ellington, S.; Strid, P.; Galang, R.R.; Oduyebo, T.; Tong, V.T.; Woodworth, K.R.; Nahabedian, J.F., 3rd; Azziz-Baumgartner, E.; Gilboa, S.M.; et al. Update: Characteristics of Symptomatic Women of Reproductive Age with Laboratory-Confirmed SARS-CoV-2 Infection by Pregnancy Status—United States, 22 January–3 October 2020. *MMWR Morb. Mortal. Wkly. Rep.* **2020**, *69*, 1641–1647. [CrossRef] [PubMed]
27. Kassir, R. Risk of COVID-19 for patients with obesity. *Obes. Rev.* **2020**, *21*, e13034. [CrossRef]
28. Petrakis, D.; Margina, D.; Tsarouhas, K.; Tekos, F.; Stan, M.; Nikitovic, D.; Kouretas, D.; Spandidos, D.A.; Tsatsakis, A. Obesity—A risk factor for increased COVID-19 prevalence, severity and lethality (Review). *Mol. Med. Rep.* **2020**, *22*, 9–19. [CrossRef]
29. Leal, M.d.C.; Esteves-Pereira, A.P.; Nakamura-Pereira, M.; Torres, J.A.; Theme-Filha, M.; Domingues, R.M.S.M.; Dias, M.A.B.; Moreira, M.E.; Gama, S.G. Prevalence and risk factors related to preterm birth in Brazil. *Reprod. Health* **2016**, *13*, 127. [CrossRef]
30. Hapshy, V.; Aziz, D.; Kahar, P.; Khanna, D.; Johnson, K.E.; Parmar, M.A.-O. COVID-19 and Pregnancy: Risk, Symptoms, Diagnosis, and Treatment. *SN Compr. Clin. Med.* **2021**, *3*, 1–7. [CrossRef]
31. Basu, J.K.; Chauke, L.; Magoro, T. Maternal mortality from COVID 19 among South African pregnant women. *J. Matern.-Fetal Neonatal Med.* **2021**, 1–3. [CrossRef] [PubMed]
32. Park, L.S.; Rentsch, C.T.; Sigel, K.; Rodriguez-Barradas, M.; Brown, S.T.; Bidwell Goetz, M.; Williams, E.C.; Althoff, K.; Brau, N.; Aoun-Barakat, L.; et al. LBPEC23. COVID-19 in the largest US HIV Cohort. In Proceedings of the 23rd International AIDS Conference, Mexico City, Mexico, 6–10 July 2020.
33. US Department of Health & Human Services. *Interim Guidance for COVID-19 and Persons with HIV Updated 19 June 2020*; AIDS Info: Washington, DC, USA, 2020.
34. Gervasoni, C.; Meraviglia, P.; Riva, A.; Giacomelli, A.; Oreni, L.; Minisci, D.; Atzori, C.; Ridolfo, A.; Cattaneo, D. Clinical features and outcomes of HIV patients with coronavirus disease 2019. *Clin. Infect Dis.* **2020**. [CrossRef]
35. Cooper, T.; Woodward, B.; Alom, S.; Harky, A. Coronavirus Disease 2019 (COVID-19) Outcomes in HIV/AIDS Patients: A Systematic Review. *HIV Med.* **2020**, *21*, 567–577. [CrossRef]

36. Iida, M.; Tanaka, M. Screening maternity populations during the COVID-19 pandemic. *BJOG* **2020**, *127*, 1557. [CrossRef] [PubMed]
37. Melo, G.C.D.; Araújo, K.C.G.M.D. COVID-19 infection in pregnant women, preterm delivery, birth weight, and vertical transmission: A systematic review and meta-analysis. *Cad. Saúde Pública* **2020**, *36*, e00087320. [CrossRef] [PubMed]
38. CDC. *Infection Control Guidance for Healthcare Professionals about Coronavirus (COVID-19)*; CDC: Atlanta, GA, USA, 2020.

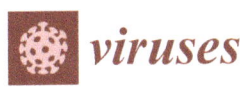 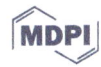

Article

Pregnancy Outcomes and SARS-CoV-2 Infection: The Spanish Obstetric Emergency Group Study

Sara Cruz Melguizo [1], María Luisa de la Cruz Conty [2,*], Paola Carmona Payán [3], Alejandra Abascal-Saiz [4], Pilar Pintando Recarte [5], Laura González Rodríguez [6], Celia Cuenca Marín [7], Alicia Martínez Varea [8], Ana Belén Oreja Cuesta [9], Pilar Prats Rodríguez [10], Irene Fernández Buhigas [11], María Victoria Rodríguez Gallego [12], Ana María Fernández Alonso [13], Rocío López Pérez [14], José Román Broullón Molanes [15], María Begoña Encinas Pardilla [1], Mercedes Ramírez Gómez [16], María Joaquina Gimeno Gimeno [17], Antonio Sánchez Muñoz [18], Oscar Martínez-Pérez [1,*] and on behalf of the Spanish Obstetric Emergency Group (S.O.E.G.) [†]

1 Department of Gynecology and Obstetrics, Puerta de Hierro University Hospital of Majadahonda, 28222 Majadahonda, Spain; saracruz.gine@yahoo.es (S.C.M.); beenpar@yahoo.es (M.B.E.P.)
2 Fundación de Investigación Biomédica, Puerta de Hierro University Hospital of Majadahonda, 28222 Majadahonda, Spain
3 Department of Gynecology and Obstetrics, University Hospital 12 de Octubre, 28041 Madrid, Spain; paolacp1993@gmail.com
4 Department of Gynecology and Obstetrics, La Paz University Hospital, 28046 Madrid, Spain; alejandra_as@hotmail.com
5 Department of Gynecology and Obstetrics, Gregorio Marañón University Hospital, 28007 Madrid, Spain; ppintadorec@yahoo.es
6 Department of Gynecology and Obstetrics, Hospital Alvaro Cunqueiro, 36213 Vigo, Spain; laura_gr_@hotmail.com
7 Department of Gynecology and Obstetrics, Regional Hospital of Málaga, 29010 Málaga, Spain; celia.cuenca.sspa@juntadeandalucia.es
8 Department of Gynecology and Obstetrics, La Fe University and Polytechnic Hospital, 46026 Valencia, Spain; martinez.alicia.v@gmail.com
9 Department of Gynecology and Obstetrics, Hospital del Tajo, 28300 Aranjuez, Spain; anaoreja@yahoo.es
10 Department of Gynecology and Obstetrics, QuirónSalud Dexeus University Hospital, 08028 Barcelona, Spain; pilpra@dexeus.com
11 Department of Gynecology and Obstetrics, Torrejón University Hospital, 28850 Torrejón de Ardoz, Spain; ibuhigas80@gmail.com
12 Department of Gynecology and Obstetrics, San Millán-San Pedro Hospital Complex, 26006 Logroño, Spain; marivirg80@gmail.com
13 Department of Gynecology and Obstetrics, Torrecárdenas University Hospital, 04009 Almería, Spain; anafernandez.alonso@gmail.com
14 Department of Gynecology and Obstetrics, Santa Lucía University Hospital, 30202 Cartagena, Spain; rocio.lopez.perez@gmail.com
15 Department of Gynecology and Obstetrics, Puerta del Mar University Hospital, 11009 Cádiz, Spain; jrbroullon@gmail.com
16 Maternal-fetal Medicine Unit, Department of Gynecology and Obstetrics, La Mancha Centro General Hospital, 13600 Alcázar de San Juan, Spain; mercebon@hotmail.com
17 Maternal-fetal Medicine Unit, Department of Gynecology and Obstetrics, Reina Sofía University Hospital, 14004 Córdoba, Spain; qgimenog@gmail.com
18 Department of Gynecology and Obstetrics, Ciudad Real University Hospital, 13005 Ciudad Real, Spain; asanchezm@sescam.jccm.es
* Correspondence: farmcruz@gmail.com (M.L.d.l.C.C.); oscarmartinezgine@gmail.com (O.M.-P.)
† A list of the Spanish Obstetric Emergency Group collaborators appears in the Acknowledgements section.

Citation: Cruz Melguizo, S.; de la Cruz Conty, M.L.; Carmona Payán, P.; Abascal-Saiz, A.; Pintado Recarte, P.; González Rodríguez, L.; Cuenca Marín, C.; Martínez Varea, A.; Oreja Cuesta, A.B.; Rodríguez, P.P.; et al. Pregnancy Outcomes and SARS-CoV-2 Infection: The Spanish Obstetric Emergency Group Study. *Viruses* 2021, *13*, 853. https://doi.org/10.3390/v13050853

Academic Editors: David Baud and Léo Pomar

Received: 31 March 2021
Accepted: 4 May 2021
Published: 7 May 2021

Publisher's Note: MDPI stays neutral with regard to jurisdictional claims in published maps and institutional affiliations.

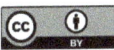

Copyright: © 2021 by the authors. Licensee MDPI, Basel, Switzerland. This article is an open access article distributed under the terms and conditions of the Creative Commons Attribution (CC BY) license (https://creativecommons.org/licenses/by/4.0/).

Abstract: Pregnant women who are infected with SARS-CoV-2 are at an increased risk of adverse perinatal outcomes. With this study, we aimed to better understand the relationship between maternal infection and perinatal outcomes, especially preterm births, and the underlying medical and interventionist factors. This was a prospective observational study carried out in 78 centers (Spanish Obstetric Emergency Group) with a cohort of 1347 SARS-CoV-2 PCR-positive pregnant women registered consecutively between 26 February and 5 November 2020, and a concurrent sample of PCR-negative mothers. The patients' information was collected from their medical records, and the association of SARS-CoV-2 and perinatal outcomes was evaluated by univariable and multivariate analyses. The data from 1347 SARS-CoV-2-positive pregnancies were compared with those from 1607 SARS-CoV-2-negative pregnancies. Differences were observed between both groups in premature rupture of membranes (15.5% vs. 11.1%, $p < 0.001$); venous thrombotic events (1.5% vs. 0.2%, $p < 0.001$); and severe pre-eclampsia incidence (40.6 vs. 15.6%, $p = 0.001$), which could have been overestimated in the infected cohort due to the shared analytical signs between this hypertensive disorder and COVID-19. In addition, more preterm deliveries were observed in infected patients (11.1% vs. 5.8%, $p < 0.001$) mainly due to an increase in iatrogenic preterm births. The prematurity in SARS-CoV-2-affected pregnancies results from a predisposition to end the pregnancy because of maternal disease (pneumonia and pre-eclampsia, with or without COVID-19 symptoms).

Keywords: SARS-CoV-2; coronavirus; COVID-19; pregnancy; delivery; perinatal outcomes; premature birth; maternal complications

1. Introduction

With more than 126,000,000 confirmed cases, the SARS-COV-2 pandemic is a life-threatening health problem, especially in high-risk individuals [1].

Due to the physiological changes of pregnancy, pregnant women are more vulnerable to respiratory infections [2] and for this reason, pregnancy should be considered a high-risk condition during the COVID-19 pandemic.

We currently know that pregnant women are at an increased risk of developing more severe COVID-19 symptoms compared to the general population, but also may suffer increased adverse perinatal outcomes [3]. Compared to non-infected pregnant women, SARS-CoV-2-positive pregnant women have increased odds of maternal death, of needing admission to the intensive care unit (ICU), and of preterm birth, leading to more neonatal intensive care unit admissions [4,5]. How obstetric intervention may influence the clinical course of the disease in these patients has also been described [6].

The Spanish Obstetric Emergency Group (SOEG), which has one of the largest series of SARS-CoV-2-infected pregnant women in the world, has contributed to the previous findings. With the present study, which includes a complete cohort of infected patients and a concurrent sample of non-infected patients and encompasses the first two high-incidence waves of SARS-CoV-2 (1 March to 5 May 2020, and 14 July to 5 November 2020) [7], we aim to better understand the relationship between maternal infection and perinatal outcomes, with a focus on preterm birth and the underlying medical and interventionist factors.

2. Materials and Methods

This was a multicenter prospective study of a cohort of SARS-CoV-2-infected pregnant women registered consecutively by the SOEG in 78 hospitals (Supplementary Materials Table S1) [8]. All procedures were approved by the Drug Research and Clinical Research Ethics Committee of Puerta de Hierro University Hospital (Madrid, Spain) on 23 March 2020 (protocol registration number, 55/20). Each collaborating center subsequently obtained protocol approval locally (ethics committees of the participant hospitals listed in the Supplementary Materials Table S1). The registry protocol is available on ClinicalTrials.gov, identifier: NCT04558996. Upon recruitment, mothers consented to participate in the study by either signing a document when possible, or by giving permission verbally, which was recorded in the patient's chart in the electronic clinical recording system. Ethics committees approved the possibility of verbal consent during the first three months of the pandemic given the contagiousness of the disease and the lack of personal protection equipment. Afterwards, written consent (using the patient consent form) was collected from every patient who had previously given permission verbally.

A specific database was designed for recording information regarding SARS-CoV-2 infection in pregnancy, and the lead researcher for each center entered the data after delivery. We developed an analysis plan using recommended contemporaneous methods and followed existing STROBE guidelines for cohort studies (Supplementary Materials Table S2) [9].

During the period of the study, from 26 February to 5 November 2020, we selected all SARS-CoV-2-positive obstetric patients detected by testing suspicious cases that came into hospital due to compatible COVID-19 symptoms and by universal screening for a SARS-CoV-2 infection at admission to the delivery ward (starting on 1 April 2020). A SARS-CoV-2 infection was diagnosed by a positive double-sampling polymerase chain reaction (PCR) from nasopharyngeal swabs. The patients of the cohort were classified as asymptomatic and symptomatic, with the latter stratified into three groups: mild–moderate symptoms (cough, anosmia, fatigue/discomfort, fever, dyspnea, etc.), pneumonia, and complicated pneumonia/shock (with ICU admission and/or mechanical ventilation and/or septic shock).

Non-infected patients were those defined as having a negative PCR at admission to delivery, and with no symptoms pre- or postpartum. In order to have a representative non-infected comparison group, each center provided between one and two PCR-negative asymptomatic pregnancies per infected mother by providing either a standardized randomization table or by selecting negative pregnancies that delivered immediately before or after each infected mother. This method was deployed to adjust for center conditions and management at the time of delivery, and to decrease the risk of selection bias.

Information regarding the demographic characteristics of each pregnant woman, co-morbidities, and previous and current obstetric history was extracted from the clinical and verbal history of the patient. Subsequently, age and race were categorized following the classifications used by the CDC (Centers for Disease Control and Prevention) [10]. For perinatal events, we recorded gestational age at delivery, the onset of labor and the type of delivery, preterm delivery (below 37 weeks), premature rupture of membranes (PROM), preterm premature rupture of membranes (PPROM), ICU admission, obstetrical complications (pre-eclampsia, hemorrhagic and thrombotic events), stillbirth, and maternal mortality. Neonatal data included a five-minute Apgar score, umbilical artery pH, birth weight, neonatal intensive care unit (NICU) admission, and neonatal mortality. Definitions of clinical and obstetric conditions followed international criteria [11–13]. Preterm deliveries were classified as spontaneous (including those resulting from a PPROM), induced labor/C-section due to PPROM, and iatrogenic (due to maternal or fetal reasons). Patients were followed until six weeks postpartum. Neonatal events were recorded until 14 days postpartum.

The numerical variables of maternal age, gestational age at delivery, gestational age at PPROM, days in ICU, and birth weight of newborns were tested for normal distribution using the Kolmogorov–Smirnov test. Descriptive data of the infected cohort and the non-infected comparison group are presented as median (interquartile range, IQR) for the numerical variables (mentioned above), or number (percentage) for the categorical variables (the remaining ones). p-values of the univariable analysis (comparison between infected and non-infected) were obtained by Mann–Whitney's U test for the numerical variables and by the Pearson's chi-squared test or the Fisher's exact test for the categorical variables. Statistical tests were two-sided and were performed with SPSS V.20 (IBM Inc., Chicago, IL, USA); a p-value below 0.05 was considered statistically significant.

In order to elucidate the reasons underlying iatrogenic delivery (no PPROM) among SARS-CoV-2-infected singleton preterm deliveries, the influence of COVID-19 mild–moderate symptoms, pneumonia (including complicated pneumonia), pre-eclampsia (moderate and severe) and their interactions were analyzed with multivariable logistic regression modeling, deriving the adjusted odds ratio (aOR) with a 95% confidence interval (95% CI) of these factors. These variables were selected after verifying their statistical association with iatrogenic delivery among the SARS-CoV-2-infected singleton preterms. Modeling was performed after excluding pregnancies with missing data. The regression analysis was carried out using the lme4 package in R, version 3.4 (RCoreTeam, 2017) [14]. The multivariable logistic regression model created was as follows:

$$\text{Iatrogenic delivery}(a) = COVID\ symptoms(b) + pre-eclampsia(c) + interaction\ of\ both \qquad (1)$$

(a) 2 categories: non-iatrogenic delivery (reference category) and iatrogenic delivery among SARS-CoV-2-infected singleton preterms; (b) 3 categories: asymptomatic (reference category), mild–moderate symptoms, and pneumonia; (c) 2 categories: absence of pre-eclampsia (reference category) and presence of moderate/severe pre-eclampsia.

3. Results

3.1. Main Results

3.1.1. General Data

- During the study period, 2954 patients were recorded in the 78 participating hospitals and analyzed: 1347 pregnant women in the infected cohort and 1607 in the non-infected comparison group (Figure 1).
- Of the 1347 positive pregnancies, 51.1% ($n = 688$) were asymptomatic at delivery while 48.9% ($n = 659$) showed symptoms.
- Among symptomatic patients, 70.9% (467/659) showed mild–moderate symptoms, 25.2% (166/659) pneumonia and 3.9% (26/659) complicated pneumonia/shock (with ICU admission and/or mechanical ventilation and/or septic shock).

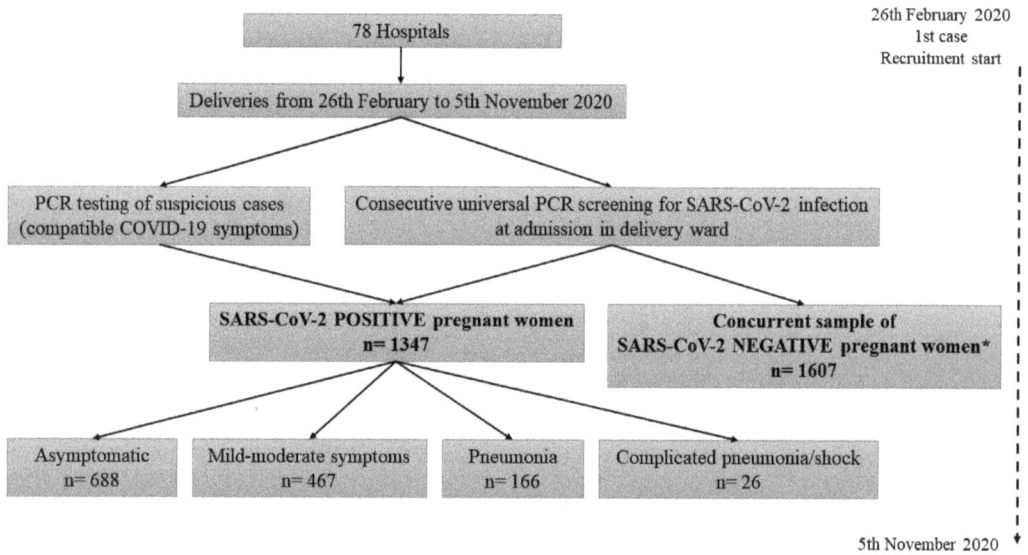

*Subsample of the screen-negative cohort from all 78 hospitals that had PCR positive mothers, deliveries before and/or after that of the positive case

Figure 1. Flow chart of the study data.

3.1.2. Baseline and Pregnancy Characteristics

- The infected cohort showed a significantly higher proportion of Latin American and Black ethnicities ($p < 0.001$) compared to the non-infected group (Table 1).
- Maternal age distribution differed between the infected cohort and the non-infected group ($p < 0.001$), being more skewed to the extremes among infected patients (higher proportion of patients under 24 and above 35 years old).

Table 1. Demographic characteristics, comorbidities, and current obstetric history of the study participants (n = 2954).

Number		Infected Cohort	Non-Infected Group	p-Value
		1347	1607	
Maternal Characteristics				
Maternal age (years; median/IQR)		33 (28–37)	33 (29–36)	0.739
Age Range	18–24	183/1336 (13.7)	165/1585 (10.4)	
	25–34	633/1336 (47.4)	850/1585 (53.6)	0.001 *
	35–49	520/1336 (38.9)	570/1585 (36.0)	
Ethnicity	White European	785/1344 (58.4)	1243/1599 (77.7)	
	Latino American	374/1344 (27.8)	155/1599 (9.7)	
	Black non-Hispanic	35/1344 (2.6)	21/1599 (1.3)	<0.001 *
	Asian non-Hispanic	40/1344 (3.0)	41/1599 (2.6)	
	Arab	110/1344 (8.2)	139/1599 (8.7)	
Nulliparous		516/1333 (38.7)	644/1596 (40.4)	0.366
Smoking [a]		131/1290 (10.2)	193/1505 (12.8)	0.028 *
Maternal Comorbidities				
Obesity (BMI > 30 kg/m^2)		245/1306 (18.8)	249/1515 (16.4)	0.105
Cardiovascular comorbidities	Baseline heart disease [b]	15/1316 (1.1)	11/1528 (0.7)	0.241
	Pre-pregnancy HBP	19/1304 (1.5)	17/1514 (1.1)	0.431
Pulmonary comorbidities	Chronic pulmonary disease (not asthma)	3/1316 (0.2)	2/1532 (0.1)	0.667
	Asthma	52/1312 (4.0)	52/1528 (3.4)	0.428
Hematologic comorbidities	Chronic hematologic disease	21/1312 (1.6)	10/1526 (0.7)	0.016 *
	Thrombophilia	25/1310 (1.9)	22/1532 (1.4)	0.325
	Antiphospholipid syndrome	7/1308 (0.5)	8/1524 (0.5)	0.970
Chronic kidney disease		5/1313 (0.4)	5/1528 (0.3)	1.000
Chronic liver disease		11/1319 (0.8)	8/1536 (0.5)	0.305
Rheumatic disease		11/1314 (0.8)	16/1524 (1.0%)	0.560
Diabetes mellitus		26 (1.9)	28 (1.7)	0.704
Depressive syndrome		15/1302 (1.2)	17/1516 (1.1)	0.939
Current Obstetric History				
Multiple pregnancies		25 (1.9)	34 (2.1)	0.615
Threatened abortion		41/1275 (3.2)	43/1,545 (2.8)	0.501
High-risk chromosomal abnormality screening		31/1288 (2.4)	37/1544 (2.4)	0.986
High-risk pre-eclampsia screening		69/1149 (6.0)	68/1438 (4.7)	0.150
Positive ultrasound prematurity screening		16/1132 (1.4)	30/1411 (2.1)	0.180
Gestational diabetes		97/1309 (7.4)	136/1584 (8.6)	0.247
Intrauterine growth restriction		48/1290 (3.7)	44/1566 (2.8)	0.170
Pregnancy-induced hypertension [c]		50 (3.7)	55 (3.4)	0.672

Data are shown as n (% of total with data), except where otherwise indicated. BMI: body mass index; HBP: high blood pressure; * statistically significant differences; [a] current smoker and ex-smoker; [b] including congenital heart disease, not hypertension; [c] hypertension + pre-eclampsia.

3.1.3. Maternal and Neonatal Outcomes

- In the SARS-CoV-2-infected cohort, gestational age at delivery was significantly lower ($p < 0.001$) and the onset of labor was less spontaneous ($p < 0.001$) compared to non-infected pregnancies (Table 2). In addition, C-section rate was higher in infected patients (27.7% vs. 20.4% non-infected, $p < 0.001$).
- A higher rate of premature rupture of membranes was observed in the SARS-CoV-2 cohort, both when we analyzed globally (PROM: 15.5% vs. 11.1%, $p < 0.001$) and in those less than 37 weeks (PPROM: 2.8% vs. 1.4%, $p = 0.012$).
- More preterm deliveries (<37 weeks of gestational age) were observed in the SARS-CoV-2-infected cohort (11.1% vs. 5.8%; OR 2.00, 95% CI 1.53–2.62; $p < 0.001$) mainly due to an increase in iatrogenic preterm births, that is, due to medical reasons different from PPROM, as nearly half of preterm births among positive pregnancies were iatrogenic (47.7% vs. 21.3% of preterm births among non-infected; OR 3.37, 95% CI 1.87–6.05; $p < 0.001$).
- Infected women were more frequently admitted to the ICU before and/or after delivery (2.7% vs. 0.1% non-infected, $p < 0.001$).
- Women infected with SARS-CoV-2 who developed pre-eclampsia met the criteria for severe pre-eclampsia significantly more than those who were not infected (40.6% vs. 15.6%; OR 3.69, 95% CI 1.62–8.39; $p < 0.001$), while in the latter, the percentage of moderate pre-eclampsia is higher.
- Higher rates of venous thrombotic events (pulmonary embolism ($p = 0.003$) and disseminated intravascular coagulation ($p = 0.043$)) were observed among infected pregnant women.
- No differences were noted between the infected cohort and the non-infected group regarding hemorrhagic events.
- There were two deaths recorded in the SARS-CoV-2-infected cohort versus none in the non-infected group.
- Higher rates of stillbirths as well as of NICU admissions were observed in the SARS-CoV-2-infected cohort; lower birth weight of newborns from infected mothers was also observed (Table 2).

Table 2. Maternal and neonatal outcomes of the study participants ($n = 2954$).

Number		Infected Cohort 1347	Non-Infected Group 1607	p-Value
PERINATAL OUTCOMES				
Gestational age at delivery (weeks + days; median/IQR)		39 + 3 (38 + 2–40 + 3)	39 + 5 (38 + 6–40 + 4)	<0.001 *
Onset of labor	Programmed C-section	142 (10.5)	85 (5.3)	<0.001 *
	Spontaneous	699 (51.9)	1000 (62.2)	
	Induced	506 (37.6)	522 (32.5)	
Type of delivery	Cesarean	373 (27.7)	328 (20.4)	<0.001 *
	Vaginal	832 (61.8)	1044 (65.0)	
	Operative vaginal	142 (10.5)	235 (14.6)	
PROM		209 (15.5)	179 (11.1)	<0.001 *
PPROM		37 (2.8)	23 (1.4)	0.012 *
Gestational age at PPROM (weeks + days; median/IQR)		35 + 0 (33 + 6–35 + 6)	35 + 1 (34 + 6–36 + 3)	0.308
Gestational age range at delivery	<28 weeks	10 (0.7)	7 (0.4)	<0.001 *
	28 to <32 weeks	21 (1.6)	8 (0.5)	
	32 to <37 weeks	118 (8.8)	79 (4.9)	
	≥37 weeks	1198 (88.9)	1513 (94.2)	

Table 2. Cont.

Number	Infected Cohort 1347	Non-Infected Group 1607	p-Value
Preterm deliveries (<37 weeks of gestational age)	149 (11.1)	94 (5.8)	<0.001 *
Spontaneous delivery (including PPROM)	58/149 (38.9)	62/94 (66.0)	
Induced /C-section due to PPROM	20/149 (13.4)	12/94 (12.8)	<0.001 *
Iatrogenic delivery (no PPROM)	71/149 (47.7)	20/94 (21.3)	
Causes of preterm iatrogenic delivery:			
COVID-19 mild–moderate symptoms	15/71 (21.1)	0/20 (0.0)	
Pneumonia [a] (alone)	27/71 (38.0)	0/20 (0.0)	
Pre-eclampsia [b] (alone)	5 [c]/71 (7.0)	6/20 (30.0)	
COVID-19 mild-moderate symptoms + pre-eclampsia [b]	7/71 (9.9)	0/20 (0.0)	
Pneumonia [a] + pre-eclampsia [b]	7/71 (9.9)	0/20 (0.0)	
Other	10/71 (14.1)	14/20 (70.0)	
Admitted in ICU [d]	36 (2.7)	2 (0.1)	<0.001 *
Days in ICU (median/IQR)	12 (8.5–17)	3 (3–3)	0.128
Hemorrhagic events	70 (5.2)	89 (5.5)	0.682
Abruptio placentae	12 (0.9)	7 (0.4)	0.123
Postpartum hemorrhage	61 (4.5)	86 (5.4)	0.306
Pre-eclampsia	69 (5.1)	64 (4.0)	0.137
Severe pre-eclampsia	28/69 (40.6)	10/64 (15.6)	0.001 *
Admitted in ICU [a]	10/28	0/10	
Invasive ventilation	4/28	0/10	
Moderate pre-eclampsia	41/69 (59.4)	54/64 (84.4)	0.001 *
Thrombotic events	7 (0.5)	2 (0.1)	0.089
Deep venous thrombosis	10 (0.7)	1 (0.1)	0.003 *
Pulmonary embolism	4 (0.3)	0 (0.0)	0.043 *
Disseminated intravascular coagulation			
Stillbirth	10 (0.7)	3 (0.2)	0.023 *
MATERNAL MORTALITY	2 (0.1)	0 (0.0)	0.208
NEONATAL DATA			
Apgar 5 score <7	20/1335 (1.5)	21/1597 (1.3)	0.674
Umbilical artery pH < 7.10	40/1081 (3.7)	46/1248 (3.7)	0.985
Birth weight (grams; median/IQR)	3240 (2890–3550)	3290 (2970–3600)	0.001
Admitted in NICU	137 (10.2)	39 (2.4)	<0.001 *
Neonatal mortality	6 (0.4)	2 (0.1)	0.153

Data are shown as n (% of total with data), except where otherwise indicated; * statistically significant differences; PROM: premature rupture of membranes; PPROM: preterm premature rupture of membranes; ICU: intensive care unit; NICU: neonatal intensive care unit; [a] both pneumonia and complicated pneumonia/shock; [b] both moderate and severe pre-eclampsia; [c] asymptomatic patients; [d] before and/or after delivery.

3.1.4. Reasons for Iatrogenic Delivery among SARS-CoV-2-Infected Singleton Preterm Deliveries

Among the SARS-CoV-2-infected pregnancies, there was a total of 149 preterm deliveries of which 138 were singletons. The multivariable logistic regression modeling results showed that the following conditions significantly increased the risk of interventionism in preterm deliveries among these patients: pneumonia (aOR 10.83, 95% CI 3.82–34.15; $p < 0.001$), pre-eclampsia (aOR 9.38, 95% CI 1.69–74.76; $p = 0.016$), and pre-eclampsia with COVID-19 mild–moderate symptoms (aOR 15.00, 95% CI 1.90–316.47; $p = 0.022$).

4. Discussion

In this multicenter prospective study, we investigated the association between SARS-CoV-2 infections and obstetric and neonatal outcomes. We found out that pregnant women with a SARS-CoV-2 infection had more premature rupture of membranes, more preterm births and, therefore, their neonates had more NICU admissions, compared to the pregnant women who were not infected [5,15]. The higher risk of premature rupture of membranes (overall as well as preterm) observed in the infected cohort can be explained by the fact that infections in pregnancy may be associated with this condition by various mechanisms, such as the activation of inflammation [16].

When the reasons for preterm births were analyzed in depth, it was observed that the proportion of preterm births resulting from PPROM (both spontaneous and induced/C-section due to this outcome) did not significantly differ between infected (37/149, 24.8%) and non-infected (23/94, 24.5%) mothers ($p = 0.949$). However, it was the medical intervention due to maternal disease that explained the decision to prematurely end the pregnancy; obstetrical interventionism in order to improve the mothers' health conditions was the main factor for the increased rate of preterm deliveries among the SARS-CoV-2-positive women. It was observed that, not the fact of being infected, but the development of pneumonia or pre-eclampsia (with or without COVID-19 symptoms) was the cause of the increased iatrogenic prematurity in SARS-CoV-2-infected pregnancies.

Our findings are in line with those previously reported by a study carried out in asymptomatic pregnant women, where an increased risk of PROM was observed among SARS-CoV-2-infected patients when compared to non-infected patients, while this was not the case for preterm delivery [5]. This difference in preterm delivery risk between their study and our study, as explained above, is because preterm delivery is associated with maternal disease manifested in symptomatic patients. This confirms the hypothesis that many obstetric outcomes are related to maternal COVID-19 symptomatology.

The risk of pre-eclampsia was similar for infected and non-infected patients; however, those infected mothers who developed these disorders ended up with severe pre-eclampsia, rather than moderate cases as in the non-infected group. In this association between a SARS-CoV-2 infection and severe pre-eclampsia, a synergistic effect of both factors should not be ruled out [17,18]. However, it must be noted that a severe pre-eclampsia diagnosis is based on hypertensive and biochemical alterations (such as increased lactate-dehydrogenase, thrombocytopenia, and elevated liver enzymes) that can be mixed up with the ones observed in COVID-19 in the general population, apart from the inflammatory status present in both conditions (COVID-19 and pre-eclampsia). Therefore, we must bear in mind that there could be an overestimation of cases of severe pre-eclampsia in the infected cohort since the analytical signs of COVID-19 could have been interpreted as alterations due to pre-eclampsia instead.

No differences were noted between the infected cohort and the non-infected comparison group regarding obstetric hemorrhagic events, while a higher incidence of venous thrombotic events was noted in our SARS-CoV-2-infected pregnancies (1.5%, compared to 0.2% in non-infected), which can be explained by the hemostatic and thromboembolic complications reported in COVID-19 [19]. Even so, the extended heparin prophylaxis policy, which was established in April 2020, may have decreased the expected venous thromboembolism and pulmonary embolism rates in infected patients [20,21]. On the other hand, disseminated intravascular coagulation cases corresponded to the SARS-CoV-2-infected cohort, and this was the underlying cause of a maternal death.

As a limitation of this study, it should be highlighted that symptomatic patients are over-represented in our study population since not all participating hospitals had a universal antenatal screening program for SARS-CoV-2 infections (so only identified symptomatic cases by passive surveillance), or implemented the program later.

Moreover, the data point to an increased risk of iatrogenic preterm delivery in SARS-CoV-2-infected mothers who developed pneumonia together with pre-eclampsia, but the small number of patients who met these criteria may have penalized the power of analysis. Another limitation of our study is the absence of an in-depth analysis of the biochemical results of the patients who developed pre-eclampsia.

Among the strengths of our study is the large cohort of SARS-CoV-2-positive deliveries (1347 from 78 centers across Spain). In addition, the SARS-CoV-2-negative comparison group was selected from the same centers where the infected mothers delivered and within the same timeframe in order to have similar conditions, thereby minimizing selection and performance biases. We acknowledge as a limitation the absence of the complete screened cohort. However, the concurrent method applied for the selection of a non-infected group (subsample of the screen-negative cohort from all 78 hospitals that had PCR-positive mothers) allowed for a comparison unaffected by the differences in time of exposure and outcome assessment. Therefore, we believe our findings are trustworthy, and the multicenter nature of the study adds to its generalizability.

5. Conclusions

Pregnant SARS-CoV-2-infected patients are a population at risk of suffering preterm births, mainly due to iatrogenic deliveries in women with pneumonia and/or pre-eclampsia. Venous thromboembolism and disseminated intravascular coagulation were more frequent in SARS-CoV-2-infected pregnancies.

There is an urgent need for an in-depth analysis of the influence of SARS-CoV-2 infection on the development of pre-eclampsia, and of the risk factors for ICU admittance of pregnant women infected with SARS-CoV-2.

Supplementary Materials: The following are available online at https://www.mdpi.com/article/10.3390/v13050853/s1, Table S1: List of hospitals members of the Spanish Obstetric Emergency Group included in this study ($n = 78$), Table S2: STROBE Statement—checklist of items that should be included in reports of observational studies.

Author Contributions: Conceptualization, O.M.-P.; methodology, M.L.d.l.C.C. and O.M.-P.; software, M.L.d.l.C.C.; validation, S.C.M., M.L.d.l.C.C., P.C.P., A.A.-S., P.P.R. (Pilar Pintando Recarte), L.G.R., C.C.M., A.M.V., A.B.O.C., P.P.R. (Pilar Prats Rodríguez), I.F.B., M.V.R.G., A.M.F.A., R.L.P., J.R.B.M., M.B.E.P., M.R.G., M.J.G.G., A.S.M. and O.M.-P.; formal analysis, M.L.d.l.C.C.; investigation, S.C.M., M.L.d.l.C.C., P.C.P., A.A.-S., P.P.R. (Pilar Pintando Recarte), L.G.R., C.C.M., A.M.V., A.B.O.C., P.P.R. (Pilar Prats Rodríguez), I.F.B., M.V.R.G., A.M.F.A., R.L.P., J.R.B.M., M.B.E.P., M.R.G., M.J.G.G., A.S.M., O.M.-P. and S.O.E.G.; resources, O.M.-P.; data curation, M.L.d.l.C.C.; writing—original draft preparation, S.C.M., M.L.d.l.C.C. and O.M.-P.; writing—review and editing, S.C.M.; visualization, S.C.M., M.L.d.l.C.C., P.C.P., A.A.-S., P.P.R. (Pilar Pintando Recarte), L.G.R., C.C.M., A.M.V., A.B.O.C., P.P.R. (Pilar Prats Rodríguez), I.F.B., M.V.R.G., A.M.F.A., R.L.P., J.R.B.M., M.B.E.P., M.R.G., M.J.G.G., A.S.M., O.M.-P. and S.O.E.G.; supervision, O.M.-P.; project administration, O.M.-P.; funding acquisition, O.M.-P. All authors have read and agreed to the published version of the manuscript.

Funding: This project was supported by public funds obtained in competitive calls: Grant COV20/00021 (EUR 43,000 from the Instituto de Salud Carlos III—Spanish Ministry of Health and co-financed with Fondo Europeo de Desarrollo Regional (FEDER) funds.

Institutional Review Board Statement: The study was conducted according to the guidelines of the Declaration of Helsinki and approved by the Institutional Review Board (or Ethics Committee) of Puerta de Hierro University Hospital (PE 55/20; 23 March 2020).

Informed Consent Statement: Informed consent was obtained from all subjects involved in the study.

Data Availability Statement: The data presented in this study are available on request from the corresponding author. The data are not publicly available due to the multicenter nature of the study.

Acknowledgments: Authors thank Ana Royuela Vicente (Biostatistics Unit, Puerta de Hierro Biomedical Research Institute, IDIPHISA-CIBERESP) for her scientific advice. Spanish Obstetric Emergency Group (S.O.E.G.): María Belén Garrido Luque (Hospital Axarquia), Camino Fernández Fernández (Complejo Asistencial de León), Ana Villalba Yarza (Complejo Asistencial Universitario de Salamanca), Esther María Canedo Carballeira (Complexo Hospitalario Universitario A Coruña), María Begoña Dueñas Carazo (Hospital Clínico Universitario de Santiago de Compostela), Rosario Redondo Aguilar (Complejo Hospitalario Jaén), Esther Álvarez Silvares (Complejo Hospitalario Universitario de Ourense), María Isabel Pardo Pumar (Complejo Hospitalario Universitario de Pontevedra), Macarena Alférez Álvarez-Mallo (HM Hospitales), Víctor Muñoz Carmona (Hospital Alto Guadalquivir, Andújar), Noelia Pérez Pérez (Hospital Clínico San Carlos), Cristina Álvarez Colomo

(Hospital Clínico Universitario de Valladolid), Onofre Alomar Mateu (Hospital Comarcal d'Inca), Claudio Marañon Di Leo (Hospital Costa del Sol), María del Carmen Parada Millán (Hospital da Barbanza), Adrián Martín García (Hospital de Burgos), José Navarrina Martínez (Hospital de Donostia), Anna Mundó Fornell (Hospital Universitario Santa Creu i Sant Pau), Elena Pascual Salvador (Hospital de Minas de Riotinto), Tania Manrique Gómez (Hospital de Montilla y Quirón Salud Córdoba), Marta Ruth Meca Casbas (Hospital de Poniente), Noemí Freixas Grimalt (Hospital Universitari Son Llàtzer), Adriana Aquise and María del Mar Gil (Hospital de Torrejón), Eduardo Cazorla Amorós (Hospital de Torrevieja), Alberto Armijo Sánchez (Hospital de Valme), María Isabel Conca Rodero (Hospital de Vinalopó), Ana Belén Oreja Cuesta (Hospital del Tajo), Cristina Ruiz Aguilar (Hospital Doctor Peset, Valencia), Susana Fernández García (Hospital General de L'Hospitalet), Carmen Baena Luque (Hospital Infanta Margarita de Cabra), Luz María Jiménez Losa (Hospital Infanta Sofía), Susana Soldevilla Pérez (Hospital Jerez de la Frontera), María Reyes Granell Escobar (Hospital Juan Ramón Jiménez), Manuel Domínguez González (Hospital La Línea), Flora Navarro Blaya (Hospital Universitario Rafael Méndez), Juan Carlos Wizner de Alva (Hospital San Pedro de Alcántara), Rosa Pedró Carulla (Hospital Sant Joan de Reus), Encarnación Carmona Sánchez (Hospital Santa Ana. Motril), Judit Canet Rodríguez (Hospital Santa Caterina de Salt), Eva Morán Antolín (Hospital Son Espases), Montse Macià (Hospital Universitari Arnau de Vilanova), Laia Pratcorona (Hospital Universitari Germans Trias i Pujol), Irene Gastaca Abásolo (Hospital Universitario Araba), Begoña Martínez Borde (Hospital Universitario de Bilbao), Óscar Vaquerizo Ruiz (Hospital Universitario de Cabueñes), José Ruiz Aragón (Hospital Universitario de Ceuta), Raquel González Seoane (Hospital Universitario de Ferrol), María Teulón González (Hospital Universitario de Fuenlabrada), Lourdes Martín González (Hospital Joan XXIII de Tarragona), Cristina Lesmes Heredia (Hospital Universitario Parc Taulí de Sabadell), Rut Bernardo (Hospital Universitario Río Hortega), Otilia González Vanegas (Hospital Universitario San Cecilio, Instituto de Investigación Biosanitaria, Granada), Lucía Díaz Meca (Hospital Universitario Virgen de la Arrixaca, Murcia), Alberto Puerta Prieto (Hospital Universitario Virgen de las Nieves, Instituto de Investigación Biosanitaria, Granada), María del Pilar Guadix Martín (Hospital Universitario Virgen Macarena), Carmen María Orizales Lago (Hospital Universitario Severo Ochoa, Leganés), José Antonio Sainz Bueno (Hospital Viamed, Grupo Chacón), Mónica Catalina Coello (Hospital Virgen Concha de Zamora), María José Núñez Valera (Hospital Virgen de la Luz), Lucas Cerrillos González (Hospital Virgen del Rocío), José Adanez García (Hospital Universitario Central de Asturias), Elena Ferriols-Pérez (Hospital del Mar), Marta Roqueta (Hospital Universitario Josep Trueta), Marta García Sánchez (Hospital Universitario Quirónsalud de Málaga), Emilio Couceiro Naveira (Hospital Álvaro Cunqueiro de Vigo), Mar Muñoz Chapuli (Hospital Universitario Gregorio Marañón), Elena Pintado Paredes (Hospital Universitario de Getafe), Inmaculada Mejía Jiménez (Hospital Universitario 12 de Octubre).

Conflicts of Interest: The authors declare no conflict of interest. The funders had no role in the design of the study; in the collection, analyses, or interpretation of data; in the writing of the manuscript, or in the decision to publish the results.

References

1. WHO Coronavirus Disease (COVID-19) Dashboard. Available online: https://covid19.who.int/?gclid=EAIaIQobChMI0bPAdSh6gIVyoKyCh0u9A2mEAAYASAAEgJjsvD_BwE (accessed on 29 March 2021).
2. Mehta, N.; Chen, K.; Hardy, E.; Powrie, R. Respiratory disease in pregnancy. *Best Pract. Res. Clin. Obstet. Gynaecol.* **2015**, *29*, 598–611. [CrossRef] [PubMed]
3. Zambrano, L.D.; Ellington, S.; Strid, P.; Galang, R.R.; Oduyebo, T.; Tong, V.T. Update: Characteristics of Symptomatic Women of Reproductive Age with Laboratory-Confirmed SARS-CoV-2 Infection by Pregnancy Status—United States, 22 January–3 October 2020. *Morb. Mortal. Wkly Rep.* **2020**, *69*, 1641–1647. [CrossRef] [PubMed]
4. Allotey, J.; Stallings, E.; Bonet, M.; Yap, M.; Chatterjee, S.; Kew, T.; Debenham, L.; Llavall, A.C.; Dixit, A.; Zhou, D.; et al. Clinical manifestations, risk factors, and maternal and perinatal outcomes of coronavirus disease 2019 in pregnancy: Living systematic review and meta-analysis. *BMJ* **2020**, *370*, m3320. [CrossRef] [PubMed]
5. Martinez Perez, O.; Prats Rodriguez, P.; Hernandez, M.M.; Pardilla, M.B.E.; Perez, N.P.; Hernandez, M.R.V. The association between COVID-19 and preterm delivery: A cohort study with multivariate analysis. *medRxiv* **2020**. [CrossRef]
6. Martínez-Perez, O.; Vouga, M.; Melguizo, S.C.; Acebal, L.F.; Panchaud, A.; Muñoz-Chápuli, M.; Baud, D. Association Between Mode of Delivery Among Pregnant Women With COVID-19 and Maternal and Neonatal Outcomes in Spain. *JAMA* **2020**, *324*, 296–299. [CrossRef] [PubMed]
7. Centro de Coordinación de Alertas y Emergencias Sanitarias, Ministerio de Sanidad, Gobierno de España. Actualización n° 239. Enfermedad por el coronavirus (COVID-19). 29 October 2020. Available online: https://www.mscbs.gob.es/profesionales/saludPublica/ccayes/alertasActual/nCov/documentos/Actualizacion_239_COVID-19.pdfCDC (accessed on 1 December 2020).

8. Encinas Pardilla, M.B.; Caño Aguilar, Á.; Marcos Puig, B.; Sanz Lorenzana, A.; Rodríguez de la Torre, I.; Hernando López de la Manzanara, P.; Fernández Bernardo, A.; Martínez Pérez, Ó. Spanish registry of Covid-19 screening in asymptomatic pregnants. *Rev. Esp. Salud Publica* **2020**, *94*, e202009092. [PubMed]
9. von Elm, E.; Altman, D.G.; Egger, M.; Pocock, S.J.; Gotzsche, P.C.; Vandenbroucke, J.P. The Strengthening the Reporting of Observational Studies in Epidemiology (STROBE) Statement: Guidelines for reporting observational studies. *Int. J. Surg.* **2014**, *12*, 1495–1499. [CrossRef] [PubMed]
10. Ellington, S.; Strid, P.; Tong Van, T.; Woodworth, K.; Galang, R.G.; Zambrano, L.D.; Nahabedian, J.; Anderson, K.; Gilboa, S.M. Characteristics of Women of Reproductive Age with Laboratory-Confirmed SARS-CoV-2 Infection by Pregnancy Status. *Morb. Mortal. Wkly Rep.* **2020**, *69*, 769–775. [CrossRef] [PubMed]
11. American College of Obstetricians and Gynecologists, Committee on Practice B-O. Prelabor Rupture of Membranes: ACOG Practice Bulletin, Number 217. *Obstet. Gynecol.* **2020**, *135*, e80–e97. [CrossRef] [PubMed]
12. Brown, M.A.; Magee, L.A.; Kenny, L.C.; Karumanchi, S.A.; McCarthy, F.P.; Saito, S.; Hall, D.R.; Warren, C.E.; Adoyi, G.; Ishaku, S.; et al. Hypertensive Disorders of Pregnancy: ISSHP Classification, Diagnosis, and Management Recommendations for International Practice. *Hypertension* **2018**, *72*, 24–43. [CrossRef] [PubMed]
13. Thomson, A.J.; Royal College of Obstetricians and Gynaecologists. Care of Women Presenting with Suspected Preterm Prelabour Rupture of Membranes from 24(+0) Weeks of Gestation: Green-top Guideline No. 73. *BJOG* **2019**, *126*, e152–e166. [CrossRef] [PubMed]
14. Bates, D.; Mächler, M.; Bolker, B.; Walker, S. Fitting Linear Mixed-Effects Models Using lme4. *J. Stat. Softw.* **2015**, *67*, 48. [CrossRef]
15. Cruz-Lemini, M.; Ferriols Perez, E.; de la Cruz Conty, M.L.; Caño Aguilar, A.; Encinas Pardilla, M.B.; Prats Rodríguez, P.; Muner Hernando, M.; Forcen Acebal, L.; Pintado Recarte, P.; Medina Mallen, M.D.C.; et al. Obstetric Outcomes of SARS-CoV-2 Infection in Asymptomatic Pregnant Women. *Viruses* **2021**, *13*, 112. [CrossRef]
16. Goldenberg, R.L.; Culhane, J.F.; Iams, J.D.; Romero, R. Epidemiology and causes of preterm birth. *Lancet* **2008**, *371*, 75–84. [CrossRef]
17. Coronado-Arroyo, J.C.; Concepción-Zavaleta, M.J.; Zavaleta-Gutiérrez, F.E.; Concepción-Urteaga, L.A. Is COVID-19 a risk factor for severe preeclampsia? Hospital experience in a developing country. *Eur. J. Obstet. Gynecol. Reprod. Biol.* **2021**, *256*, 502–503. [CrossRef] [PubMed]
18. Mendoza, M.; Garcia-Ruiz, I.; Maiz, N.; Rodo, C.; Garcia-Manau, P.; Serrano, B.; Lopez-Martinez, R.M.; Balcells, J.; Fernandez-Hidalgo, N.; Carreras, E.; et al. Pre-eclampsia-like syndrome induced by severe COVID-19: A prospective observational study. *BJOG* **2020**, *127*, 1374–1380. [CrossRef] [PubMed]
19. Servante, J.; Swallow, G.; Thornton, J.G.; Myers, B.; Munireddy, S.; Malinowski, A.K.; Othman, M.; Li, W.; O'Donoghue, K.; Walker, K.F. Haemostatic and thrombo-embolic complications in pregnant women with COVID-19: A systematic review and critical analysis. *BMC Pregnancy Childbirth* **2021**, *21*, 108. [CrossRef] [PubMed]
20. Juan, J.; Gil, M.M.; Rong, Z.; Zhang, Y.; Yang, H.; Poon, L.C. Effect of coronavirus disease 2019 (COVID-19) on maternal, perinatal and neonatal outcome: Systematic review. *Ultrasound Obstet. Gynecol.* **2020**, *56*, 15–27. [CrossRef] [PubMed]
21. Breslin, N.; Baptiste, C.; Gyamfi-Bannerman, C.; Miller, R.; Martinez, R.; Bernstein, K.; Ring, L.; Landau, R.; Purisch, S.; Friedman, A.M.; et al. Coronavirus disease 2019 infection among asymptomatic and symptomatic pregnant women: Two weeks of confirmed presentations to an affiliated pair of New York City hospitals. *Am. J. Obstet. Gynecol. MFM* **2020**, *2*, 100118. [CrossRef] [PubMed]

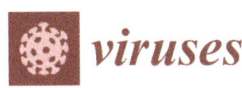

Brief Report

Novel Ratio Soluble Fms-like Tyrosine Kinase-1/Angiotensin-II (sFlt-1/ANG-II) in Pregnant Women Is Associated with Critical Illness in COVID-19

Salvador Espino-y-Sosa [1,2,†], Raigam Jafet Martinez-Portilla [1,2,†], Johnatan Torres-Torres [1,2,3,*], Juan Mario Solis-Paredes [1], Guadalupe Estrada-Gutierrez [1], Jose Antonio Hernandez-Pacheco [1], Aurora Espejel-Nuñez [1], Paloma Mateu-Rogell [1,2], Angeles Juarez-Reyes [3], Francisco Eduardo Lopez-Ceh [3], Jose Rafael Villafan-Bernal [2,4], Lourdes Rojas-Zepeda [5], Iris Paola Guzman-Guzman [6] and Liona C. Poon [7]

1. Clinical Research Deparment, Instituto Nacional de Perinatologia Isidro Espinosa de los Reyes, Mexico City 11400, Mexico; salvadorespino@gmail.com (S.E.-y.-S.); raifet@hotmail.com (R.J.M.-P.); juan.mario.sp@gmail.com (J.M.S.-P.); gpestrad@gmail.com (G.E.-G.); dr.antoniohernandezp@gmail.com (J.A.H.-P.); auro.espejel@gmail.com (A.E.-N.); dramateurogell@gmail.com (P.M.-R.)
2. Iberoamerican Research Network in Obstetrics, Gynecology and Translational Medicine, Mexico City 06720, Mexico; joravibe@gmail.com
3. Maternal Fetal Medicine Department, Hospital General de Mexico, "Dr. Eduardo Liceaga", Mexico City 06720, Mexico; dra.angejuarez@gmail.com (A.J.-R.); doctorceh.mx@gmail.com (F.E.L.-C.)
4. Laboratory of Immunogenomics and Metabolic Diseases, Instituto Nacional de Medicina Genomica, Mexico City 14610, Mexico
5. Maternal Fetal Medicine Department, Instituto Materno Infantil del Estado de Mexico, Mexico City 50170, Mexico; dra.rojaszepeda@gmail.com
6. Faculty of Chemical-Biological Sciences, Autonomous University of Guerrero, Chilpancingo 39086, Mexico; ipguzman2@gmail.com
7. Department of Obstetrics and Gynaecology, The Chinese University of Hong Kong, Hong Kong, China; liona.poon@cuhk.edu.hk
* Correspondence: torresmmf@gmail.com; Tel.: +52-55-5-520-9900 (ext. 317)
† These authors contributed equally to this work.

Abstract: Background: In healthy pregnancies, components of the Renin-Angiotensin system (RAS) are present in the placental villi and contribute to invasion, migration, and angiogenesis. At the same time, soluble fms-like tyrosine kinase 1 (sFlt-1) production is induced after binding of ANG-II to its receptor (AT-1R) in response to hypoxia. As RAS plays an essential role in the pathogenesis of COVID-19, we hypothesized that angiogenic marker (sFlt-1) and RAS components (ANG-II and ACE-2) may be related to adverse outcomes in pregnant women with COVID-19; Methods: Prospective cohort study. Primary outcome was severe pneumonia. Secondary outcomes were ICU admission, intubation, sepsis, and death. Spearman's Rho test was used to analyze the correlation between sFlt-1 and ANG-II levels. The sFlt-1/ANG-II ratio was determined and the association with each adverse outcome was explored by logistic regression analysis and the prediction was assessed using receiver-operating-curve (ROC); Results: Among 80 pregnant women with COVID-19, the sFlt-1/ANG-II ratio was associated with an increased probability of severe pneumonia (odds ratio [OR]: 1.31; $p = 0.003$), ICU admission (OR: 1.05; $p = 0.007$); intubation (OR: 1.09; $p = 0.008$); sepsis (OR: 1.04; $p = 0.008$); and death (OR: 1.04; $p = 0.018$); Conclusion: sFlt-1/ANG-II ratio is a good predictor of adverse events such as pneumonia, ICU admission, intubation, sepsis, and death in pregnant women with COVID-19.

Keywords: COVID-19; maternal death; angiotensin-II; sFlt-1

1. Introduction

SARS-CoV-2 infection and its symptomatic disease (COVID-19) are nowadays one of the leading causes of death worldwide. Different studies have shown that pregnant

---

Citation: Espino-y-Sosa, S.; Martinez-Portilla, R.J.; Torres-Torres, J.; Solis-Paredes, J.M.; Estrada-Gutierrez, G.; Hernandez-Pacheco, J.A.; Espejel-Nuñez, A.; Mateu-Rogell, P.; Juarez-Reyes, A.; Lopez-Ceh, F.E.; et al. Novel Ratio Soluble Fms-like Tyrosine Kinase-1/Angiotensin-II (sFlt-1/ANG-II) in Pregnant Women Is Associated with Critical Illness in COVID-19. *Viruses* **2021**, *13*, 1906. https://doi.org/10.3390/v13101906

Academic Editors: David Baud and Leó Pomar

Received: 22 August 2021
Accepted: 16 September 2021
Published: 23 September 2021

Publisher's Note: MDPI stays neutral with regard to jurisdictional claims in published maps and institutional affiliations.

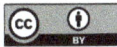

Copyright: © 2021 by the authors. Licensee MDPI, Basel, Switzerland. This article is an open access article distributed under the terms and conditions of the Creative Commons Attribution (CC BY) license (https://creativecommons.org/licenses/by/4.0/).

women with COVID-19 are at increased risk of serious illness, such as pneumonia (relative risk [RR]: 1.97; 95% CI: 1.82–2.13) and death (RR: 1.68; 95% CI: 1.36–2.08), than matched reproductive-age non-pregnant women [1,2].

The Renin-Angiotensin system (RAS) is now known to play an essential role in the pathogenesis of COVID-19 [3]. Typically, renin cleaves angiotensinogen into Angiotensin-I (ANG-l), ANG-l (physiologically inactive) is converted into Angiotensin-II (ANG-II) by the Angiotensin-Converting Enzyme-1 (ACE-1), and ANG-II is transformed into ANG 1–7 by Angiotensin-Converting Enzyme-2 (ACE-2), regulating the cardiovascular and renal function [4]. In target tissues (alveolar epithelial cells, intestinal epithelial cells, and endothelial cells), SARS-CoV-2 spike (S) protein binds to ACE-2, causing a reduction of the ACE-2 receptor in the membrane, potentially impairing ANG-II balance [5,6].

In healthy pregnancies, RAS components are present in the placental villi and contribute to placental invasion, migration, and angiogenesis [7]. Furthermore, RAS components help promote placental circulation and blood flow, facilitating fetal oxygenation [8]. Expression of ACE-2 and TMPRSS2 decreases in late gestation [9]. This downregulation of RAS is associated with adverse maternal-perinatal outcomes, particularly pre-eclampsia and fetal growth restriction [10]. To date, there are no original studies in pregnant women with COVID-19 reporting blood concentrations of ACE-2 and ANG-II, two molecules that are potentially involved in the pathogenesis of severe disease in COVID-19 [11,12].

On the other hand, soluble fms-like tyrosine kinase 1 (sFlt-1) is a protein related to placental hypoxia, endothelial damage, sepsis, and acute lung injury (15) [13]. sFlt-1 production is induced when ANG-II binds to its receptor (AT1) as a response to hypoxia [14]. It is known that sFlt-1 causes endothelial dysfunction, sensitizing the endothelial cells to the effect of ANG-II in the whole endothelium and placenta [15]. In critically ill non-pregnant COVID-19 patients, there is an upregulation of sFlt-1, suggesting that this protein might play a role in the COVID-19-associated systemic endothelial dysfunction [16,17].

We hypothesized that the primary endothelial dysfunction component characterized by an imbalance between sFlt-1 as an angiogenic marker and RAS components (ANG-II and ACE-2) may be related to adverse outcomes in pregnant women with COVID-19.

Therefore, this study aims to investigate the association between serum concentrations of sFlt-1 and RAS components to adverse outcomes in pregnant women with COVID-19.

2. Materials and Methods

2.1. Study Design and Participants

We conducted a prospective cohort study at the National Institute of Perinatology "Isidro Espinosa de los Reyes" and the General Hospital of Mexico "Dr. Eduardo Liceaga", both third reference hospitals in Mexico City. Inclusion criteria were all pregnant women who arrived at the emergency department with respiratory symptoms and a positive RTqPCR for SARS-CoV-2 between December 2020 and July 2021. The study protocol was prospectively approved by the Ethics and Research Committee of the National Institute of Perinatology (2020–1-32). All enrolled women provided written informed consent.

2.2. Data Collection

The following data were collected from the medical records: age, gestational age, pregestational body mass index (pBMI [kg/m^2]), chronic hypertension, pre-gestational diabetes, mean arterial pressure (MAP), pneumonia, sepsis, acute renal failure, organ dysfunction, ICU admission, intubation, and mortality. The following pregnancy outcomes were recorded: preeclampsia (defined according to The American College of Obstetricians and Gynecologists) [18], preterm birth (birth < 37 weeks' gestation), birth weight, Apgar score at the 1st and 5th min, neonatal asphyxia, respiratory distress syndrome (RDS), neonatal sepsis, the requirement of neonatal intensive care unit (NICU) admission, and neonatal death. Blood samples were obtained at hospital admission, and the following laboratory results were recorded: leukocytes, neutrophils, lymphocytes, hemoglobin, hematocrit, platelets, glucose, creatinine, uric acid, aspartate aminotransferase (AST), alanine aminotransferase (ALT), direct bilirubin, indirect bilirubin, triglycerides, cholesterol, D-dimer, fibrinogen, partial thromboplastin time (PTT), prothrombin time (PT), C-reactive protein (C-RP), and procalcitonin. These parameters are routinely tested in pregnant women with COVID-19.

2.3. Plasma Measurements of ACE-2, ANG-II, and sFlt-1

Upon admission, an additional blood sample was obtained specifically for research purposes. The blood sample was centrifuged for 10 min at $1000 \times g$. Plasma was separated, aliquoted, and stored at $-70\,^\circ$C until analysis. ELISA commercial kits were used to measure ACE-2 (Aviscera Bioscience, Santa Clara, CA. USA. cat SK00707-01) and ANG-II (Enzo Life Sciences, Farmingdale, NY. USA. cat ADI-900-204) according to the manufacturer's instructions and analyzed in a Synergy HT plate reader (BioTek, Winooski, VT, USA). PlGF (Elecsys PlGF, Roche®) and sFlt-1 (Elecsys sFlt-1, Roche®) levels were measured by electrochemiluminescence using an automated analyzer cobas-e411 (Roche Diagnostics®, CH) according to the manufacturer's instructions.

2.4. Outcome

The primary outcome was pregnant women with severe pneumonia. Secondary outcomes were ICU admission, intubation, viral sepsis, and maternal death as a direct result of SARS-CoV-2 infection. Severe pneumonia was defined according to the American Thoracic Society criteria, which include either one major criterion (septic shock with need for vasopressors, or respiratory failure requiring mechanical ventilation) or three or more minor criteria (respiratory rate $\geq$ 30 breaths/min; PaO_2/FIO_2 ratio $\leq$ 250; multilobar infiltrates; confusion/disorientation; uremia [blood urea nitrogen level $\geq$ 20 mg/dL]; leukopenia [white blood cell count < 4000 cells/µL]; thrombocytopenia [platelet count < 100,000/µL]; hypothermia [core temperature < 36 $^\circ$C]; hypotension requiring aggressive fluid resuscitation) [19,20]. ICU admission was decided according to the Quick Sequential Organ Failure Assessment (qSOFA) score, where a score of $\geq$2 points would require ICU admission [21]. Viral sepsis was defined according to the Sepsis-3 International Consensus [22] associated with SARS-CoV-2 infection [23].

2.5. Statistical Analysis

Descriptive and inferential statistics were used. Quantitative variables were reported as the median and interquartile range (IQR), while qualitative data were reported as numbers and percentages. Differences between variables among COVID-19-severity were compared using the Mann–Whitney U test or X^2 test. We performed a correlation between all biochemical parameters to explore possible candidates for multiple logistic regression. All significant candidates were explored in an adjusted logistic regression to establish independent predictors for adverse outcomes. To explore a possible endothelial dysfunction, we performed sFlt-1/PlGF and sFlt-1/ANG-II ratios. Forward and backward stepwise logistic regression analyses were performed to assess the association between independent variables and primary and secondary outcomes including all possible candidates in the correlation analysis. The adjusted model's performance after logistic regression was evaluated by receiver-operating-curve (ROC) analysis to estimate the area under the curve. p-values < 0.05 were considered statistically significant. (StataCorp. 2020. Stata Statistical Software: Release 17. College Station, TX, USA: StataCorp LLC.).

3. Results

3.1. Description of the Cohort and Characteristics of the Study Population

A total of 80 pregnant women with SARS-CoV-2 infection were included for the analysis. Twenty-five (31.25%) had severe COVID-19 disease and 55 were classified as non-severe. There were two (2.5%) maternal deaths. Baseline characteristics were similar between groups (Table 1).

There were no significant differences in the rate of preeclampsia between severe and non-severe COVID-19. Among the 25 severe cases, 24 (96%) were delivered by Cesarean section, 6 (24%) had neonatal asphyxia, 10 (40%) had RDS, and 11 (44%) required NICU admission, including 7 (28%) neonatal deaths (Table S1).

Table 1. Clinical characteristics of the study population.

Characteristic	Non-Severe COVID-19 $n = 55$	Severe COVID-19 $n = 25$	p-Value
Maternal age (years)	29.05 (24.94–33.5)	30.56 (28.40–33.73)	0.185
Gestational age at diagnosis (weeks)	33.4 (28.0–38.1)	32.0 (27.2–36.1)	0.557
pBMI (kg/m^2)	29.72 (25.0–33.8)	28.2 (23.4–33.5)	0.739
MAP (mmHg)	87.7 (82.7–95.0)	86.0 (80.0–89.7)	0.301
Smoking	1 (1.82%)	0	0.497
Chronic hypertension	3 (5.45%)	1 (4.00%)	0.782
Pre-gestational diabetes	3 (5.45%)	0	0.234
Asthma	1 (1.82%)	0	0.497
Chronic renal disease	4 (7.27%)	1 (4.00%)	0.575
SpO2%	94.5 (92.5–96.0)	92.5 (78–97.5)	0.713
Preeclampsia (clinical diagnosis)	11 (20.75%)	5 (20.0%)	0.939
True preeclampsia (Suspected preeclampsia + anormal sFlt-1/PlGF ratio)	6 (10.9%)	2 (8.0%)	0.118
Threatened preterm labor	2 (3.77%)	1 (4.00%)	0.961
Fetal growth restriction	4 (7.55%)	5 (20.0%)	0.108
Stillbirth	0	1 (4.00%)	0.143
Pneumonia	0	25 (100%)	<0.0001
ICU admission	0	11 (44.0%)	<0.0001
Intubation	0	7 (31.82%)	<0.0001
Viral sepsis	0	3 (12.0%)	0.009
Multiple organ dysfunction	0	3 (12.0%)	0.009
Maternal death	0	2 (8.00%)	0.034

pBMI: pregestational body mass index; MAP: Mean arterial pressure; SpO2: Oxygen saturation. Mann–Whitney-U test for continuous variables expressed as median and interquartile range; X^2 or Fisher's test for categorical variables expressed as number and percentage.

Women with severe pneumonia had higher levels of AST, direct bilirubin, C-RP, sFlt-1, procalcitonin, sFlt-1/PlGF ratio, and sFlt-1/ ANG-II ratio. The severe group had lower levels of lymphocytes, total cholesterol, and ANG-II (Table 2).

Table 2. Biochemical characteristics of the included population.

Characteristic	Non-Severe COVID-19 n = 55	Severe COVID-19 n = 25	p-Value
Leukocytes ($\times 10$/L)	8.15 (7.2–10.1)	8.5 (7.1–13.5)	0.339
Neutrophils ($\times 10$/L)	6.40 (5.30–7.60)	7.1 (5.6–12.6)	0.093
Lymphocytes ($\times 10$/L)	1.30 (1.0–1.5)	1.0 (0.6–1.4)	0.071
Hemoglobin (g/dL)	12.4 (11.3–13.9)	11.9 (11–12.7)	0.086
Hematocrit %	37.6 (34.0–41.6)	35.7 (32.6–38.7)	0.245
Platelets ($\times 10^3$/L)	212 (184–270)	227 (170–271)	0.975
Glucose (mg/dL)	78.0 (73–85)	84 (72–120)	0.260
Creatinine (mg/dL)	0.55 (0.49–0.64)	0.54 (0.46–0.67)	0.624
Uric acid (mg/dL)	4.4 (3.8–5.8)	3.9 (3.4–5.0)	0.285
AST (U/L)	20.5 (17–28)	26 (21–36)	0.042
ALT (U/L)	17.5 (12–25)	23 (17–40)	0.082
LDH (U/L)	173 (146–212)	197 (152–295)	0.112
Direct bilirubin (mg/dL)	0.10 (0.06–0.14)	0.19 (0.07–0.42)	0.029
Indirect bilirubin (mg/dL)	0.32 (0.25–0.43)	0.34 (0.28–0.48)	0.464
Triglycerides (mg/dL)	263 (203–313)	265 (210–312)	0.885
Total cholesterol (mg/dL)	197 (172–235)	154 (118–217)	0.017
D-dimer (ng/mL)	1549 (1242–2981)	1438 (1248–2511)	0.302
Fibrinogen (mg/dL)	526 (481–591)	570 (428–611)	0.521
PTT (seconds)	26.2 (24.8–29.2)	26.9 (24.8–28.9)	0.949
PT (seconds)	10.8 (10.55–11.4)	10.3 (9.9–11)	0.398
C-RP (mg/L)	21.1 (6.45–81.7)	61.15 (16.5–188)	0.014
Procalcitonin (ng/mL)	0.05 (0.03–0.13)	0.2 (0.07–0.53)	0.0006
PlGF (pg/mL)	150.1 (56–215.6)	114.3 (32.29–212.3)	0.186
sFlt-1 (pg/mL)	1424 (1054–2099)	6119 (2099–7900)	0.0001
ACE-2 (pg/mL)	8754 (6040–27480)	7904 (5928–14216)	0.324
ANG-II (pg/mL)	1479 (915.3–7873)	404.3 (180.8–471)	0.0001
sFlt1/PlGF ratio	11.21 (5.43–26.38)	53.72 (31.87–126.12)	0.0001
sFlt-1/ANG-II ratio	0.92 (0.25–2.03)	14.27 (4.47–42.46)	0.0001

AST: Aspartate aminotransferase; ALT: Alanine aminotransferase; LDH: Lactate dehydrogenase; PTT: Partial thromboplastin time; PT: prothrombin time; C-RP: C-reactive protein; PlGF: Placental growth factor; sFlt-1: Soluble fms-like tyrosine kinase-1; ACE-2: Angiotensin-converting enzyme-2; ANG-II: Angiotensin-II. Mann-Whitney-U test for continuous variables expressed as median and interquartile range.

3.2. Correlation between sFlt-1 and ANG-II

Spearman´s Rho test was used to identify the relationship of sFlt-1 and ANG-II, and a significant correlation was found among severe pneumonia (r = −0.453; $p < 0.001$) (Figure 1).

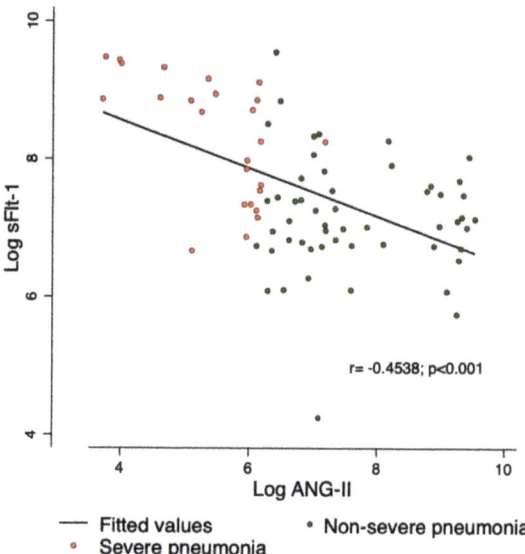

Figure 1. Relationship of sFlt-1 and ANG-II. A significant negative correlation was identified, between lower plasma concentrations of ANG-II, and very high plasma concentrations of sFlt-1.

3.3. Association with the Primary and Secondary Outcomes

There was a significant association between severe pneumonia in women with SARS-CoV-2 infection and sFlt-1/ANG-II ratio (OR: 1.31; 95% CI: 1.09–1.56; p = 0.003) (Table 3). Among secondary outcomes, sFlt-1/ANG-II ratio was associated with ICU admission (OR: 1.05; 95% CI: 1.01–1.09; p = 0.007); intubation (OR: 1.09; 95% CI: 1.02–1.16; p = 0.008); viral sepsis (OR: 1.04; 95% CI: 1.01–1.08; p = 0.008); and maternal death (OR: 1.04; 95% CI: 1.00–1.07; p = 0.018) (Table S2).

Table 3. Association between biochemical markers and severe COVID-19.

Biochemical Marker	OR	95% CI	p-Value
AST (U/L)	1.00	0.99–1.00	0.636
Direct bilirubin (mg/dL)	15.69	0.81–303.44	0.069
Total cholesterol (mg/dL)	0.99	0.98–1.00	0.064
C-RP (mg/L)	1.01	1.00–1.02	0.025
Procalcitonin (ng/mL)	1.12	0.67–1.88	0.651
sFlt1 (pg/mL)	1.01	1.00–1.01	<0.0001
ANG-II (pg/mL)	0.99	0.98–0.99	0.001
sFlt1/PlGF	1.02	1.00–1.03	0.002
sFlt-1/ANG-II	1.31	1.09–1.56	0.003

C-RP: C-reactive protein; sFlt-1: Soluble fms-like tyrosine kinase-1; ANG-II: Angiotensin-II; PlGF: Placental growth factor; OR: Odds ratio; CI: Confidence interval.

3.4. sFlt-1/ANG-II Ratio for the Prediction of Adverse Outcomes in COVID-19

The AUC of sFlt-1/ANG-II ratio for the prediction of severe pneumonia by COVID-19 was 0.9608 (95% CI: 0.807–0.981). The detection rates for severe pneumonia at 5% and 10% false-positive-rate were 52% and 88%, respectively (Figure 2). The best cut-off value of the sFlt-1/ANG-II ratio was 3.06 showing a sensitivity (Se) of 96% and specificity (Sp) of 88.6%

for severe pneumonia. The Se and Sp were 100% and 71.6% for ICU admission and 100% and 70.5% for intubation, respectively (Table 4).

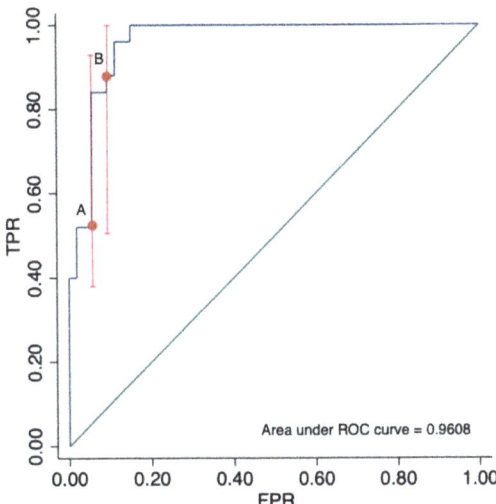

Figure 2. Area under the receiver-operating-curve (ROC) of sFlt1-1/ANG-II ratio for the prediction of severe pneumonia by COVID-19. ROC 0.9608. The detection rate (true-positive rate [TPR]) for severe pneumonia, at (A) 5% and (B) 10% false-positive rate (FPR) were 52% and 88%, respectively.

Table 4. Performance of sFlt-1/ANG-II ratio $\geq$ 3.06 for the prediction of adverse maternal outcomes.

Outcome	Se (95% CI)	Sp 95% CI	Positive LR 95% CI	Negative LR (95% CI)
Severe pneumonia	0.96 (0.88–1.0)	0.886 (0.80–0.972)	8.48 (3.97–18)	0.045 (0.01–0.31)
ICU admission	1.0 (1.0–1.0)	0.716 (0.443–0.789)	3.52 (2.26–4.95)	0.01 (0.01–0.88)
Intubation	1.0 (1.0–1.0)	0.705 (0.567–0.784)	3.4 (1.93–4.20)	0.01 (0.01–1.54)
Viral sepsis	1.0 (1.0–1.0)	0.64 (0.531–0.748)	2.77 (1.50–3.89)	0.01 (0.01–2.63)
Maternal death	1.0 (1.0–1.0)	0.631 (0.523–0.74)	2.71 (1.26–4.04)	0.01 (0.01–3.34)

sFlt-1: Soluble fms-like tyrosine kinase-1; ANG-II: Angiotensin-II; ICU: Intensive care unit; Se: sensitivity; Sp: specificity; LR: Likelihood ratio; CI: Confidence interval.

3.5. Hypothetical Molecular Mechanisms Contributing to the Pathogenesis of Severe COVID-19 in Pregnant Women

In pregnant women with severe pneumonia by COVID-19, plasma levels of ANG-II are reduced, and plasma levels of sFlt-1 are increased, compared to those with non-severe disease. This leads to an imbalance in the sFlt-1/ANG-II ratio. Although the molecular mechanisms involved in the production of ANG-II and sFlt-1 were not explored in our work, current evidence allows us to propose a hypothetical pathway on how SARS-CoV-2 infection in the placenta affects the RAS signaling pathway contributing to the pathogenesis of severe COVID-19 in pregnant women (Figure 3).

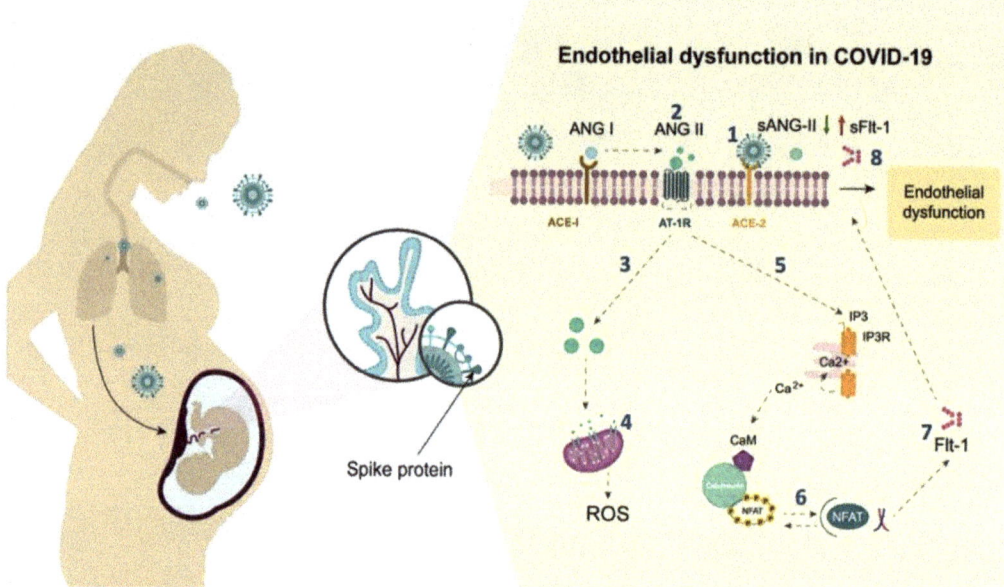

Figure 3. Hypothetical molecular mechanisms contributing to the pathogenesis of severe COVID-19 in pregnant women. Spike protein of SARS-CoV-2 virus binds to trophoblastic cells expressing ACE-2, (1) blocking the conversion of ANG-II into ANG 1-7 [3]. (2) Accumulation of ANG-II on the cell surface enhances its binding to the AT-1 receptor (AT-1R), promoting downstream signaling, followed by rapid endocytosis of the ANG-II/AT-1R complex [24]. (3) By avoiding the endosome/lysosome degradation, the excess of ANG-II is accumulated in endothelial cells [25]. (4) ANG-II binds to mitochondrial AT-1R [26], inducing cellular senescence with positive regulation of reactive oxygen species (ROS) [27]. (5) Over-activation of AT-1R on the cell membrane leads to increased PKC and calcineurin activity [25]. (6) Transcription factors NF-kB and NFAT are activated and translocated to the nucleus, leading to an increase in gene expression and release of Flt-1 [25]. (7) Flt-1 alternative splicing generates sFlt-1 isoform [25]. (8) The excess of sFlt-1 protein is released into the circulation causing endothelial dysfunction.

4. Discussion

4.1. Main Findings

A high ratio of sFlt-1/ANG-II was associated with a 1.31-fold increase in severe pneumonia and higher odds of ICU admission, viral sepsis, and maternal death. So, this ratio can be considered as a high-performance prognostic marker in pregnant women with COVID-19.

4.2. Comparison with Existing Literature

Studies in non-pregnant individuals have reported higher serum levels of sFlt-1 in patients with pneumonia due to COVID-19 compared to non-COVID-19-pneumonia [28]. Negro and colleagues have reported higher levels of sFlt-1 among deceased compared to COVID-19 survivors [29]. This report has demonstrated higher sFlt-1 levels in pregnant women with COVID-19 severe pneumonia. Other studies have reported lower plasma ACE-2 levels in non-survivors than in critically ill patients that have survived COVID-19 [30], however, our study has failed to demonstrate a difference in this parameter between those with critical illness and non-critical illness. We have found lower plasma levels of ANG-II in pregnant women with severe pneumonia by COVID-19. Lower ANG-II levels have been found in previous studies among people with acute respiratory distress syndrome not related to SARS-CoV-2. Studies in non-pregnant participants with severe COVID-19 have shown lower serum levels of ANG-II among deceased patients when compared to survivors [30]. A possible explanation of the ANG-II downregulation could be a defect in the endothelial–bound ACE activity due to endothelial injury [31].

We have shown that the sFlt-1/ANG-II ratio could be a potential predictor of adverse events such as severe pneumonia, ICU admission, intubation, viral sepsis, and death among pregnant women who tested positive for SARS-CoV-2 infection. This ratio should be tested in a larger cohort to prove its utility before its clinical use.

In relation to preeclampsia, no significant differences in the incidence among patients with severe and non-severe COVID-19 have been observed; this finding is contradictory to previous studies in which higher rates of preeclampsia have been demonstrated in cases of severe COVID-19 [32–34].

4.3. Strengths and Limitations

The strength of our study is the number of adverse events that allowed us to make statistical inferences for outcomes such as severe pneumonia. Furthermore, the baseline clinical characteristics between groups were similar, which decreases the probability of selection bias.

The limitations are, despite being a cohort, the analysis was carried out cross-sectionally, which does not allow us to infer the causal relationship between the sFlt-1/ANG-II ratio and adverse outcomes, and the ORs could be overestimated. Although the sFlt-1/ANG-II ratio has a positive predictive value for predicting the severity of COVID-19 in the short term, the results need clinical validation in a new cohort.

4.4. Clinical Interpretation

In this study, a negative correlation has been found between the plasma concentrations of ANG-II and sFlt-1. A high sFlt-1/ANG-II ratio is associated with several adverse outcomes related to COVID-19, such as severe pneumonia, ICU admission, intubation, viral sepsis, and death. The sFlt-1/ANG-II ratio may allow the development of predictive models for the identification of high-risk pregnant women in need of intensive surveillance and aggressive supportive treatment upon admission to the hospital, thus preventing clinical deterioration.

5. Conclusions

sFlt-1/ANG-II ratio is a promising predictor for adverse outcomes such as pneumonia, ICU admission, intubation, viral sepsis, and death in pregnant women with COVID-19. However, further research in a larger prospective cohort is needed to validate the association and accuracy of the sFlt-1/ANG-II ratio for the prediction of adverse events among pregnant women with COVID-19.

Supplementary Materials: The following are available online at https://www.mdpi.com/article/10.3390/v13101906/s1, Table S1: Pregnancy outcome of the study population, Table S2: Association between sFlt-1/ANG-II ratio and each adverse outcome of COVID-19.

Author Contributions: Conceptualization: S.E.-y.-S., R.J.M.-P., J.R.V.-B., J.M.S.-P., and J.T.-T.; methodology: J.T.-T., and R.J.M.-P.; formal analysis: S.E.-y.-S., J.R.V.-B., and J.T.-T.; writing—original draft: J.T.-T., S.E.-y.-S., L.C.P., and J.M.S.-P.; resources: A.J.-R., F.E.L.-C., J.A.H.-P., P.M.-R., L.R.-Z. and I.P.G.-G.; writing—review and editing, G.E.-G., A.E.-N., R.J.M.-P., J.T.-T. and L.C.P.; funding acquisition: J.T.-T., J.R.V.-B., R.J.M.-P. and G.E.-G. All authors have read and agreed to the published version of the manuscript.

Funding: sFlt-1 and PlGF assays for this study were donated by Roche Diagnostics® and did not have any influence on the design of this study, analysis, results, or interpretation of the results.

Institutional Review Board Statement: The study was conducted according to the guidelines of the Declaration of Helsinki and approved by the Institutional Review Board of Instituto Nacional de Perinatología (Register number 2020-1-32) on 16 December 2020.

Informed Consent Statement: Informed consent was obtained from all subjects involved in the study.

Data Availability Statement: The data presented in this study are available on request from the corresponding author. The data are not publicly available due to privacy.

Acknowledgments: This work would not have been possible without the effort of the healthcare workers in the COVID areas (Epidemiology, Nursery, Obstetrics and Gynecology, Researchers, Residents, Interns, Attendings, Postgraduate Students, Medical Students, and the Molecular Diagnosis teams) in the Instituto Nacional de Perinatologia, and Hospital General de Mexico "Dr. Eduardo Liceaga".

Conflicts of Interest: The authors declare no conflict of interest.

References

1. Martinez-Portilla, R.J.; Sotiriadis, A.; Chatzakis, C.; Torres-Torres, J.; Espino, Y.S.S.; Sandoval-Mandujano, K.; Castro-Bernabe, D.A.; Medina-Jimenez, V.; Monarrez-Martin, J.C.; Figueras, F.; et al. Pregnant women with SARS-CoV-2 infection are at higher risk of death and pneumonia: Propensity score matched analysis of a nationwide prospective cohort (COV19Mx). *Ultrasound Obstet. Gynecol.* **2021**, *57*, 224–231. [CrossRef]
2. Zambrano, L.D.; Ellington, S.; Strid, P.; Galang, R.R.; Oduyebo, T.; Tong, V.T.; Woodworth, K.R.; Nahabedian, J.F., 3rd; Azziz-Baumgartner, E.; Gilboa, S.M.; et al. Update: Characteristics of Symptomatic Women of Reproductive Age with Laboratory-Confirmed SARS-CoV-2 Infection by Pregnancy Status-United States, 22 January–3 October 2020. *MMWR Morb. Mortal. Wkly. Rep.* **2020**, *69*, 1641–1647. [CrossRef] [PubMed]
3. Zhang, H.; Penninger, J.M.; Li, Y.; Zhong, N.; Slutsky, A.S. Angiotensin-converting enzyme 2 (ACE2) as a SARS-CoV-2 receptor: Molecular mechanisms and potential therapeutic target. *Intensive Care Med.* **2020**, *46*, 586–590. [CrossRef] [PubMed]
4. Santos, R.A.S.; Sampaio, W.O.; Alzamora, A.C.; Motta-Santos, D.; Alenina, N.; Bader, M.; Campagnole-Santos, M.J. The ACE2/Angiotensin-(1-7)/MAS Axis of the Renin-Angiotensin System: Focus on Angiotensin-(1-7). *Physiol. Rev.* **2018**, *98*, 505–553. [CrossRef] [PubMed]
5. Luther, J.M.; Gainer, J.V.; Murphey, L.J.; Yu, C.; Vaughan, D.E.; Morrow, J.D.; Brown, N.J. Angiotensin II induces interleukin-6 in humans through a mineralocorticoid receptor-dependent mechanism. *Hypertension* **2006**, *48*, 1050–1057. [CrossRef] [PubMed]
6. Sargiacomo, C.; Sotgia, F.; Lisanti, M.P. COVID-19 and chronological aging: Senolytics and other anti-aging drugs for the treatment or prevention of corona virus infection? *Aging* **2020**, *12*, 6511–6517. [CrossRef]
7. Pringle, K.G.; Tadros, M.A.; Callister, R.J.; Lumbers, E.R. The expression and localization of the human placental prorenin/renin-angiotensin system throughout pregnancy: Roles in trophoblast invasion and angiogenesis? *Placenta* **2011**, *32*, 956–962. [CrossRef]
8. Irani, R.A.; Xia, Y. The functional role of the renin-angiotensin system in pregnancy and preeclampsia. *Placenta* **2008**, *29*, 763–771. [CrossRef]
9. Pavličev, M.; Wagner, G.P.; Chavan, A.R.; Owens, K.; Maziarz, J.; Dunn-Fletcher, C.; Kallapur, S.G.; Muglia, L.; Jones, H. Single-cell transcriptomics of the human placenta: Inferring the cell communication network of the maternal-fetal interface. *Genome Res.* **2017**, *27*, 349–361. [CrossRef]
10. Powe, C.E.; Levine, R.J.; Karumanchi, S.A. Preeclampsia, a disease of the maternal endothelium: The role of antiangiogenic factors and implications for later cardiovascular disease. *Circulation* **2011**, *123*, 2856–2869. [CrossRef]
11. AlGhatrif, M.; Cingolani, O.; Lakatta, E.G. The Dilemma of Coronavirus Disease 2019, Aging, and Cardiovascular Disease: Insights From Cardiovascular Aging Science. *JAMA Cardiol.* **2020**, *5*, 747–748. [CrossRef]
12. Ni, W.; Yang, X.; Yang, D.; Bao, J.; Li, R.; Xiao, Y.; Hou, C.; Wang, H.; Liu, J.; Yang, D.; et al. Role of angiotensin-converting enzyme 2 (ACE2) in COVID-19. *Crit. Care* **2020**, *24*, 422. [CrossRef]
13. Sacks, D.; Baxter, B.; Campbell, B.C.V.; Carpenter, J.S.; Cognard, C.; Dippel, D.; Eesa, M.; Fischer, U.; Hausegger, K.; Hirsch, J.A.; et al. Multisociety Consensus Quality Improvement Revised Consensus Statement for Endovascular Therapy of Acute Ischemic Stroke. *Int. J. Stroke* **2018**, *13*, 612–632. [CrossRef]
14. Campbell, N.; LaMarca, B.; Cunningham, M.W., Jr. The Role of Agonistic Autoantibodies to the Angiotensin II Type 1 Receptor (AT1-AA) in Pathophysiology of Preeclampsia. *Curr. Pharm. Biotechnol.* **2018**, *19*, 781–785. [CrossRef]
15. Murphy, S.R.; Cockrell, K. Regulation of soluble fms-like tyrosine kinase-1 production in response to placental ischemia/hypoxia: Role of angiotensin II. *Physiol. Rep.* **2015**, *3*, e12310. [CrossRef] [PubMed]
16. Flores-Pliego, A.; Miranda, J.; Vega-Torreblanca, S.; Valdespino-Vázquez, Y.; Helguera-Repetto, C.; Espejel-Nuñez, A.; Borboa-Olivares, H.; Espino, Y.S.S.; Mateu-Rogell, P.; León-Juárez, M.; et al. Molecular Insights into the Thrombotic and Microvascular Injury in Placental Endothelium of Women with Mild or Severe COVID-19. *Cells* **2021**, *10*, 364. [CrossRef] [PubMed]
17. Mehta, P.; McAuley, D.F.; Brown, M.; Sanchez, E.; Tattersall, R.S.; Manson, J.J. COVID-19: Consider cytokine storm syndromes and immunosuppression. *Lancet* **2020**, *395*, 1033–1034. [CrossRef]
18. Gestational Hypertension and Preeclampsia: ACOG Practice Bulletin, Number 222. *Obstet. Gynecol.* **2020**, *135*, e237–e260. [CrossRef] [PubMed]
19. Metlay, J.P.; Waterer, G.W.; Long, A.C.; Anzueto, A.; Brozek, J.; Crothers, K.; Cooley, L.A.; Dean, N.C.; Fine, M.J.; Flanders, S.A.; et al. Diagnosis and Treatment of Adults with Community-acquired Pneumonia. An Official Clinical Practice Guideline of the American Thoracic Society and Infectious Diseases Society of America. *Am. J. Respir. Crit. Care Med.* **2019**, *200*, e45–e67. [CrossRef] [PubMed]

20. Poon, L.C.; Yang, H.; Kapur, A.; Melamed, N.; Dao, B.; Divakar, H.; McIntyre, H.D.; Kihara, A.B.; Ayres-de-Campos, D.; Ferrazzi, E.M.; et al. Global interim guidance on coronavirus disease 2019 (COVID-19) during pregnancy and puerperium from FIGO and allied partners: Information for healthcare professionals. *Int. J. Gynaecol. Obstet.* **2020**, *149*, 273–286. [CrossRef] [PubMed]
21. Jiang, J.; Yang, J.; Mei, J.; Jin, Y.; Lu, Y. Head-to-head comparison of qSOFA and SIRS criteria in predicting the mortality of infected patients in the emergency department: A meta-analysis. *Scand. J. Trauma Resusc. Emerg. Med.* **2018**, *26*, 56. [CrossRef]
22. Singer, M.; Deutschman, C.S.; Seymour, C.W.; Shankar-Hari, M.; Annane, D.; Bauer, M.; Bellomo, R.; Bernard, G.R.; Chiche, J.D.; Coopersmith, C.M.; et al. The Third International Consensus Definitions for Sepsis and Septic Shock (Sepsis-3). *JAMA* **2016**, *315*, 801–810. [CrossRef] [PubMed]
23. Li, H.; Liu, L.; Zhang, D.; Xu, J.; Dai, H.; Tang, N.; Su, X.; Cao, B. SARS-CoV-2 and viral sepsis: Observations and hypotheses. *Lancet* **2020**, *395*, 1517–1520. [CrossRef]
24. Cunningham, M.W., Jr.; Castillo, J.; Ibrahim, T.; Cornelius, D.C.; Campbell, N.; Amaral, L.; Vaka, V.R.; Usry, N.; Williams, J.M.; LaMarca, B. AT1-AA (Angiotensin II Type 1 Receptor Agonistic Autoantibody) Blockade Prevents Preeclamptic Symptoms in Placental Ischemic Rats. *Hypertension* **2018**, *71*, 886–893. [CrossRef]
25. Xia, Y.; Ramin, S.M.; Kellems, R.E. Potential roles of angiotensin receptor-activating autoantibody in the pathophysiology of preeclampsia. *Hypertension* **2007**, *50*, 269–275. [CrossRef] [PubMed]
26. Li, X.C.; Zhou, X.; Zhuo, J.L. Evidence for a Physiological Mitochondrial Angiotensin II System in the Kidney Proximal Tubules: Novel Roles of Mitochondrial Ang II/AT(1a)/O(2)(-) and Ang II/AT(2)/NO Signaling. *Hypertension* **2020**, *76*, 121–132. [CrossRef]
27. Kawai, T.; Forrester, S.J.; O'Brien, S.; Baggett, A.; Rizzo, V.; Eguchi, S. AT1 receptor signaling pathways in the cardiovascular system. *Pharmacol. Res.* **2017**, *125*, 4–13. [CrossRef]
28. Giardini, V.; Carrer, A.; Casati, M.; Contro, E.; Vergani, P.; Gambacorti-Passerini, C. Increased sFLT-1/PlGF ratio in COVID-19: A novel link to angiotensin II-mediated endothelial dysfunction. *Am. J. Hematol.* **2020**, *95*, e188–e191. [CrossRef]
29. Negro, A.; Fama, A.; Penna, D.; Belloni, L.; Zerbini, A.; Giuri, P.G. SFLT-1 levels in COVID-19 patients: Association with outcome and thrombosis. *Am. J. Hematol.* **2021**, *96*, e41–e43. [CrossRef] [PubMed]
30. Eleuteri, D.; Montini, L.; Cutuli, S.L.; Rossi, C.; Alcaro, F.; Antonelli, M. Renin-angiotensin system dysregulation in critically ill patients with acute respiratory distress syndrome due to COVID-19: A preliminary report. *Crit. Care* **2021**, *25*, 91. [CrossRef]
31. Orfanos, S.E.; Armaganidis, A.; Glynos, C.; Psevdi, E.; Kaltsas, P.; Sarafidou, P.; Catravas, J.D.; Dafni, U.G.; Langleben, D.; Roussos, C. Pulmonary capillary endothelium-bound angiotensin-converting enzyme activity in acute lung injury. *Circulation* **2000**, *102*, 2011–2018. [CrossRef] [PubMed]
32. Gurol-Urganci, I.; Jardine, J.E.; Carroll, F.; Draycott, T.; Dunn, G.; Fremeaux, A.; Harris, T.; Hawdon, J.; Morris, E.; Muller, P.; et al. Maternal and perinatal outcomes of pregnant women with SARS-CoV-2 infection at the time of birth in England: National cohort study. *Am. J. Obstet. Gynecol.* **2021**, *2021*. [CrossRef]
33. Mendoza, M.; Garcia-Ruiz, I.; Maiz, N.; Rodo, C.; Garcia-Manau, P.; Serrano, B.; Lopez-Martinez, R.M.; Balcells, J.; Fernandez-Hidalgo, N.; Carreras, E.; et al. Pre-eclampsia-like syndrome induced by severe COVID-19: A prospective observational study. *BJOG Int. J. Obstetr. Gynaecol.* **2020**, *127*, 1374–1380. [CrossRef] [PubMed]
34. Papageorghiou, A.T.; Deruelle, P.; Gunier, R.B.; Rauch, S.; García-May, P.K.; Mhatre, M.; Usman, M.A.; Abd-Elsalam, S.; Etuk, S.; Simmons, L.E.; et al. Preeclampsia and COVID-19: Results from the INTERCOVID prospective longitudinal study. *Am. J. Obstet. Gynecol.* **2021**, *225*, 289.e1–289.e17. [CrossRef]

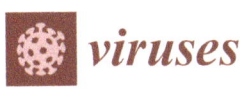

Communication

Letter to the Editor: SFlt-1 and PlGF Levels in Pregnancies Complicated by SARS-CoV-2 Infection

Valentina Giardini [1,*], Sara Ornaghi [1], Eleonora Acampora [1], Maria Viola Vasarri [1], Francesca Arienti [1], Carlo Gambacorti-Passerini [2], Marco Casati [3], Andrea Carrer [2] and Patrizia Vergani [1]

1. Department of Obstetrics and Gynecology, MBBM Foundation, San Gerardo Hospital, University of Milano-Bicocca, 20900 Monza, Italy; sara.ornaghi@gmail.com (S.O.); e.acampora@campus.unimib.it (E.A.); m.vasarri@campus.unimib.it (M.V.V.); f.arienti9@campus.unimib.it (F.A.); patrizia.vergani@unimib.it (P.V.)
2. Hematology Division, ASST-Monza, San Gerardo Hospital, University of Milano-Bicocca, 20900 Monza, Italy; carlo.gambacorti@unimib.it (C.G.-P.); mail.carrer@gmail.com (A.C.)
3. Laboratory Medicine, ASST-Monza, San Gerardo Hospital, University of Milano-Bicocca, 20900 Monza, Italy; m.casati@asst-monza.it
* Correspondence: valentinagiardini1985@gmail.com

Keywords: COVID-19; SARS-CoV-2; angiogenic factors; sFlt-1; endothelial dysfunction

Dear Editor

We read with interest the work by Espino-y-Sosa and colleagues [1], who recently reported that the Soluble Fms-like Tyrosine Kinase-1/Angiotensin-II (sFlt-1/ANG-II) ratio could be a good predictor of adverse outcomes, including pneumonia, intensive care unit (ICU) admission, intubation, viral sepsis, and death, among pregnant women with COVID-19.

COVID-19 is a respiratory infection characterized by signs and symptoms associated with the dysfunction of the renin–angiotensin system (RAS). RAS activation leads to the formation of ANG II, a powerful vasoconstrictor and promotor of inflammation, fibrosis, and coagulation [2]; it also induces the release of sFlt-1 in case of hypoxia [3]. sFlt-1 is the soluble receptor of placental growth factor (PlGF), a potent angiogenic factor, and it antagonizes PlGF's activity in the circulation, thus creating an anti-angiogenic state and ensuing endothelial dysfunction (ED) [4].

SARS-CoV-2 invades the respiratory mucosa of the host via the Angiotensin-Converting Enzyme 2 (ACE2) receptor. ACE2 is an important element of RAS [5], and catalyzes ANG II into angiotensin 1–7 (ANG 1–7), a vasodilator with the opposite function of ANG II. Use of the ACE2 receptor for viral entry leads to the downregulation of its synthesis, with the subsequent amplification of ANG II actions and, in turn, vasospasm, inflammation, microvascular thrombosis, and organ damage. In line with these observations, a linear association between serum ANG II levels and viral load and lung damage in COVID-19 patients has been reported [6].

Preeclampsia (PE), a pregnancy-specific hypertensive disorder with multisystem involvement, is characterized by increased sensitivity to ANG II and ED, with high sFlt-1 and low PlGF values. Currently, the sFlt1/PlGF ratio is used as a clinical biomarker for the early detection and prognosis of PE [7].

Considering the common RAS-mediated underlying etiopathogenesis, we initially investigated the sFlt1/PlGF ratio in non-pregnant patients with COVID-19 pneumonia. We originally identified the presence of an angiogenic imbalance in COVID-19 patients, similar to that identified in PE women [8]. Precisely, levels of sFlt-1 were significantly higher in COVID-19-related pneumonia cases compared to those with pneumonia due to other causes and to healthy controls. PlGF values were not significantly affected by COVID-19, but the sFlt1/PlGF ratio was substantially higher in COVID-19-positive compared with COVID-19-negative pneumonia. Subsequently, other authors confirmed the increased

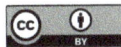

sFlt-1 values in severe COVID-19 and identified sFlt-1 as a biomarker to predict survival and thrombotic accidents in COVID-19 patients [9].

The role of angiogenic markers in pregnancies complicated by SARS-CoV-2 infection is still unclear, possibly because of the interference of the placenta, the major extrarenal RAS site during pregnancy [10].

We then proceeded to assess the sFlt1/PlGF ratio in pregnant women with SARS-CoV-2 infection. Assessment of this ratio could be helpful in guiding the management of these patients and improving the understanding of the pathophysiology of SARS-CoV-2 infection in pregnancy. In fact, an increased incidence of PE among COVID-19 mothers has been reported, although such association is still incompletely elucidated [11,12]. In addition, a study showed that a PE-like syndrome can be induced by severe COVID-19 during pregnancy [13].

Precisely, we conducted a retrospective analysis of positive SARS-CoV-2 pregnant women admitted to our center from April 2020 to October 2021. SARS-CoV-2 infection was diagnosed by RT-PCR assay on nasopharyngeal swabs. Serum dosage of sFlt-1 and PlGF (Cobas e801 analyzer Roche platform, Roche Diagnostics) was performed at the time of diagnosis of SARS-CoV-2 infection, before the beginning of any therapy. Patients already on therapy (enoxaparin sodium, steroids, or hydroxychloroquine) as well as patients without a chest X-ray performed at the time of hospital admission were excluded. The study population included 57 pregnant women, who were divided into two groups (Table 1): women with signs and symptoms of COVID-19 at hospital presentation ($n = 20$, 35%) and asymptomatic women ($n = 37$, 65%). sFlt-1/PlGF ratio was stratified using cut-off values clinically utilized for PE prediction (low risk < 38, high risk > 85 if before 34 weeks' gestation or > 110 if after 34 weeks' gestation) [14].

Asymptomatic women were identified at a surveillance swab required before hospital admission for obstetric reasons in 86% of cases ($n = 32$). The mean gestational age at diagnosis of SARS-CoV-2 infection was $37^{5/7}$ weeks in asymptomatic women and $32^{0/7}$ weeks in symptomatic women ($p = 0.089$). Of note, 4 (11%) asymptomatic women had radiological evidence of pneumonia compared to 16 (80%) in the symptomatic group. In Espino-y-Sosa's work [1], none of the pregnant women with non-severe COVID-19 had pneumonia; it is not clear whether patients underwent radiological examination upon hospital admission.

Among our 20 COVID-19 symptomatic cases, 7 (35%) required high-dependency/intensive care with 3 of them undergoing endotracheal intubation. Continuous positive airway pressure was applied in five cases (25%). Eight (40%) women delivered by cesarean section but only in two cases (10%) for respiratory failure. The mean gestational age at delivery was $38^{2/7}$ weeks with a mean latency time between symptom onset and delivery of 48 ± 44 days. All women received therapy with enoxaparin sodium, 14 (70%) were given steroids, and 2 (10%) hydroxychloroquine (first pandemic wave). Of note, there were no stillbirths, or maternal or neonatal deaths, among these symptomatic patients; additionally, no cases of PE, fetal growth restriction, or small for gestational age neonates were diagnosed. Espino-y-Sosa et al. reported worse maternal and neonatal outcomes compared with our results.

Additionally, differently from Espino-y-Sosa et al., we identified higher sFlt-1 levels in asymptomatic patients compared to symptomatic patients (4899 ± 4357 vs. 3187 ± 2426 pg/mL, $p = 0.005$). sFlt-1/PlGF ratio at admission was ≤ 38 in 18 of the 20 symptomatic women compared to 22 (59%) of the asymptomatic patients (mean gestational age at admission $32^{1/7}$ weeks versus $38^{3/7}$ weeks) ($p = 0.018$). In turn, rates of patients with sFlt-1/PlGF ratio at admission > 85/110 were similar between symptomatic and asymptomatic group ($n = 0$ versus $n = 4$, 11%; $p = 0.286$).

This difference in the increase in sFlt-1 between our data and those reported by Espino-y-Sosa and colleagues may be due to the higher gestational age at hospital admission of our asymptomatic patients. An additional explanation might be the delayed hospital access of Espino-y-Sosa's severe COVID-19 patients, leading to increased sFlt-1 levels due to prolonged exposure to hypoxia [3]. In our study, the mean number of days between symptom onset and hospital admission was five. Furthermore, we performed the assay of sFlt-1 and PlGF on serum according to the instructions of Roche Diagnostics; in Espino-y-Sosa's work, it is unclear whether sFlt-1 and PlGF tests were performed on plasma or serum and whether these women received pre-hospital treatment that may have affected the markers analyzed.

No significant differences in the incidence of PE were identified between severe and non-severe COVID-19 patients in Espino-y-Sosa's work, as well as in our cohort. A recent sub-analysis from the INTERCOVID study population showed that COVID-19 during pregnancy is independently associated with PE. Interestingly, this association is not modified by COVID-19 severity [15]. sFlt-1/PlGF ratio results among SARS-CoV-2-infected asymptomatic women are of particular interest. If the increase in sFlt-1 levels we observed is the consequence of viral infection, and not just of the higher gestational age at its evaluation, then the identification of asymptomatically infected pregnant women might be important since they may benefit from more intensive antenatal surveillance of fetal growth and blood pressure due to a potential increased risk of developing PE. Furthermore, the data from this study provide further reason to push pregnant women to be vaccinated, given the possible obstetric complications in the case of asymptomatic SARS-CoV-2 infection. In conclusion, our data suggest that SARS-CoV-2 infection during pregnancy could influence the angiogenic profile, but likely with a different effect according to the type of viral infection (symptomatic versus asymptomatic). Further research in a larger prospective cohort is needed.

Table 1. Population characteristics comparing positive SARS-CoV-2 pregnant women with signs and symptoms of COVID-19 at admission to asymptomatic women.

SARS-CoV-2 Pregnant Women Variables	All n = 57	Asymptomatic 37 (65)	Symptomatic 20 (35)	p Value
Anamnestic Characteristics				
Age (years)	33 ± 5	33 ± 5	33 ± 4	0.667
Italian	30 (53)	20 (54)	10 (50)	0.788
Nulliparous	23 (40)	14 (38)	6 (30)	0.772
Obesity (BMI > 30 kg/m^2)	12 (21)	7 (19)	5 (25)	0.736
Diabetes/Gestational diabetes mellitus	15 (26)	10 (27)	5 (25)	0.580
Chronic hypertension	2 (4)	2 (5)	0	0.536
SARS-CoV-2 infection				
GA at positive swab (weeks.days ± weeks)	35.5 ± 6	37.5 ± 5	32 ± 6	0.089
Respiratory symptoms at admission	16 (28)	0	16 (80)	0.0001
Pneumonia on chest x-ray	20 (35)	4 (11)	16 (80)	0.0001
High dependency unit admission	6 (11)	0	6 (30)	0.001
ICU admission	3 (5)	0	3 (15)	0.039
Oxygen supplementation	14 (25)	0	14 (70)	0.0001
Continuous positive airway pressure (CPAP)	5 (9)	0	5 (25)	0.004
Intubation	3 (5)	0	3 (15)	0.039
Maternal/fetal/neonatal death	0	0	0	NA

Table 1. Cont.

SARS-CoV-2 Pregnant Women Variables	All n = 57	Asymptomatic 37 (65)	Symptomatic 20 (35)	p Value
Angiogenic factors				
GA at blood test (weeks.days ± weeks)	36.2 ± 6	38.3 ± 4	32.1 ± 6	0.208
Latency timeCOVID-19 symptoms—blood test (days)	14 ± 24	27 ± 34	5 ± 4	0.038
sFlt-1 (pg/mL)	4948 ± 3988	4899 ± 4357	3187 ± 2426	0.005
PlGF (pg/mL)	237 ± 178	178 ± 104	346 ± 232	0.099
sFlt1/PlGF ratio	38 ± 50	50 ± 58	17 ± 23	0.099
sFlt1/PlGF < 38	40 (70)	22 (59)	18 (90)	0.018
sFlt1/PlGF > 85/110 (if before/after 34 weeks)	4 (7)	4 (11)	0	0.286
Pregnancy				
Hypertensive disorders of pregnancy/post-partum	5 (9)	4 (11)	1 (5)	0.647
Fetal growth restriction	3 (5)	3 (8)	0	0.545
Premature birth < 37 weeks	4 (7)	0	4 (20)	0.012
Small for gestational age newborn	6 (11)	6 (16)	0	0.081

Data presented as mean ± standard deviation or n (%). GA: gestational age. Fetal growth restriction: Delphi consensus methodology [16]. Small for gestational age newborn: birthweight below the 10th percentile (INeS charts) [17].

Author Contributions: Conceptualization, V.G.; methodology, V.G.; formal analysis, V.G.; writing—original draft preparation, V.G.; writing—review and editing, S.O., P.V., C.G.-P., M.C. and A.C.; supervision, P.V.; data collection, V.G., E.A., M.V.V. and F.A. All authors have read and agreed to the published version of the manuscript.

Funding: This research received no external funding.

Institutional Review Board Statement: The study was conducted according to the guidelines of the Declaration of Helsinki, and approved by the Ethics Committee of MBBM Foundation (AMICO study—16 July 2020).

Informed Consent Statement: Informed consent was obtained from all subjects involved in the study.

Data Availability Statement: The data that support the findings of this study are available on request from the corresponding author.

Conflicts of Interest: The authors declare no conflisct of interest.

References

1. Espino-y-Sosa, S.; Martinez-Portilla, R.J.; Torres-Torres, J.; Solis-Paredes, J.M.; EstradaGutierrez, G.; Hernandez-Pacheco, J.A.; Espejel-Nuñez, A.; Mateu-Rogell, P.; Juarez-Reyes, A.; Lopez-Ceh, F.E.; et al. Novel Ratio Soluble Fms-like Tyrosine Kinase-1/Angiotensin-II (sFlt1/ANG-II) in Pregnant Women Is Associated with Critical Illness in COVID-19. *Viruses* **2021**, *13*, 1906. [CrossRef] [PubMed]
2. Benigni, A.; Cassis, P.; Remuzzi, G. Angiotensin II revisited: New roles in inflammation, immunology and aging. *EMBO Mol. Med.* **2010**, *2*, 247–257. [CrossRef] [PubMed]
3. Murphy, S.R.; Cockrell, K. Regulation of soluble fms-like tyrosine kinase-1 production in response to placental ischemia/hypoxia: Role of angiotensin II. *Physiol. Rep.* **2015**, *3*, e12310. [CrossRef] [PubMed]
4. Maynard, S.E.; Min, J.Y.; Merchan, J.; Lim, K.H.; Li, J.; Mondal, S.; Libermann, T.A.; Morgan, J.P.; Sellke, F.W.; Stillman, I.E.; et al. Excess placental soluble fms-like tyrosine kinase 1 (sFlt1) may contribute to endothelial dysfunction, hypertension, and proteinuria in preeclampsia. *J. Clin. Investig.* **2003**, *111*, 649–658. [CrossRef] [PubMed]
5. Cheng, H.; Wang, Y.; Wang, G.Q. Organ-protective effect of angiotensin-converting enzyme 2 and its effect on the prognosis of COVID-19. *J. Med. Virol.* **2020**, *92*, 726–730. [CrossRef] [PubMed]
6. Liu, Y.; Yang, Y.; Zhang, C.; Huang, F.; Wang, F.; Yuan, J.; Wang, Z.; Li, J.; Li, J.; Feng, C.; et al. Clinical and biochemical indexes from 2019-nCoV infected patients linked to viral loads and lung injury. *Sci. China Life Sci.* **2020**, *63*, 364–374. [CrossRef] [PubMed]
7. Stepan, H.; Hund, M.; Andraczek, T. Combining Biomarkers to Predict Pregnancy Complications and Redefine Preeclampsia: The Angiogenic-Placental Syndrome. *Hypertension* **2020**, *75*, 918–926. [CrossRef] [PubMed]

8. Giardini, V.; Carrer, A.; Casati, M.; Contro, E.; Vergani, P.; Gambacorti-Passerini, C. Increased sFLT-1/PlGF ratio in COVID-19: A novel link to angiotensin II-mediated endothelial dysfunction. *Am. J. Hematol.* **2020**, *95*, E188–E191. [CrossRef] [PubMed]
9. Negro, A.; Fama, A.; Penna, D.; Belloni, L.; Zerbini, A.; Giuri, P.G. SFLT-1 levels in COVID-19 patients: Association with outcome and thrombosis. *Am. J. Hematol.* **2021**, *96*, E41–E43. [CrossRef] [PubMed]
10. Verdonk, K.; Visser, W.; Van Den Meiracker, A.H.; Danser, A.H. The renin-angiotensin-aldosterone system in pre-eclampsia: The delicate balance between good and bad. *Clin. Sci.* **2014**, *126*, 537–544. [CrossRef] [PubMed]
11. Ahlberg, M.; Neovius, M.; Saltvedt, S.; Söderling, J.; Pettersson, K.; Brandkvist, C.; Stephansson, O. Association of SARS-CoV-2 Test Status and Pregnancy Outcomes. *JAMA* **2020**, *324*, 1782–1785. [CrossRef] [PubMed]
12. Wei, S.Q.; Bilodeau-Bertrand, M.; Liu, S.; Auger, N. The impact of COVID-19 on pregnancy outcomes: A systematic review and meta-analysis. *CMAJ* **2021**, *193*, E540–E548. [CrossRef] [PubMed]
13. Mendoza, M.; Garcia-Ruiz, I.; Maiz, N.; Rodo, C.; Garcia-Manau, P.; Serrano, B.; Lopez-Martinez, R.M.; Balcells, J.; Fernandez-Hidalgo, N.; Carreras, E.; et al. Pre-eclampsia-like syndrome induced by severe COVID-19: A prospective observational study. *BJOG* **2020**, *127*, 1374–1380. [CrossRef] [PubMed]
14. Herraiz, I.; Llurba, E.; Verlohren, S.; Galindo, A.; Spanish Group for the Study of Angiogenic Markers in Preeclampsia. Update on the Diagnosis and Prognosis of Preeclampsia with the Aid of the sFlt-1/PlGF Ratio in Singleton Pregnancies. *Fetal Diagn. Ther.* **2018**, *43*, 81–89. [CrossRef] [PubMed]
15. Papageorghiou, A.T.; Deruelle, P.; Gunier, R.B.; Rauch, S.; García-May, P.K.; Mhatre, M.; Usman, M.A.; Abd-Elsalam, S.; Etuk, S.; Simmons, L.E.; et al. Preeclampsia and COVID-19: Results from the INTERCOVID prospective longitudinal study. *Am. J. Obstet. Gynecol.* **2021**, *225*, e1–e289. [CrossRef] [PubMed]
16. Gordijn, S.J.; Beune, I.M.; Thilaganathan, B.; Papageorghiou, A.; Baschat, A.A.; Baker, P.N.; Silver, R.M.; Wynia, K.; Ganzevoort, W. Consensus definition of fetal growth restriction: A Delphi procedure. *Ultrasound Obstet. Gynecol.* **2016**, *48*, 333–339. [CrossRef] [PubMed]
17. Bertino, E.; Di Nicola, P.; Varalda, A.; Occhi, L.; Giuliani, F.; Coscia, A. Neonatal growth charts. *J. Matern. Fetal Neonatal Med.* **2012**, *25* (Suppl. 1), 67–69. [CrossRef] [PubMed]

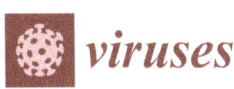

Article

Maternal Death by COVID-19 Associated with Elevated Troponin T Levels

Johnatan Torres-Torres [1,2,3,†], Raigam Jafet Martinez-Portilla [1,2,3,†], Salvador Espino y Sosa [1,2,3,*], Juan Mario Solis-Paredes [1], Jose Antonio Hernández-Pacheco [1], Paloma Mateu-Rogell [1,3], Anette Cravioto-Sapien [1], Adolfo Zamora-Madrazo [1], Guadalupe Estrada-Gutierrez [1], Miguel Angel Nares-Torices [1], Norma Patricia Becerra-Navarro [2], Virginia Medina-Jimenez [3], Jose Rafael Villafan-Bernal [3,4], Lourdes Rojas-Zepeda [5], Diana Hipolita Loya-Diaz [6] and Manuel Casillas-Barrera [7]

1. Clinical Research Branch, Instituto Nacional de Perinatología Isidro Espinosa de los Reyes, Mexico City 11000, Mexico; torresmmf@gmail.com (J.T.-T.); raifet@hotmail.com (R.J.M.-P.); juan.mario.sp@gmail.com (J.M.S.-P.); antonhernp@yahoo.com.mx (J.A.H.-P.); dramateurogell@gmail.com (P.M.-R.); cravioto.anette@gmail.com (A.C.-S.); adolfozm84@gmail.com (A.Z.-M.); gpestrad@gmail.com (G.E.-G.); drnarestorices@hotmail.com (M.A.N.-T.)
2. ABC Medical Center, Medical Association, Mexico City 05330, Mexico; npatriciabn@hotmail.com
3. Iberoamerican Research Network in Obstetrics, Gynecology and Translational Medicine, Mexico City 06720, Mexico; dravirginiamedina@gmail.com (V.M.-J.); joravibe@gmail.com (J.R.V.-B.)
4. Laboratory of Immunogenomics and Metabolic Diseases, INMEGEN, Mexico City 14610, Mexico
5. Instituto Materno Infantil del Estado de México, Toluca 50170, Mexico; dra.rojaszepeda@gmail.com
6. Maternal Fetal Medicine Department, Hospital General de Mexico "Dr. Eduardo Liceaga", Mexico City 06720, Mexico; dianitaldiaz@gmail.com
7. Hospital de la Mujer, Mexico City 11340, Mexico; mcasillasbarrera@gmail.com
* Correspondence: salvadorespino@gmail.com
† These authors contributed equally to this work.

Abstract: Cardiomyocyte injury and troponin T elevation has been reported within COVID-19 patients and are associated with a worse prognosis. Limited data report this association among COVID-19 pregnant patients. Objective: We aimed to analyze the association between troponin T levels in severe COVID-19 pregnant women and risk of viral sepsis, intensive care unit (ICU) admission, or maternal death. Methods: We performed a prospective cohort of all obstetrics emergency admissions from a Mexican National Institute. All pregnant women diagnosed by reverse transcription-polymerase chain reaction (RT-qPCR) for SARS-CoV-2 infection between October 2020 and May 2021 were included. Clinical data were collected, and routine blood samples were obtained at hospital admission. Seric troponin T was measured at admission. Results: From 87 included patients, 31 (35.63%) had severe COVID-19 pneumonia, and 6 (6.89%) maternal deaths. ROC showed a significant relationship between troponin T and maternal death (AUC 0.979, CI 0.500–1.000). At a cutoff point of 7 ng/mL the detection rate for severe pneumonia was 83.3% (95%CI: 0.500–0.100) at 10% false-positive rate. Conclusion: COVID-19 pregnant women with elevated levels of troponin T present a higher risk of death and severe pneumonia.

Keywords: COVID-19; maternal death; troponin T

1. Introduction

COVID-19 is currently the leading cause of maternal death in Mexico; during 2021, it was responsible for 46% of maternal deaths, double the maternal mortality ratio compared with the pre-pandemic stage (31.1 vs. 54.5 per 100 thousand births) [1]. Pregnant women are more susceptible to severe pneumonia and death due to physiological changes of pregnancy and systemic inflammation induced by the SARS-CoV2 infection [2–4]. In addition, the high prevalence of comorbidities such as obesity, diabetes, hypertension, and chronic kidney disease are major risk factors for death in pregnant women with COVID-19 [5].

One of the main characteristics of COVID-19 is its capacity to evolve into a severe disease affecting multiple organs, including the endothelium and the heart [6]. Myocardiocyte damage due to SARS-CoV-2 is frequent and has been described in up to 8–20% of infected patients, particularly in severe forms of the disease [7]. It has also been described that patients infected with SARS-CoV-2 may develop cardiac injury with long-time consequences that may even require cardiac rehabilitation, leading to cardiac dysfunction and arrhythmias [8]. Several mechanisms could explain how SARS-CoV-2 infection affects the myocardium and how a clinical heart disease may be expected from severe COVID-19 [8]. SARS-CoV-2 can directly injure myocardial cells by inducing a cytokine rush resulting in myocardial oxygen (supply/demand). This mechanism has been described as a common way of myocardial injury in other diseases related to inflammatory response syndrome [7]. This hypothesis is supported by increased serum cardiac enzymes such as troponin I, troponin T, and bNP, which are logical markers of a worse prognosis in COVID-19 [9,10].

There are scarce reports on the association between cardiac enzymes (troponin I, troponin T, and bNP) with severe pneumonia, viral sepsis, ICU admission, and death in pregnant women. We hypothesized that cardiac enzymes may be elevated in pregnant women with COVID-19, compared with those without COVID-19, and that they could also be associated with severe clinical outcomes among women with COVID-19. Thus, this study aimed to evaluate the association between troponin T and the risk of severe adverse maternal outcomes in pregnant women with COVID-19.

2. Materials and Methods

2.1. Study Design and Participants

We conducted a prospective cohort study in the National Institute of Perinatology "Isidro Espinosa de los Reyes" and General Hospital of Mexico "Dr. Eduardo Liceaga", in Mexico City. All symptomatic pregnant women with positive SARS-CoV-2 tests were included between December 2020 and September 2021. The Ethics and Research Internal Review Board of the National Institute of Perinatology approved the protocol (2020-1-32). All enrolled women signed informed consent.

2.2. Data Collection

The criterion for performing PCR was the identification of suggestive symptoms in the evaluation of emergency services, and blood samples were taken upon admission without taking into account the days of evolution of the symptoms. Medical data such as age, gestational age, pregestational body mass index (pBMI (kg/m^2)), the status of chronic hypertension, pre-gestational diabetes, chronic renal disease, mean arterial pressure (MAP), oxygen saturation (SpO2), preeclampsia, threatened preterm labor, fetal growth restriction, stillbirth, pneumonia, viral sepsis, and mortality were collected from medical records. Rutinary blood samples were obtained at hospital admission. Troponin T and D-dimer serum levels were measured by an automated analyzer (Cobas-t511, Roche®, Mexico City, Mexico), whereas C-reactive protein serum levels were measured using an automated analyzer (Cobas-501, Roche®, Mexico City, Mexico) according to the manufacturer's instructions.

2.3. Outcome

The primary outcome was maternal death as a direct cause of COVID-19. Secondary outcomes were severe pneumonia, the requirement of ICU admission, and viral sepsis.

Severe pneumonia was defined according to the American Thoracic Society criteria, which include either one major criterion (septic shock with the need for vasopressors or respiratory failure requiring mechanical ventilation) or three or more minor criteria (respiratory rate $\geq$ 30 breaths/min; PaO_2/FIO_2 ratio $\leq$ 250; multilobar infiltrates; confusion/disorientation; uremia (blood urea nitrogen level $\geq$ 20 mg/dL); leukopenia (white blood cell count < 4000 cells/µL); thrombocytopenia (platelet count < 100,000/µL); hypothermia (core temperature < 36 °C); hypotension requiring aggressive fluid resuscitation) [11,12]. ICU admission was decided according to the Quick Sequential Organ Failure

Assessment (qSOFA) score, where a score ≥ 2 points would require ICU admission [13]. Viral sepsis is defined as life-threatening organ dysfunction caused by a dysregulated host response to infection, following the Third International Consensus Definitions for Sepsis and Septic Shock (Sepsis-3), organ dysfunction can be identified as an acute change in total SOFA score ≥2 points consequent to the confirmed SARS-CoV-2 infection [14].

2.4. Statistical Analysis

Descriptive and inferential statistics were used. Quantitative variables were reported as the median and interquartile range (IQR), while qualitative data were reported as numbers and percentages. Among patients with pneumonia, differences between variables were compared with maternal death using the Mann–Whitney U test or X^2 test. Forward and backward stepwise logistic regression analyses were performed to assess the association between independent variables and the primary and secondary outcomes. After logistic regression, the adjusted model's performance was evaluated by receiver-operating curve (ROC) analysis estimating the area under the curve (AUC). A p-value < 0.05 was considered significant. (StataCorp, 2020, Stata Statistical Software: Release 17; StataCorp LLC., College Station, TX, USA).

3. Results

3.1. Description of the Cohort

A total of 115 pregnant women with suspected SARS-CoV-2 infection were included in the original cohort. In total, 28 were excluded because although they were COVID positive, they did not warrant hospital admission or additional biochemical evaluation, as they were asymptomatic. Consequently, 87 symptomatic pregnant women with SARS-CoV-2 infection were included in the statistical analysis: of those, 31 (35.63%) had severe COVID-19 pneumonia, including 6 (6.89%) maternal deaths.

3.2. Comparison of Women with Severe and Non-Severe Pneumonia by COVID-19

In baseline characteristics, there were some differences between women with severe and non-severe pneumonia by COVID-19. Women with severe pneumonia had lower median gestational age at hospital admission (30.3 vs. 35.3; p = 0.002) and lower oxygen saturation (O2Sat%) (91.1 vs. 95.6; p = 0.005) than those with non-severe pneumonia. Women with severe pneumonia had significantly higher troponin T serum levels and other hematological and biochemical parameters than non-severe pneumonia. There was no significant correlation between the results of D-dimer with severity. Compared with non-severe pneumonia, those patients with severe pneumonia had a higher frequency of fetal growth restriction, stillbirth, ICU admission, viral sepsis, multiple organ dysfunction, and maternal death (Table 1).

3.3. Clinical and Biochemical Profile of Deceased Patients and Survivors

Among 31 pregnant women with severe pneumonia by COVID-19, there were six maternal deaths. Compared with survivors, the patients who died exhibit higher frequency of smoking habit, stillbirth (33.3% vs. 4%; p = 0.029), ICU admission (100% vs. 50%; p = 0.025), and viral sepsis (66.6% vs. 8%; p = 0.001). Additionally, they had higher levels of troponin T (p = 0.001) (70.45 vs. 92.25.; p = 0.009) and myoglobin (Table 1).

3.4. Association of Troponin and Maternal Outcome

Compared with non-severe COVID-19 (1.2 ng/mL), the median of troponin T serum levels in patients required ICU admission (5.7 ng/mL), with viral sepsis (12.3 ng/mL) and deceased (17.8 ng/mL) were significantly higher (Figure 1).

Table 1. Clinical characteristics of the included population.

Characteristics	COVID-19		p-Value
	Non-Severe Pneumonia n = 56	Severe Pneumonia n = 31	
Maternal age	30.46 (26.38–33.47)	31.19 (26.38–35.55)	0.361
Gestational age at diagnosis	35.3 (30–39.1)	30.3 (25.1–33.3)	0.002
pBMI (kg/m^2)	31.42 (26.7–34.25)	26.83 (25.39–33.05)	0.135
MAP (mmHg)	85.5 (80.16–92)	87.66 (80–95.33)	0.657
Smoking	0 (0%)	2 (6.45%)	0.054
Chronic hypertension	2 (3.57%)	1 (3.33%)	0.954
Pre-gestational diabetes	3 (5.36%)	0 (0%)	0.190
Chronic kidney disease	2 (3.57%)	0 (0%)	0.287
SpO2%	95.6 (93–96.4)	91.1 (79.4–95.4)	0.005
Leukocytes (x10/L)	8.15 (7–10)	9.8 (7.8–13.5)	0.017
Neutrophils (x10/L)	6.35 (5.3–7.4)	8.8 (6.9–13)	0.0003
Glucose (mg/dL)	77.5 (73–85)	87 (75–116)	0.006
Troponin T (ng/mL)	1.2 (0.3–2.05)	2.7 (1.3–7.1)	0.0001
Myoglobin	17.8 (13.4–27.1)	29.3 (19.2–48)	0.010
D-dimer (ng/mL)	1916 (1262–2953)	1425 (1184–4083)	0.532
C-RP	16.25 (7.04–60.6)	110.5 (63.8–200)	0.0001
AST (U/L)	19 (15–32)	31 (24–49)	0.0001
ALT (U/L)	16 (11–28)	26 (18–40)	0.003
LDH (U/L)	173 (140–201)	249 (192–375)	0.0001
Direct bilirubin	0.1 (0.07–0.18)	0.22 (0.13–0.38)	0.001
Indirect bilirubin	0.32 (0.24–0.44)	0.42 (0.31–0.49)	0.075
Cholesterol	206.5 (171–240)	155 (128–187)	0.0003
Procalcitonin	0.05 (0.03–0.13)	0.39 (0.18–0.68)	0.0001
Preeclampsia (clinical diagnosis)	9 (16.36%)	8 (25.81%)	0.291
Threatened preterm labor	3 (5.56%)	3 (9.68%)	0.475
Fetal growth restriction	4 (7.41%)	7 (23.33%)	0.038
Stillbirth	0 (0%)	3 (9.68%)	0.020
ICU admission	0 (0%)	18 (60%)	<0.0001
Viral sepsis	0 (0%)	6 (19.35%)	0.001
Multiple organ dysfunction	0 (0%)	4 (12.9%)	0.006
Maternal death	0 (0%)	6 (19.35%)	0.001

pBMI: pre-gestational body mass index; MAP: mean arterial pressure; MoM: multiples of the median; SpO2: oxygen saturation; Mann–Whitney U test for continuous variables is expressed as median and interquartile range; X^2 or Fisher's test for categorical variables is expressed as number and percentage.

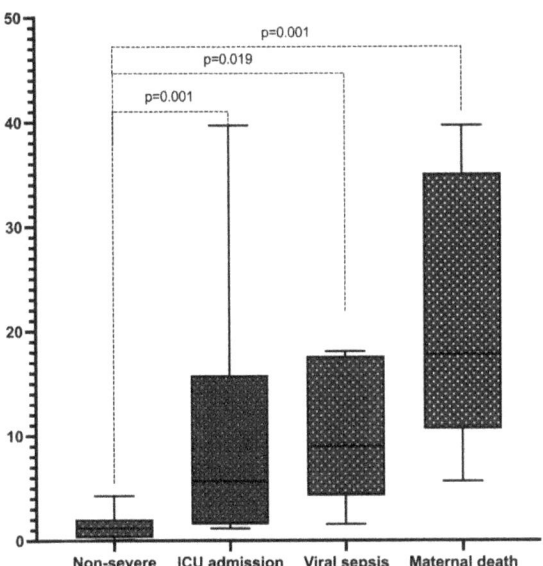

Figure 1. Troponin T levels in severe COVID-19 pregnant women with adverse outcomes. Non-severe n = 56 (1.2 ng/mL (0.3–2.05 ng/mL)); ICU admission n = 18 (5.7 ng/mL (1.25–14.9 ng/mL)); viral sepsis n = 6 (12.3 ng/mL (5.7–17.5 ng/mL)); maternal death n = 6 (17.8 ng/mL (12.3–33.6 ng/mL)).

In ROC analysis, (n = 87) the troponin T predicted maternal death (AUC 0.833, CI 0.500–1.000). At a 10% false-positive rate, a cutoff point of 7 ng/mL predicted maternal death with a sensibility of 83.3% (Figure 2), which means that troponin T had an excellent predictive value for maternal death in the pregnant population with PCR positive for SARS-CoV-2 who presented symptomatically to the emergency department. This adequate balance between sensitivity and specificity for the analyzed outcomes motivated us to explore its predictive performance.

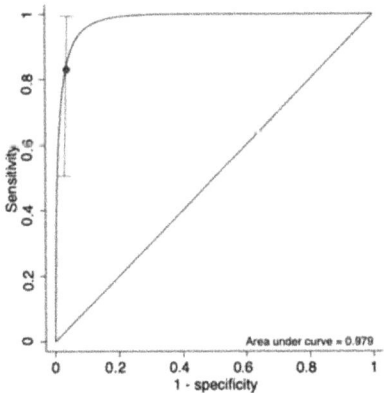

Figure 2. Area under the receiver-operating curve (ROC) of troponin T for the prediction of maternal death by COVID-19. Detection rate for maternal death at a 10% false-positive rate was 83.3% (95%CI:0.500–0.100).

Through a multinomial logistic regression, we further analyzed the relationship of elevated troponin T with maternal outcomes. A troponin T value higher than 7 ng/mL was significantly related to severe pneumonia (OR 1.51, CI95% 1.15–1.98, $p < 0.003$), viral sepsis (OR 1.12, CI95% 1.008–1.254, $p = 0.035$), ICU admission (OR 1.17, CI95% 1.054–1.311, $p = 0.004$), and maternal death (OR 1.42, CI95% 1.13–1.784, $p = 0.003$) (Table 2).

Table 2. COVID-19 complications associated with elevated troponin.

	OR	95%CI	p-Value	aOR	95%CI	p-Value
Severe pneumonia	1.52	1.156–1.991	0.003	1.51	1.151–1.983	0.003
Viral sepsis	1.08	1.003–1.169	0.039	1.12	1.008–1.254	0.035
ICU admission	1.17	1.037–1.319	0.01	1.17	1.054–1.311	0.004
Maternal death	1.27	1.084–1.498	0.003	1.42	1.13–1.784	0.003

OR: odds ratio; aOR: adjusted odds ratio with BMI; ICU: intensive care unit.

4. Discussion

4.1. Main Findings

The principal findings of this study are that higher levels of troponin in pregnant women with severe pneumonia by COVID-19 are associated with a 1.17-fold increase in ICU admission, a 1.12-fold increase in viral sepsis, and a 1.42-fold increase in maternal death.

4.2. Comparison with Existing Literature

Cardiac troponins are used in clinical practice to study cardiac damage in acute coronary syndrome (ACS), septic shock, and more recently, in SARS-CoV-2 infection [15,16]. Elevated troponin levels are frequently found in patients with COVID-19 as a result of viral myocarditis, cytokine-driven myocardial damage, microangiopathy, and unmasked coronary artery disease [17].

Ruiz Mercedes et al. reported the elevation of serum troponins resulting from myocardial injury and left ventricular dysfunction in a case series of 15 pregnant women diagnosed with COVID-19, with a 13.3% mortality rate [18]. However, they did not study the relationship of troponin T with adverse maternal outcomes. Cortes-Telles et al. conducted a cohort of 200 Mexican patients where troponin T elevation was associated with an OR for mortality of 6.3 (CI95% 3.30–12.05) $p < 0.001$ [19]. Thus, our results in pregnant women with severe pneumonia reinforce the utility of troponin T as a prognostic marker related to death in pregnant women testing positive for COVID-19. In addition, levels higher than 7 ng/mL are related to the risk of sepsis, severe pneumonia, and admission to ICU.

Our results are supported by observations in non-pregnant critical COVID-19 patients for whom cardiac biomarkers (troponin I, troponin T, creatine kinase-MB, and myoglobin) predict poor prognosis [20].

Cardiomyocytes infection by SARS-CoV2 occurs through ACE 2 receptors, which are highly expressed in these cells. Under normal circumstances, ACE2 activity confers cardiovascular protection [21], because its peptidase activity cleaves angiotensin II (Ang II) into angiotensin 1–7 (Ang 1–7) [22,23]. As a result of infection, ACE2 activity decreases because it binds to SARS-CoV-2, and the complex is internalized to the cell. [24] In consequence, ACE activity is increased, producing an elevation of Ang II serum levels, which promotes cardiac damage/injury through vasoconstriction [21].

In those diagnosed with COVID-19, Ang II serum levels are lower in deceased patients, compared with surviving patients [25]. A hypothetical mechanism leading to this relative decrease in Ang II levels in non-surviving patients is through a greater binding of Ang II to cell surface AT1 (AT1a) receptors, which induces downstream signaling responses, followed by quicker endocytosis of the Ang II/AT1. Excess cytoplasmic Ang II induces overproduction of mitochondrial reactive oxygen species (ROS) [26].

Oxidative damage of cardiomyocytes causes an alteration to the membrane integrity leaking cardiac troponin T. It also seems that COVID-19 reduces blood flow to coronary arteries resulting in myocardial damage. SARS-CoV-2 may lead to severe endothelial inflammation, leading to atherosclerotic plaque instability and rupture [27]. Aside from vasoconstriction and hypercoagulable state, all these mechanisms contribute to myocardial damage [28].

4.3. Strengths and Limitations

Some limitations should be reported. Firstly, due to the span of the study, the sample was relatively small; therefore, analysis of a larger patient's sample will be needed for external validation and replication in other populations. In addition, some other specific myocardial damage biomarkers such as troponin I and pro-BNP could not be measured, and therefore, an improved approach that includes the analysis of these cardiac enzymes is suggested in future research.

4.4. Clinical Interpretation

Decision-making can benefit from the evaluation of functional and/or structural cardiovascular damage through monitoring and surveillance with electrocardiography and echocardiography, screening of inflammatory and cardiac biomarkers, mainly troponin T, and inflammatory markers of the acute phase of the disease such as water balance, together with SOFA, APACHE, MEWT, MEOWS scores at hospital admission of all pregnant women with COVID-19.

From the fetal point of view, carditis is one of the components of multiple organ failure due to SARS-CoV-2, (which causes inflammation of the myocardium with troponin release) that leads to heart failure and arrhythmias, decreasing cardiac output, which affects the uteroplacental flow, and it would have repercussions on the efficiency of the exchange membrane; this causal relationship has not been studied. This supports fetal surveillance during the critical period of COVID-19 with an emphasis on characterizing the area of exchange and redistribution of fetal vascular flows.

5. Conclusions

Elevated levels of troponin T among pregnant women with COVID-19 present a higher risk of death. Therefore, myocardial biomarkers should be evaluated in pregnant patients with COVID-19 that require hospital admission for risk stratification purposes.

Author Contributions: Conceptualization, S.E.yS., J.T.-T., R.J.M.-P. and J.M.S.-P.; methodology, J.T.-T., G.E.-G. and J.M.S.-P.; formal analysis, J.T.-T., G.E.-G., S.E.yS., J.A.H.-P., R.J.M.-P. and J.M.S.-P.; investigation, J.A.H.-P., P.M.-R., A.C.-S., A.Z.-M., D.H.L.-D., M.C.-B., M.A.N.-T. and N.P.B.-N.; resources, J.T.-T. and G.E.-G.; writing—original draft preparation, P.M.-R., A.C.-S., A.Z.-M. and V.M.-J.; writing—review and editing, J.T.-T., G.E.-G., S.E.yS., J.A.H.-P., R.J.M.-P., L.R.-Z., V.M.-J., J.R.V.-B. and J.M.S.-P.; visualization, S.E.yS., J.T.-T., J.M.S.-P., R.J.M.-P. and G.E.-G.; supervision J.T.-T., J.M.S.-P. and S.E.yS.; project administration, M.C.-B., J.T.-T. and G.E.-G.; funding acquisition, J.T.-T. and G.E.-G. All authors have read and agreed to the published version of the manuscript.

Funding: This research was funded by the Instituto Nacional de Perinatología (grant 2020-1-32).

Institutional Review Board Statement: The study was conducted according to the guidelines of the Declaration of Helsinki and approved by the Institutional Review Board of Instituto Nacional de Perinatología. (Register Number 2020-1-32, date of approval 16 December 2020).

Informed Consent Statement: Informed consent was obtained from all subjects involved in the study.

Data Availability Statement: The data presented in this study are available on request from the corresponding author. The data are not publicly available due to privacy.

Acknowledgments: This work would not have been possible without the effort of the healthcare workers in the COVID areas (epidemiology, nursery, obstetrics and gynecology, researchers, residents, interns, attendings, postgraduate students, medical students, and the molecular diagnosis teams) in the Instituto Nacional de Perinatologia, and Hospital General de Mexico "Eduardo Liceaga".

Conflicts of Interest: The authors declare no conflict of interest.

References

1. Observatorio de Mortalidad Materna de México. Paperpile. Available online: https://paperpile.com/app/p/10cf28f7-a201-0bdd-891b-a4f1cff572eb (accessed on 19 November 2021).
2. Martinez-Portilla, R.J.; Sotiriadis, A.; Chatzakis, C.; Torres-Torres, J.; Espino Y Sosa, S.; Sandoval-Mandujano, K.; Castro-Bernabe, D.A.; Medina-Jimenez, V.; Monarrez-Martin, J.C.; Figueras, F.; et al. Pregnant women with SARS-CoV-2 infection are at higher risk of death and pneumonia: Propensity score matched analysis of a nationwide prospective cohort (COV19Mx). *Ultrasound Obstet. Gynecol.* **2021**, *57*, 224–231. [CrossRef]
3. Zambrano, L.D.; Ellington, S.; Strid, P.; Galang, R.R.; Oduyebo, T.; Tong, V.T.; Woodworth, K.R.; Nahabedian, J.F.; Azziz-Baumgartner, E.; Gilboa, S.M.; et al. Update: Characteristics of Symptomatic Women of Reproductive Age with Laboratory-Confirmed SARS-CoV-2 Infection by Pregnancy Status—United States, January 22–October 3, 2020. *MMWR. Morb. Mortal. Wkly. Rep.* **2020**, *69*, 1641–1647. [CrossRef]
4. Wang, Z.; Wang, Z.; Xiong, G. Clinical characteristics and laboratory results of pregnant women with COVID-19 in Wuhan, China. *Int. J. Gynecol. Obstet.* **2020**, *150*, 312–317. [CrossRef]
5. La Peña, J.E.-D.; Rascón-Pacheco, R.A.; Ascencio-Montiel, I.D.J.; González-Figueroa, E.; Fernández-Gárate, J.E.; Medina-Gómez, O.S.; Borja-Bustamante, P.; Santillán-Oropeza, J.A.; Borja-Aburto, V.H. Hypertension, Diabetes and Obesity, Major Risk Factors for Death in Patients with COVID-19 in Mexico. *Arch. Med Res.* **2021**, *52*, 443–449. [CrossRef]
6. Flaumenhaft, R.; Enjyoji, K.; A Schmaier, A. Vasculopathy in COVID-19. *Blood* **2022**. [CrossRef] [PubMed]
7. Lippi, G.; Plebani, M. Laboratory abnormalities in patients with COVID-2019 infection. *Clin. Chem. Lab. Med.* **2020**, *58*, 1131–1134. [CrossRef] [PubMed]
8. Yuan, H.; Liu, J.; Gao, Z.; Hu, F. Clinical Features and Outcomes of Acute Kidney Injury in Patients Infected with COVID-19 in Xiangyang, China. *Blood Purif.* **2020**, *50*, 513–519. [CrossRef] [PubMed]
9. Piccioni, A.; Brigida, M.; Loria, V.; Zanza, C.; Longhitano, Y.; Zaccaria, R.; Racco, S.; Gasbarrini, A.; Ojetti, V.; Franceschi, F.; et al. Role of troponin in COVID-19 pandemic: A review of literature. *Eur. Rev. Med. Pharmacol. Sci.* **2020**, *24*, 10293–10300. [PubMed]
10. Guo, T.; Fan, Y.; Chen, M.; Wu, X.; Zhang, L.; He, T.; Wang, H.; Wan, J.; Wang, X.; Lu, Z. Cardiovascular Implications of Fatal Outcomes of Patients With Coronavirus Disease 2019 (COVID-19). *JAMA Cardiol.* **2020**, *5*, 811–818. [CrossRef] [PubMed]
11. Moberg, A. *Diagnosing Pneumonia in Primary Care: Aspects of the Value of Clinical and Laboratory Findings and the Use of Chest X-Ray*; Linköping University: Linköping, Sweden, 2020.
12. Poon, L.C.; Yang, H.; Kapur, A.; Melamed, N.; Dao, B.; Divakar, H.; McIntyre, H.D.; Kihara, A.B.; Ayres-De-Campos, D.; Ferrazzi, E.M.; et al. Global interim guidance on coronavirus disease 2019 (COVID-19) during pregnancy and puerperium from FIGO and allied partners: Information for healthcare professionals. *Int. J. Gynecol. Obstet.* **2020**, *149*, 273–286. [CrossRef] [PubMed]
13. Jiang, J.; Yang, J.; Mei, J.; Jin, Y.; Lu, Y. Head-to-head comparison of qSOFA and SIRS criteria in predicting the mortality of infected patients in the emergency department: A meta-analysis. *Scand. J. Trauma Resusc. Emerg. Med.* **2018**, *26*, 1–11. [CrossRef] [PubMed]
14. Murphy, S.R.; Cockrell, K. Regulation of soluble fms-like tyrosine kinase-1 production in response to placental ischemia/hypoxia: Role of angiotensin II. *Physiol. Rep.* **2015**, *3*, e12310. [CrossRef]
15. Li, H.; Liu, L.; Zhang, D.; Xu, J.; Dai, H.; Tang, N.; Su, X.; Cao, B. SARS-CoV-2 and viral sepsis: Observations and hypotheses. *Lancet* **2020**, *395*, 1517–1520. [CrossRef]
16. Maeder, M.; Fehr, T.; Rickli, H.; Ammann, P. Sepsis-Associated Myocardial Dysfunction. *Chest* **2006**, *129*, 1349–1366. [CrossRef]
17. Tersalvi, G.; Vicenzi, M.; Calabretta, D.; Biasco, L.; Pedrazzini, G.; Winterton, D. Elevated Troponin in Patients with Coronavirus Disease 2019: Possible Mechanisms. *J. Card. Fail.* **2020**, *26*, 470–475. [CrossRef] [PubMed]
18. Mercedes, B.R.; Serwat, A.; Naffaa, L.; Ramirez, N.; Khalid, F.; Steward, S.B.; Feliz, O.G.C.; Kassab, M.B.; Karout, L. New-onset myocardial injury in pregnant patients with coronavirus disease 2019: A case series of 15 patients. *Am. J. Obstet. Gynecol.* **2021**, *224*, 387.e1–387.e9. [CrossRef]
19. Cortés-Téllés, A.; López-Romero, S.; Mancilla-Ceballos, R.; Ortíz-Farías, D.L.; Núñez-Caamal, N.; Figueroa-Hurtado, E. Risk Factors for Mortality in Hospitalized Patients with COVID-19: An Overview in a Mexican Population. *Tuberc. Respir. Dis.* **2020**, *83*, S46–S54. [CrossRef]
20. An, W.; Kang, J.-S.; Wang, Q.; Kim, T.-E. Cardiac biomarkers and COVID-19: A systematic review and meta-analysis. *J. Infect. Public Heal.* **2021**, *14*, 1191–1197. [CrossRef]
21. Kalra, R.S.; Tomar, D.; Meena, A.S.; Kandimalla, R. SARS-CoV-2, ACE2, and Hydroxychloroquine: Cardiovascular Complications, Therapeutics, and Clinical Readouts in the Current Settings. *Pathogens* **2020**, *9*, 546. [CrossRef] [PubMed]
22. Eleuteri, D.; Montini, L.; Cutuli, S.L.; Rossi, C.; Alcaro, F.; Antonelli, M. Renin–angiotensin system dysregulation in critically ill patients with acute respiratory distress syndrome due to COVID-19: A preliminary report. *Crit. Care* **2021**, *25*, 1–3. [CrossRef]

23. Santos, R.A.S.; Sampaio, W.O.; Alzamora, A.C.; Motta-Santos, D.; Alenina, N.; Bader, M.; Campagnole-Santos, M.J. The ACE2/Angiotensin-(1–7)/MAS Axis of the Renin-Angiotensin System: Focus on Angiotensin-(1–7). *Physiol. Rev.* **2018**, *98*, 505–553. [CrossRef] [PubMed]
24. Zhang, H.; Penninger, J.M.; Li, Y.; Zhong, N.; Slutsky, A.S. Angiotensin-converting enzyme 2 (ACE2) as a SARS-CoV-2 receptor: Molecular mechanisms and potential therapeutic target. *Intensive Care Med.* **2020**, *46*, 586–590. [CrossRef] [PubMed]
25. Espino-Y-Sosa, S.; Martinez-Portilla, R.J.; Torres-Torres, J.; Solis-Paredes, J.M.; Estrada-Gutierrez, G.; Hernandez-Pacheco, J.A.; Espejel-Nuñez, A.; Mateu-Rogell, P.; Juarez-Reyes, A.; Lopez-Ceh, F.E.; et al. Novel Ratio Soluble Fms-like Tyrosine Kinase-1/Angiotensin-II (sFlt-1/ANG-II) in Pregnant Women Is Associated with Critical Illness in COVID-19. *Viruses* **2021**, *13*, 1906. [CrossRef] [PubMed]
26. Li, X.C.; Zhou, X.; Zhuo, J.L. Evidence for a Physiological Mitochondrial Angiotensin II System in the Kidney Proximal Tubules. *Hypertens.* **2020**, *76*, 121–132. [CrossRef]
27. Yang, C.; Liu, F.; Liu, W.; Cao, G.; Liu, J.; Huang, S.; Zhu, M.; Tu, C.; Wang, J.; Xiong, B. Myocardial injury and risk factors for mortality in patients with COVID-19 pneumonia. *Int. J. Cardiol.* **2021**, *326*, 230–236. [CrossRef]
28. Ogungbe, O.; Kumbe, B.; Fadodun, O.; Latha, T.; Meyer, D.; Asala, A.; Davidson, P.M.; Himmelfarb, C.R.D.; Post, W.S.; Commodore-Mensah, Y. Subclinical myocardial injury, coagulopathy, and inflammation in COVID-19: A meta-analysis of 41,013 hospitalized patients. *Int. J. Cardiol. Heart Vasc.* **2022**, 100950. [CrossRef]

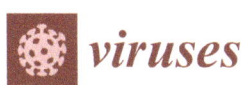

Case Report

Decreased Fetal Movements: A Sign of Placental SARS-CoV-2 Infection with Perinatal Brain Injury

Guillaume Favre [1,†], Sara Mazzetti [2,†], Carole Gengler [3,†], Claire Bertelli [4], Juliane Schneider [5], Bernard Laubscher [2,6], Romina Capoccia [7], Fatemeh Pakniyat [7], Inès Ben Jazia [7], Béatrice Eggel-Hort [8], Laurence de Leval [3], Léo Pomar [1,9], Gilbert Greub [4,10], David Baud [1,*,†] and Eric Giannoni [5,†]

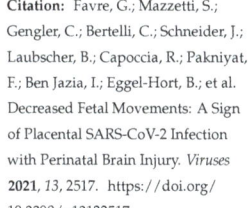

1. Materno-Fetal and Obstetrics Research Unit, Department Woman-Mother-Child, Lausanne University Hospital, University of Lausanne, 1011 Lausanne, Switzerland; guillaume.favre@chuv.ch (G.F.); leo.pomar@chuv.ch (L.P.)
2. Clinic of Pediatrics, Department Mother-Woman-Child, Lausanne University Hospital, University of Lausanne, 1011 Lausanne, Switzerland; sara.mazzetti@chuv.ch (S.M.); Bernard.Laubscher@chuv.ch (B.L.)
3. Department of Laboratory Medicine and Pathology, Institute of Pathology, Lausanne University Hospital, University of Lausanne, 1011 Lausanne, Switzerland; carole.gengler@chuv.ch (C.G.); Laurence.DeLeval@chuv.ch (L.d.L.)
4. Institute of Microbiology, Lausanne University Hospital, University of Lausanne, 1011 Lausanne, Switzerland; Claire.Bertelli@chuv.ch (C.B.); Gilbert.Greub@chuv.ch (G.G.)
5. Clinic of Neonatology, Department Mother-Woman-Child, Lausanne University Hospital, University of Lausanne, 1011 Lausanne, Switzerland; juliane.schneider@chuv.ch (J.S.); eric.giannoni@chuv.ch (E.G.)
6. Department of Pediatrics, Réseau Hospitalier Neuchâtelois, 2000 Neuchâtel, Switzerland
7. Department of Obstetrics and Gynecology, Réseau Hospitalier Neuchâtelois, 2000 Neuchatel, Switzerland; romina.capoccia-brugger@rhne.ch (R.C.); Fatemeh.Pakniyat@rhne.ch (F.P.); ines.ben-jazia@rhne.ch (I.B.J.)
8. Department of Obstetrics and Gynecology, Hôpital du Valais—Centre Hospitalier du Valais Romand—Site de Sion, 1951 Sion, Switzerland; Beatrice.Eggel-Hort@hopitalvs.ch
9. Midwifery Department, School of Health Sciences (HESAV), University of Applied Sciences and Arts Western Switzerland, 1011 Lausanne, Switzerland
10. Infectious Diseases Service, Department of Internal Medicine, Lausanne University Hospital, University of Lausanne, 1011 Lausanne, Switzerland
* Correspondence: david.baud@chuv.ch; Tel.: +41-79-556-13-51
† These authors contributed equally to this work.

Abstract: Neonatal COVID-19 is rare and mainly results from postnatal transmission. Severe acute respiratory syndrome coronavirus 2 (SARS-CoV-2), however, can infect the placenta and compromise its function. We present two cases of decreased fetal movements and abnormal fetal heart rhythm 5 days after mild maternal COVID-19, requiring emergency caesarean section at 29 + 3 and 32 + 1 weeks of gestation, and leading to brain injury. Placental examination revealed extensive and multifocal chronic intervillositis, with intense cytoplasmic positivity for SARS-CoV-2 spike antibody and SARS-CoV-2 detection by RT-qPCR. Vertical transmission was confirmed in one case, and both neonates developed extensive cystic peri-ventricular leukomalacia.

Keywords: SARS-CoV-2; COVID-19; perinatal; placental; brain injury; fetal movements; neurosonography; MRI

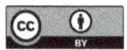

1. Introduction

Severe acute respiratory syndrome coronavirus 2 (SARS-CoV-2) is causing a major and devastating pandemic, with pregnant women representing a group at increased risk of severe coronavirus disease 2019 (COVID-19) [1–4], as with other infectious disease [5]. Nevertheless, neonates are relatively spared, with the majority of infants from COVID-19-affected pregnant women exhibiting a favorable short-term outcome [6,7]. SARS-CoV-2, however, can infect the placenta and compromise its function, leading to fetal distress, intrauterine death, or perinatal asphyxia [6,8–11]. Case reports have described severe neonatal disease in infants from COVID-19-affected mothers, with respiratory failure and/or brain damage [8–10,12]. These findings, however, could not be unambiguously attributed to SARS-CoV-2 infection, due to the absence of documentation of vertical transmission and the presence of comorbidities, in particular prematurity. Vertical transmission is proven when the following criteria from the World Health Organization (WHO) are met: evidence of maternal SARS-CoV-2 infection during pregnancy, in utero fetal SARS-CoV-2 exposure, and SARS-CoV-2 persistence or immune response in the neonate [13].

Here, we present two women who developed mild COVID-19 confirmed by nasopharyngeal PCR during their third trimester of pregnancy. Both presented with decreased fetal movements five days after the onset of symptoms requiring an emergency caesarean section (C-section). The two cases of confirmed and strongly suspected congenital SARS-CoV-2 infection were associated with brain damage in neonates.

2. Methods

2.1. Patients' Consent and Ethical Approval

We obtained institutional review board approval and written informed consent from both patients.

2.2. Sample Collection and Microbiological Investigation

Within minutes of placental extraction by C-section, the fetal surface of the placenta was disinfected and incised with a sterile scalpel, and 2 swabs and biopsies were obtained as previously described [14]. For the first case, we collected cord blood in the sterile surgical field immediately after clamping the umbilical cord, and collected neonatal endotracheal secretions using a sterile procedure. RNA was extracted using a MagNA-Pure 96 instrument (Roche, Basel, Switzerland), and quantitative SARS-CoV-2 reverse transcriptase–polymerase chain reaction (RT-qPCR) was performed using an automated platform [15,16] on samples from mothers, placentas, and infants. Quantification was performed using calibrated positive plasmid controls and a calibrated SARS-CoV-2 cell culture supernatant [16]. No amniotic fluid samples were collected for SARS-CoV-2 screening.

2.3. Placental Examination and In Situ SARS-CoV-2 Detection

Placentas were fixed in 4% buffered formalin. Sampling was performed as previously described [17]. After hematoxylin and eosin staining of paraffin-embedded tissues, we stained samples for immunohistochemical studies with CD68-PGM1, ACE2, and SARS-CoV-2 spike antibodies. We performed in situ detection of SARS-CoV-2 mRNA by RNAScope technology on 4 µm sections from selected formalin-fixed, paraffin-embedded (FFPE) tissue blocks. SARS-CoV-2 detection and quantification by RT-qPCR was performed for both cases, starting from total RNA extracted from 10 µm thick sections of placental FFPE tissue blocks containing foci of chronic intervillositis.

2.4. SARS-CoV-2 Genome Sequencing

The CleanPlex SARS-CoV-2 Panel (Paragon Genomics, Hayward, CA, USA) were used according to the manufacturer's protocol to amplify the SARS-CoV-2 genome from the RNA used for RT-qPCR, as detailed previously [18]. Tiled amplicon libraries were analyzed using a Fragment Analyzer (standard sensitivity NGS, AATI) and quantified with a Qubit Standard Sensitivity NGS dsDNA kit (Invitrogen, Waltham, MA, USA) before sequencing on an Illumina MiSeq (San Diego, CA, USA). We analyzed sequence reads using GENCOV (https://github.com/metagenlab/GENCOV/releases/tag/1.0, accessed on 1 December 2021), a modified version of CoVpipe (https://gitlab.com/RKIBioinformaticsPipelines/ncov_minipipe, accessed on 1 December 2021). SARS-CoV-2 lineages were assigned with pangolin [19].

3. Case Description

3.1. Case 1

A primiparous 34-year-old previously healthy pregnant woman presented to a regional hospital at 28 + 4 weeks of gestation with chills, fever, myalgia, ageusia, and anosmia. She tested positive for SARS-CoV-2. As the obstetrical examination was unremarkable, she was discharged home the same day, and symptoms resolved rapidly. Five days later, she presented again for reduced fetal movements, confirmed by ultrasound, which motivated transfer to a tertiary center after a first dose of Betamethasone, 12 mg, for fetal lung maturation. Urine and blood tests were normal, with the exception of thrombocytopenia at 63 G/L (first trimester platelet count was in the normal range) and elevated D-dimers (14,860 ng/mL). Due to non-reassuring fetal heart rate (FHR) (Figure S1 in the Supplementary Materials), absence of fetal movements, and abnormal fetal Doppler (inversed cerebroplacental ratio) suggestive of fetal distress, an emergency C-section without trial of labor and intact amniotic membranes was performed at 29 + 1 weeks' gestation.

3.2. Case 2

A 29-year-old primigravida with gestational diabetes on diet presented to a regional hospital with fever and flu-like symptoms at 31 + 0 weeks' gestation. She tested positive for SARS-CoV-2 two days after the onset of symptoms and quarantined at home. Five days later, she presented with decreased fetal movements. As the obstetrical examination was unremarkable, the patient was discharged home. Three days later, she was admitted, complaining of absent fetal movements. Abnormal FHR pattern led to an emergency C-section. Basic laboratory tests were within the normal range.

4. Results

4.1. Maternal Outcomes

Both mothers recovered well after delivery. Case 1 had persistent anosmia and ageusia, and her platelet count and D-dimers normalized spontaneously. Both were discharged home at 5 days after C-section.

4.2. Placenta Analysis

The weight of the two placentas were normal (50–70th percentile) for gestational age. Gross examination of cross sections showed massive transplacental changes with trabeculae and lattice-like deposition of fibrin, affecting more than 80% of the total placental volume (Figure S2 in the Supplementary Materials). Extensive and multifocal chronic intervillositis, characterized by clusters of CD68-positive histiocytes, filled up the intervillous space (Figure 1). Chorionic villi were largely spared from the inflammatory process. The histiocytic intervillous infiltrate was associated with peri-villous fibrin deposition and extensive placental infarction. Intervillous inflammation closely encircled the chorionic villi, and their trophoblastic cells showed a membranous staining for ACE2, as well as an intense cytoplasmic positivity for SARS-CoV-2 spike antibody in both cases. Areas of villi not expressing the SARS-CoV-2 spike protein were not surrounded by CD68-positive histiocytes. SARS-CoV-2 was detected in areas of chronic intervillositis by RT-qPCR in FFPE tissue blocks of both cases. Quantification of viral E gene was 277 copies per reaction for case 1 and 289 copies per reaction for case 2, in the presence of adequate internal MSTN controls. In situ hybridization for SARS-CoV-2 spike protein mRNA visualized the presence of the virus in villous trophoblastic cells in the foci of chronic intervillositis, mirroring the immunohistochemical pattern of expression of SARS-CoV-2 spike antibody (Figure 1).

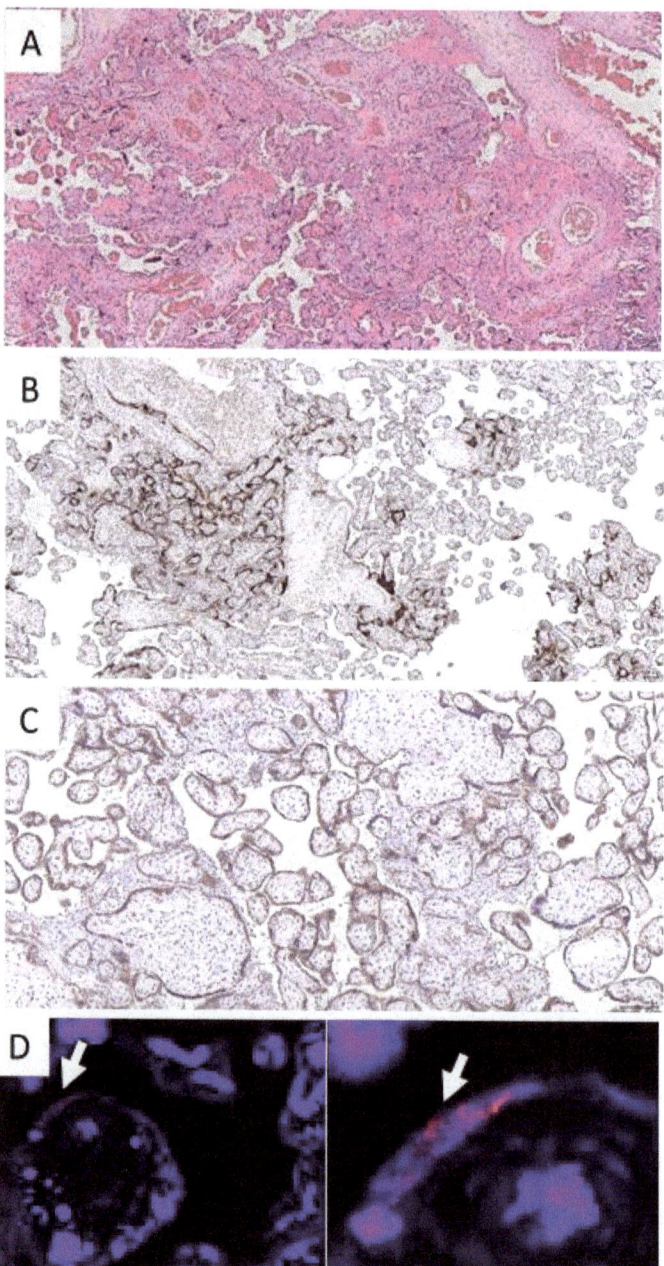

Figure 1. Placental examination—case 1. (**A**) Foci of chronic intervillositis with massive peri-villous fibrin deposition and early placental infarction (hematoxylin and eosin, original magnification ×4). (**B**) Strong cytoplasmic positivity of villous trophoblastic cells with SARS-CoV-2 spike antibody co-localized with the foci of chronic intervillous inflammation (hematoxylin and eosin, original magnification ×4). The following antibodies were used: CD68-PGM1 (Dako Monoclonal Mouse Anti-Human CD68, Clone PG-M1, dilution 1/200), ACE2 (Atlas antibodies, clone CL4035, dilution 1/1000),

and SARS-CoV-2 spike antibody (Sino Biological, SARS-CoV Spike S1 Subunit Antibody, Rabbit PAb, Antigen Affinity Purified, dilution 1/250). (**C**) Diffuse and strong membranous ACE2 expression of cytotrophoblastic cells (original magnification ×10). (**D**) In situ hybridization for SARS-CoV-2 spike protein mRNA by RNA scope. In situ detection of SARS-CoV-2 mRNA was performed on 4μm sections from selected formalin-fixed, paraffin-embedded (FFPE) tissue blocks. Actively transcribed SARS-CoV-2 was detected by RNAScope technology (ACDBio, Newark, CA, USA) using a probe specific for the SARS-CoV-2 S protein (2.5VS Probe-V-nCoV2019-S, ACDBio), as previously reported [19]. SARS-CoV-2 detection and quantification by RT-qPCR was performed for both cases, starting from total RNA extracted from 10 μm thick sections of placental FFPE tissue blocks containing foci of chronic intervillositis, using a Cobas z480 instrument (Roche Diagnostics, Basel, Switzerland); one-step RT-qPCR LightCycler® Multiplex RNA Virus Master Mix (Roche Diagnostics); and the following primers: LightMix® Modular SARS, Wuhan CoV E-gene, and LightMix® Modular MSTN extraction control (Roche Diagnostics), as previously reported. The limit of detection (LoD) for E gene was 7 copies per reaction, as previously determined in our laboratory by Probit regression analysis [20].

4.3. Neonatal Outcomes

4.3.1. Case 1

A 1370 g (50–75th percentile) female neonate was born at 29 + 3 weeks of gestation with APGAR scores of 4, 8, and 8 at 1, 5, and 10 min, respectively. She developed respiratory distress due to hyaline membrane disease, was intubated 30 min after birth, and received a dose surfactant intratracheally. A complete blood count performed at birth was within the normal range, and blood cultures remained negative (Table 1). She was mechanically ventilated for 13 h and then extubated to nasal continuous positive airway pressure (nCPAP). Umbilical cord blood collected at birth was positive for SARS-CoV-2 (2000 copies/mL). Tracheal secretions collected 11 h after birth were positive for SARS-CoV-2 (1300 copies/mL). Following extubation, additional SARS-CoV-2 PCR tests were negative.

Table 1. Case 1: neonatal, maternal, and placental microbiology.

	Before Birth	Birth	H11	H36	H48	DOL 4	DOL 7
Newborn							
Cord blood PCR	-	POSITIVE [1]	-	-	-	-	-
Tracheal secretion PCR	-	-	POSITIVE [2]	-	-	-	-
Nasopharyngeal swab PCR	-	-	-	Negative	-	-	-
Serum PCR	-	-	Negative	-	Negative	-	Negative
Serology IgG	-	-	-	Negative	-	-	-
Serology IgM	-	-	-	Negative	-	-	-
Blood culture	-	Negative	-	-	-	-	-
Mother							
Nasopharyngeal swab PCR	POSITIVE	-	-	-	-	-	-
Serology IgG	-	-	-	-	-	POSITIVE [3]	-
Placenta							
Placenta swab PCR IgM	-	POSITIVE [4]	-	-	-	-	-
SARS-CoV-2 identification	-	POSITIVE [5]	-	-	-	-	-

DOL: day of life; [1] 2.0×10^3 copies/mL; [2] 1.3×10^3 copies/mL; [3] 99.6 (ratio), negative if <4; [4] 2.8×10^7/mL; [5] RNAscope ISH assay.

Head ultrasound (HUS) performed on postnatal day 3 identified a right grade II intraventricular hemorrhage and a focal unilateral periventricular hemorrhagic infarction, which evolved to a right frontal porencephalic cyst, progressive ventricular dilatation, and heterogeneous echogenicities throughout the white matter (Figure 2). Bilateral fronto-parieto-occipital cystic peri-ventricular leukomalacia (cPVL) was observed on postnatal day 25. Brain magnetic resonance imaging (MRI) performed on postnatal day 56 (37 + 1 weeks' postmenstrual age) confirmed extensive bilateral fronto-parieto-occipital cPVL, ependymal hemorrhage sequelae, and moderate ventriculomegaly (Figure 2). At discharge home (postnatal day 75), the infant continued to have an abnormal neurological examination with axial and lower limb hypertonia.

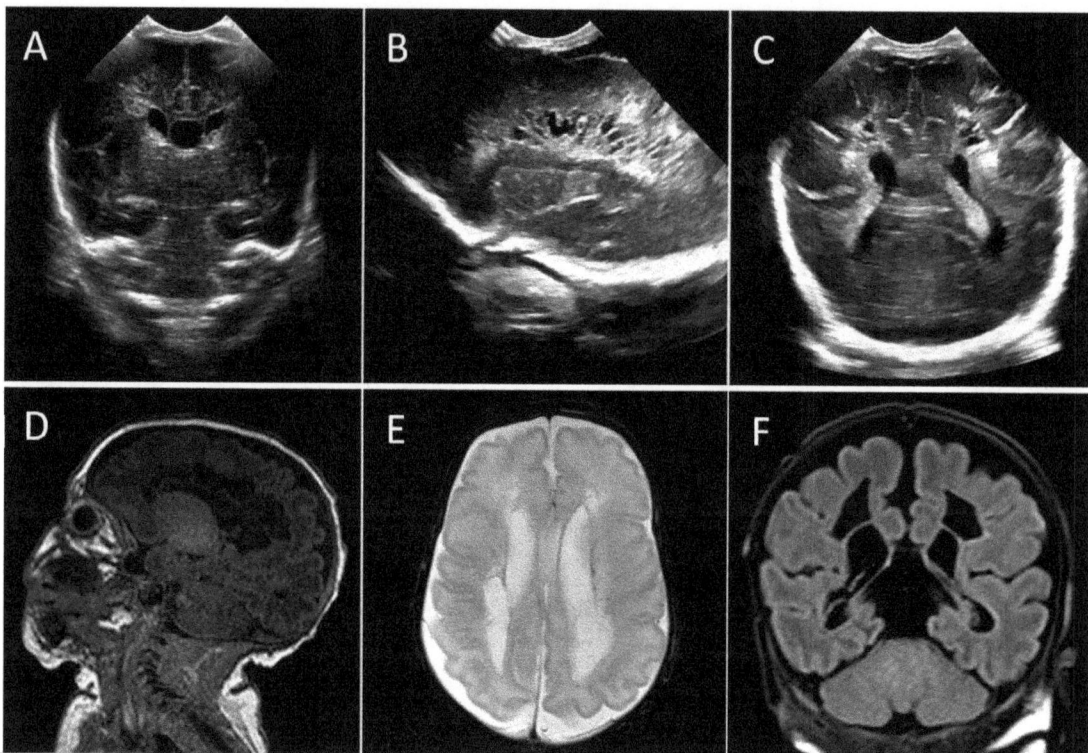

Figure 2. CASE 1: Postnatal brain imaging of the neonates. (**A**) Postnatal day 11 head ultrasound (HUS) coronal view showing a right-sided grade II intraventricular hemorrhage and a focal unilateral periventricular hemorrhagic infarction. Postnatal day 24 HUS with sagittal (**B**) and coronal (**C**) views showing extensive periventricular fronto-parieto-occipital cystic lesions. (**D**) Brain magnetic resonance imaging (MRI) on postnatal day 56 (37 + 1 weeks postmenstrual age) with sagittal T1-weighted, (**E**) axial T2-weighted, and (**F**) coronal T2-FLAIR (fluid-attenuated inversion recovery) images confirming severe periventricular cystic leukomalacia, sequelae of germinal hemorrhage, and moderate ventriculomegaly.

4.3.2. Case 2

A female neonate was delivered at 32 + 1 week's gestation, weighing 1800 g (50th percentile). APGAR scores were 2, 4, and 5 at 1, 5, and 10 min, respectively. Umbilical cord arterial pH was 6.69. Due to absence of respiratory efforts and bradycardia, the neonate required bag and mask ventilation and chest compressions during the first 5 min after birth. She was then intubated and started on invasive ventilation. Due to hyaline membrane disease, the neonate received intratracheal surfactant. Blood gas showed severe lactic acidosis. She was transferred to a tertiary care neonatal intensive care unit. Laboratory findings are reported in Table S1 in the Supplementary Materials.

The neonate fulfilled criteria for perinatal asphyxia with grade II acute hypoxic-ischemic encephalopathy, according to Sarnat score. She developed multiorgan failure, requiring catecholamine treatment, fresh frozen plasma, and platelet transfusions. Persistent pulmonary hypertension was confirmed by echocardiography and required treatment with inhaled nitric oxide for 24 h. She was extubated to nCPAP on postnatal day 4. Intravenous antibiotics, started the day of birth, were stopped after 72 h, as blood cultures were negative. Nasopharyngeal swabs collected at 16 and 76 h following birth and cerebro-spinal fluid collected on postnatal day 5 were negative for SARS-CoV-2 (Table 2).

Table 2. Case 2: neonatal, maternal, and placental microbiology.

	Before Birth	Birth	H5	H16	DOL 3	DOL 4	DOL 5
Newborn							
Nasopharyngeal swab PCR	-	-	-	Negative	Negative	-	-
Blood culture	-	-	Negative	-	-	Negative	Negative
Cerebrospinal fluid PCR	-	-	-	-	-	-	Negative
Mother							
Nasopharyngeal swab PCR	POSITIVE	-	-	-	-	-	-
Placenta							
Placental swab PCR	-	POSITIVE [1]	-	-	-	-	-
SARS-CoV-2 identification	-	POSITIVE [2]	-	-	-	-	-

DOL: day of life; [1] 3.0×10^6/mL; [2] RNAscope ISH assay.

At 18 h of life, she presented with status epilepticus lasting 3 h that resolved after 3 intravenous doses of midazolam. Recurring electrographic seizures on postnatal day 3 prompted a loading dose of phenobarbitone. The electroencephalogram showed a severely suppressed pattern.

HUS performed on postnatal days 1, 2, and 3 showed a right-sided germinal matrix hemorrhage, cerebral edema, and hyperechogenicity in the fronto-parietal white matter. Brain MRI on postnatal day 7 revealed multiple intraventricular and parenchymal hemorrhages and severe anoxic lesions affecting the white matter and basal ganglia (Figure 3). Hemorrhagic lesions were compatible with asphyxia, coagulopathy, thrombocytopenia, and thrombosis of the straight sinus. She was discharged home on postnatal day 41 (38 weeks postmenstrual age), at which time she continued to have an abnormal neurological examination with limb hypertonia. A repeat brain MRI on postnatal day 55 displayed parenchymal hemorrhagic sequelae, widespread bilateral cPVL, and a non-occlusive thrombus in the straight sinus (Figure 3).

4.4. SARS-CoV-2 Sequencing

Genome sequences obtained from nasopharyngeal swabs (case 1 and 2) and a fragment of the placenta (case 2) were attributed to the PANGO lineage B.1.221, a European lineage with increasing prevalence among sequences available in public databases from September 2020 to March 2021, concomitant with the second wave. Genome sequences from both cases only differed by one synonymous mutation. The consensus genome sequences of all three samples are available in GISAID with accession numbers EPI_ISL_2359178 for case 1, and EPI_ISL_2367310 and EPI_ISL_2367312 for case 2.

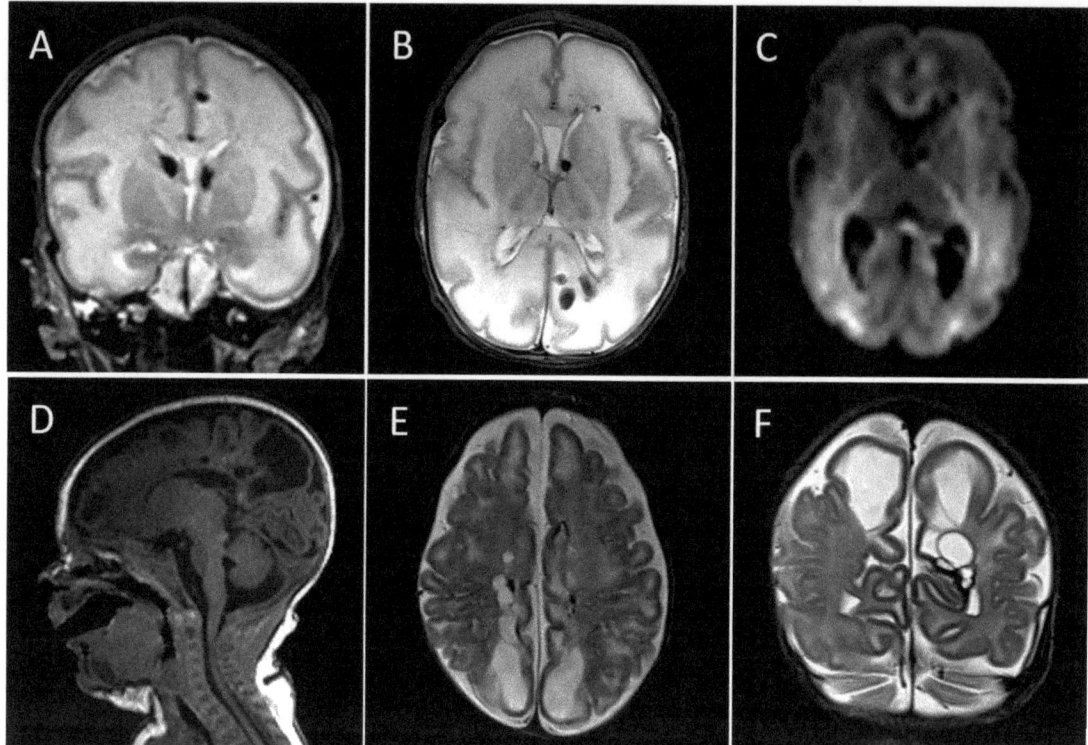

Figure 3. CASE 2: Postnatal brain imaging of the neonates. Postnatal day 7 MRI with (**A**) coronal, (**B**) axial T2-weighted, and (**C**) axial diffusion-weighted images showing germinal, intraventricular, and multiple parenchymal hemorrhages, as well as severe anoxic lesions affecting the white matter bilaterally predominantly in parieto-occipital regions and the basal ganglia. (**D**) Postnatal day 55 (40 weeks postmenstrual age) MRI with sagittal T1-weighted, (**E**) axial, (**F**) and coronal T2-weighted images showing transformation of the anoxic lesions to bilateral cystic periventricular leukomalacia, predominantly in parieto-occipital lobes and sequelae of germinal matrix and fronto-parietal white matter hemorrhage.

5. Discussion

Both cases illustrate severe neurological injury following a clinical history of decreased fetal movements five days after mild maternal COVID-19. Pregnant women and healthcare providers should be aware that even with non-severe forms of the disease, reduced fetal movements is a sign of potential placental and fetal involvement and should prompt an urgent obstetrical evaluation of fetal well-being.

According to the WHO definition [13], the first case meets criteria for transplacental transmission of SARS-CoV-2. The virus was detected by PCR in the mother–placenta–newborn triad. Vertical transmission through the placenta was supported by direct identification of SARS-CoV-2 on the fetal side of the placenta by in situ techniques (immunohistochemistry, RNA-Scope) corresponding to SARS-CoV-2-induced placental intervillositis. Negative maternal and neonatal SARS-CoV-2 IgG and IgM in case 1 does not rule out an infection in the newborn, as seroconversion can occur within the first 30 days after onset of symptoms [21,22]. The second case remains a suspected vertical transmission. Despite a positive maternal nasopharyngeal PCR and placental detection of the virus, neonatal nasopharyngeal swabs remained negative for SARS-CoV-2, which could be explained by the potential instability of viral RNA [23] or by a rapid viral clearance by the neonate, which occurred in less than two days in the first case. This raises the interesting possibility that preterm newborns can mount an effective immune response against SARS-CoV-2. It is also possible that, despite widespread SARS-CoV-2 placental infection, the virus did not reach the fetus in the second case.

Schwartz et al. [24] identified chronic intervillositis in placentas from SARS-CoV-2-infected maternal-fetal dyads. The inflammatory pattern of chronic intervillositis strongly suggests placental invasion by SARS-CoV-2 and represents a possible mechanism by which the virus can breach the maternal–fetal interface. The identification by in situ techniques of viral particles in the villous trophoblastic cells highly expressing ACE2 may explain the predominance of inflammation in the intervillous space, which differs from chronic villitis caused by other viral agents. Our cases underline the potential for placental infection by SARS-CoV-2 and demonstrate its ability to cause fulminant placental parenchymal destruction, leading to fetal distress within days of mild maternal disease [8–11,25].

Both preterm neonates developed extensive cPVL. Due to progress in perinatal care, cPVL has become extremely rare [26]. The pathogenesis of cPVL is multifactorial, involving ischemia, inflammation with or without infection, oxidative stress, and excitotoxicity [27]. Given the extent and the type of brain damage observed in our patients, we consider that SARS-CoV-2 is likely to have directly or indirectly caused cPVL. Placental dysfunction occurred in both cases, and led to perinatal asphyxia, hypoxic-ischemic encephalopathy, and severe hypoglycemia in the second case. Yet, these complications do not fully explain the nature and the severity of the brain injury. In adults and children, neurological manifestations have been reported during SARS-CoV-2 infection [28–30]. However, viral RNA was detected in the cerebrospinal fluid in a minority of adult patients with neurologic symptoms. In our study, a lumbar puncture performed in case 2 showed no evidence of central nervous system invasion by the virus. Other potential mechanisms for brain injury have been suggested, including systemic inflammation, immune-mediated damage, vasculitis, and thromboembolic events [31]. Our cases do not meet criteria for fetal inflammatory response syndrome [32], and we cannot determine whether vasculitis or thromboembolic events could have contributed to perinatal brain injury.

With a measured rate of 22.8 mutations per year [33], one mutation is expected every two transmissions. The single base difference between both cases suggests a short contact chain, although no epidemiological link could be identified (the two women lived 200 km apart). The limited number of cases does not allow testing for associations between mutations and severity of neonatal disease. It is striking, however, that the same B1.1.221 lineage was involved in both cases presenting with severe neonatal brain injury.

6. Conclusions

SARS-CoV-2 can cause severe placental damage and acute fetal distress within days of mild maternal infectious symptoms, leading to extensive cerebral lesions in the infants. The only clinical symptom was maternal perception of decreased fetal movements. Pregnant patients and healthcare professionals should be aware of rare but possibly severe outcomes related to SARS-CoV-2 infection in pregnancy. Information on severe outcomes is the basis of an effective and secure healthcare system, as demonstrated in previous viral crises [34]. Serial HUS should be performed to detect neonatal white matter damage when placental COVID-19 is confirmed. More research is needed to understand the long-term impact of COVID-19 on the developing brain, as well as to confirm whether one of the mutations present in the viral lineage B.1.221 is specifically associated with brain injury or whether this may occur with other variants.

Supplementary Materials: The following are available online at https://www.mdpi.com/article/10.3390/v13122517/s1, Figure S1: CASE 1—fetal heart rhythm (FHR) monitoring at admission. Figure S2: CASE 1—placental gross examination. Table S1: Neonatal laboratory values at birth.

Author Contributions: Conceptualization—G.F., S.M., C.G., D.B. and E.G.; patient care—G.F., S.M., J.S., B.L., R.C., F.P., I.B.J., B.E.-H. and E.G.; placental histopathology—C.G. and L.d.L.; microbiology—C.B. and G.G.; methodology—G.F., C.G., G.G., L.P., D.B. and E.G.; writing—G.F., S.M., C.G., D.B. and E.G.; review and editing, all authors. All authors have read and agreed to the published version of the manuscript.

Funding: This research received no external funding.

Institutional Review Board Statement: The study was conducted according to the guidelines of the Declaration of Helsinki and approved by the Institutional Review Board of Lausanne University Hospital (approval number CER-VD-2020-00548).

Informed Consent Statement: Informed consent was obtained from all subjects involved in the study.

Data Availability Statement: Not applicable.

Conflicts of Interest: The authors declare no conflict of interest.

References

1. Favre, G.; Pomar, L.; Musso, D.; Baud, D. 2019-nCoV epidemic: What about pregnancies? *Lancet* **2020**, *395*, e40. [CrossRef]
2. Woodworth, K.R. Birth and Infant Outcomes Following Laboratory-Confirmed SARS-CoV-2 Infection in Pregnancy—SET-NET, 16 Jurisdictions, March 29–October 14, 2020. *MMWR Morb. Mortal. Wkly. Rep.* **2020**, *69*, 1635. [CrossRef] [PubMed]
3. Allotey, J.; Stallings, E.; Bonet, M.; Yap, M.; Chatterjee, S.; Kew, T.; Debenham, L.; Llavall, A.C.; Dixit, A.; Zhou, D.; et al. Clinical manifestations, risk factors, and maternal and perinatal outcomes of coronavirus disease 2019 in pregnancy: Living systematic review and meta-analysis. *BMJ* **2020**, *370*, m3320. [CrossRef] [PubMed]
4. Vouga, M.; Favre, G.; Martinez-Perez, O.; Pomar, L.; Acebal, L.F.; Abascal-Saiz, A.; Hernandez, M.R.V.; Hcini, N.; Lambert, V.; Carles, G.; et al. Maternal outcomes and risk factors for COVID-19 severity among pregnant women. *Sci. Rep.* **2021**, *11*, 13898. [CrossRef]
5. Di Gennaro, F.; Marotta, C.; Pisani, L.; Veronese, N.; Pisani, V.; Lippolis, V.; Pellizer, G.; Pizzol, D.; Tognon, F.; Bavaro, D.F.; et al. Maternal caesarean section infection (MACSI) in Sierra Leone: A case-control study. *Epidemiol. Infect.* **2020**, *148*, e40. [CrossRef]
6. Gale, C.; Quigley, M.A.; Placzek, A.; Knight, M.; Ladhani, S.; Draper, E.S.; Sharkey, D.; Doherty, C.; Mactier, H.; Kurinczuk, J.J. Characteristics and outcomes of neonatal SARS-CoV-2 infection in the UK: A prospective national cohort study using active surveillance. *Lancet Child Adolesc. Health* **2021**, *5*, 113–121. [CrossRef]
7. Raschetti, R.; Vivanti, A.J.; Vauloup-Fellous, C.; Loi, B.; Benachi, A.; de Luca, D. Synthesis and systematic review of reported neonatal SARS-CoV-2 infections. *Nat. Commun.* **2020**, *11*, 5164. [CrossRef]
8. Schoenmakers, S.; Snijder, P.; Verdijk, R.M.; Kuiken, T.; Kamphuis, S.S.M.; Koopman, L.P.; Krasemann, T.B.; Rousian, M.; Broekhuizen, M.; Steegers, E.A.P.; et al. Severe Acute Respiratory Syndrome Coronavirus 2 Placental Infection and Inflammation Leading to Fetal Distress and Neonatal Multi-Organ Failure in an Asymptomatic Woman. *J. Pediatr. Infect. Dis. Soc.* **2020**, *10*, 556–561. [CrossRef]
9. Correia, C.R.; Marçal, M.; Vieira, F.; Santos, E.; Novais, C.; Maria, A.T.; Malveiro, D.; Prior, A.R.; Aguiar, M.; Salazar, A.; et al. Congenital SARS-CoV-2 Infection in a Neonate with Severe Acute Respiratory Syndrome. *Pediatr. Infect. Dis. J.* **2020**, *39*, e439–e443. [CrossRef]
10. Vivanti, A.J.; Vauloup-Fellous, C.; Prevot, S.; Zupan, V.; Suffee, C.; Do Cao, J.; Benachi, A.; de Luca, D. Transplacental transmission of SARS-CoV-2 infection. *Nat. Commun.* **2020**, *11*, 3572. [CrossRef]
11. Di Nicola, P.; Ceratto, S.; Dalmazzo, C.; Roasio, L.; Castagnola, E.; Sannia, A. Concomitant SARS-CoV-2 infection and severe neu-rologic involvement in a late-preterm neonate. *Neurology* **2020**, *95*, 834–835. [CrossRef] [PubMed]
12. Hopwood, A.J.; Jordan-Villegas, A.; Gutierrez, L.D.; Cowart, M.C.; Vega-Montalvo, W.; Cheung, W.L.; McMahan, M.J.; Gomez, M.R.; Laham, F.R. Severe Acute Respiratory Syndrome Coronavirus-2 Pneumonia in a Newborn Treated with Remdesivir and Coronavirus Disease 2019 Convalescent Plasma. *J. Pediatr. Infect. Dis. Soc.* **2021**, *10*, 691–694. [CrossRef]
13. Definition and Categorization of the Timing of Mother-to-Child Transmission of SARS-CoV-2. Available online: https://www.who.int/publications-detail-redirect/WHO-2019-nCoV-mother-to-child-transmission-2021.1 (accessed on 23 February 2021).
14. Baud, D.; Greub, G.; Favre, G.; Gengler, C.; Jaton, K.; Dubruc, E.; Pomar, L. Second-Trimester Miscarriage in a Pregnant Woman With SARS-CoV-2 Infection. *JAMA* **2020**, *323*, 2198–2200. [CrossRef] [PubMed]
15. Greub, G.; Sahli, R.; Brouillet, R.; Jaton, K. Ten years of R&D and full automation in molecular diagnosis. *Future Microbiol.* **2016**, *11*, 403–425. [CrossRef]
16. Opota, O.; Brouillet, R.; Greub, G.; Jaton, K. Comparison of SARS-CoV-2 RT-PCR on a high-throughput molecular diagnostic platform and the cobas SARS-CoV-2 test for the diagnostic of COVID-19 on various clinical samples. *Pathog. Dis.* **2020**, *78*, ftaa061. [CrossRef] [PubMed]
17. Khong, T.Y.; Mooney, E.E.; Ariel, I.; Balmus, N.C.M.; Boyd, T.K.; Brundler, M.-A.; Derricott, H.; Evans, M.J.; Faye-Petersen, O.M.; Gillan, J.E.; et al. Sampling and Definitions of Placental Lesions: Amsterdam Placental Workshop Group Consensus Statement. *Arch. Pathol. Lab. Med.* **2016**, *140*, 698–713. [CrossRef] [PubMed]

18. Kubik, S.; Marques, A.C.; Xing, X.; Silvery, J.; Bertelli, C.; de Maio, F.; Pournaras, S.; Burr, T.; Duffourd, Y.; Siemens, H.; et al. Recommendations for accurate genotyping of SARS-CoV-2 using amplicon-based sequencing of clinical samples. *Clin. Microbiol. Infect.* **2021**, *27*, 1036.e1–1036.e8. [CrossRef]
19. Rambaut, A.; Holmes, E.C.; O'Toole, Á.; Hill, V.; McCrone, J.T.; Ruis, C.; du Plessis, L.; Pybus, O.G. A dynamic nomenclature proposal for SARS-CoV-2 lineages to assist genomic epidemiology. *Nat. Microbiol.* **2020**, *5*, 1403–1407. [CrossRef]
20. Berezowska, S.; Lefort, K.; Ioannidou, K.; Ndiaye, D.-R.; Maison, D.; Petrovas, C.; Rotman, S.; Piazzon, N.; Milowich, D.; Sala, N.; et al. Postmortem Cardiopulmonary Pathology in Patients with COVID-19 Infection: Single-Center Report of 12 Autopsies from Lausanne, Switzerland. *Diagnostics* **2021**, *11*, 1357. [CrossRef]
21. Long, Q.X.; Liu, B.Z.; Deng, H.J.; Wu, G.C.; Deng, K.; Chen, Y.K.; Liao, P.; Qiu, J.F.; Lin, Y.; Cai, X.F.; et al. Antibody responses to SARS-CoV-2 in patients with COVID-19. *Nat. Med.* **2020**, *26*, 845–848. [CrossRef]
22. Joseph, N.T.; Dude, C.M.; Verkerke, H.P.; Irby, L.S.; Dunlop, A.L.; Patel, R.M.; Easley, K.A.; Smith, A.K.; Stowell, S.R.; Jamieson, D.J.; et al. Maternal Antibody Response, Neutralizing Potency, and Placental Antibody Transfer After Severe Acute Respiratory Syndrome Coronavirus 2 (SARS-CoV-2) Infection. *Obstet. Gynecol.* **2021**, *138*, 189–197. [CrossRef]
23. Pomar, L.; Nielsen-Saines, K.; Baud, D. Stability of severe acute respiratory syndrome coronavirus 2 RNA in placenta and fetal cells. *Am. J. Obstet. Gynecol.* **2021**, *224*, 126–127. [CrossRef] [PubMed]
24. Schwartz, D.A.; Morotti, D. Placental Pathology of COVID-19 with and without Fetal and Neonatal Infection: Trophoblast Necrosis and Chronic Histiocytic Intervillositis as Risk Factors for Transplacental Transmission of SARS-CoV-2. *Viruses* **2020**, *12*, 1308. [CrossRef] [PubMed]
25. Lorenz, N.; Treptow, A.; Schmidt, S.; Hofmann, R.; Raumer-Engler, M.; Heubner, G.; Gröber, K. Neonatal Early-Onset Infection With SARS-CoV-2 in a Newborn Presenting with Encephalitic Symptoms. *Pediatr. Infect. Dis. J.* **2020**, *39*, e212. [CrossRef] [PubMed]
26. Van Haastert, I.C.; Groenendaal, F.; Uiterwaal, C.S.; Termote, J.U.; van der Heide-Jalving, M.; Eijsermans, M.J.; Gorter, J.W.; Helders, P.J.; Jongmans, M.J.; de Vries, L.S. Decreasing incidence and severity of cerebral palsy in prematurely born children. *J. Pediatr.* **2011**, *159*, 86–91. [CrossRef] [PubMed]
27. Schneider, J.; Miller, S.P. Preterm brain Injury: White matter injury. *Handb. Clin. Neurol.* **2019**, *162*, 155–172. [CrossRef]
28. Pezzini, A.; Padovani, A. Lifting the mask on neurological manifestations of COVID-19. *Nat. Rev. Neurol.* **2020**, *16*, 636–644. [CrossRef]
29. Lin, J.E.; Asfour, A.; Sewell, T.B.; Hooe, B.; Pryce, P.; Earley, C.; Shen, M.Y.; Kerner-Rossi, M.; Thakur, K.T.; Vargas, W.S.; et al. Neurological issues in children with COVID-19. *Neurosci. Lett.* **2021**, *743*, 135567. [CrossRef]
30. Bernard-Valnet, R.; Perriot, S.; Canales, M.; Pizzarotti, B.; Caranzano, L.; Castro-Jiménez, M.; Epiney, J.-B.; Vijiala, S.; Salvioni-Chiabotti, P.; Anichini, A.; et al. Encephalopathies Associated with Severe COVID-19 Present Neurovascular Unit Alterations Without Evidence for Strong Neuroinflammation. *Neurol.—Neuroimmunol. Neuroinflammation* **2021**, *8*, e1029. Available online: https://nn.neurology.org/content/8/5/e (accessed on 27 September 2021). [CrossRef]
31. Stafstrom, C.E.; Jantzie, L.L. COVID-19: Neurological Considerations in Neonates and Children. *Children* **2020**, *7*, 133. Available online: www.ncbi.nlm.nih.gov/pmc/articles/PMC7552690/ (accessed on 7 September 2021). [CrossRef]
32. McCarty, K.L.; Tucker, M.; Lee, G.; Pandey, V. Fetal Inflammatory Response Syndrome Associated with Maternal SARS-CoV-2 Infection. *Pediatrics* **2020**, *147*, e2020010132. [CrossRef] [PubMed]
33. Hadfield, J.; Megill, C.; Bell, S.M.; Huddleston, J.; Potter, B.; Callender, C.; Sagulenko, P.; Bedford, T.; Neher, R.A. Nextstrain: Real-time tracking of pathogen evolution. *Bioinformatics* **2018**, *34*, 4121–4123. [CrossRef] [PubMed]
34. Quaglio, G.; Tognon, F.; Finos, L.; Bome, D.; Sesay, S.; Kebbie, A.; di Gennaro, F.; Camara, B.S.; Marotta, C.; Pisani, V.; et al. Impact of Ebola outbreak on reproductive health services in a rural district of Sierra Leone: A prospective observational study. *BMJ Open* **2019**, *9*, e029093. [CrossRef] [PubMed]

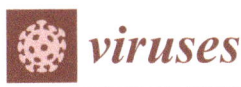

Case Report

Vertical Transmission of SARS-CoV-2 in Second Trimester Associated with Severe Neonatal Pathology

Gennady Sukhikh [1,2], Ulyana Petrova [1], Andrey Prikhodko [1], Natalia Starodubtseva [1,3], Konstantin Chingin [4], Huanwen Chen [4], Anna Bugrova [1,5], Alexey Kononikhin [1,6], Olga Bourmenskaya [1], Alexander Brzhozovskiy [1,6], Evgeniya Polushkina [1,*], Galina Kulikova [1], Alexander Shchegolev [1], Dmitry Trofimov [1], Vladimir Frankevich [1], Evgeny Nikolaev [6] and Roman G. Shmakov [1]

[1] National Medical Research Center for Obstetrics, Gynecology and Perinatology, Ministry of Healthcare of the Russian Federation, 117997 Moscow, Russia; g_sukhikh@oparina4.ru (G.S.); u_petrova@oparina4.ru (U.P.); a_prikhodko@oparina4.ru (A.P.); n_starodubtseva@oparina4.ru (N.S.); a_bugrova@oparina4.ru (A.B.); A.Kononikhin@Skoltech.ru (A.K.); o_bourmenskaya@oparina4.ru (O.B.); a_brzhozovzkiy@oparina4.ru (A.B.); g_kulikova@oparina4.ru (G.K.); ashegolev@oparina4.ru (A.S.); d_trofimov@oparina4.ru (D.T.); v_frankevich@oparina4.ru (V.F.); r_shmakov@oparina4.ru (R.G.S.)

[2] Department of Obstetrics, Gynecology, Neonatology and Reproduction, First Moscow State Medical University Named after I.M. Sechenov, 119991 Moscow, Russia

[3] Moscow Institute of Physics and Technology, 141701 Moscow, Russia

[4] Jiangxi Key Laboratory for Mass Spectrometry and Instrumentation, East China University of Technology, Nanchang 330013, China; 201360012@ecut.edu.cn (K.C.); chw@ecut.edu.cn (H.C.)

[5] Emanuel Institute for Biochemical Physics, Russian Academy of Sciences, 119334 Moscow, Russia

[6] Skolkovo Institute of Science and Technology, 121205 Moscow, Russia; E.Nikolaev@skoltech.ru

* Correspondence: e_polushkina@oparina4.ru; Tel.: +7-90-3154-7413

Citation: Sukhikh, G.; Petrova, U.; Prikhodko, A.; Starodubtseva, N.; Chingin, K.; Chen, H.; Bugrova, A.; Kononikhin, A.; Bourmenskaya, O.; Brzhozovskiy, A.; et al. Vertical Transmission of SARS-CoV-2 in Second Trimester Associated with Severe Neonatal Pathology. *Viruses* 2021, *13*, 447. https://doi.org/10.3390/v13030447

Academic Editor: David Baud

Received: 2 February 2021
Accepted: 1 March 2021
Published: 10 March 2021

Publisher's Note: MDPI stays neutral with regard to jurisdictional claims in published maps and institutional affiliations.

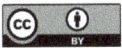

Copyright: © 2021 by the authors. Licensee MDPI, Basel, Switzerland. This article is an open access article distributed under the terms and conditions of the Creative Commons Attribution (CC BY) license (https://creativecommons.org/licenses/by/4.0/).

Abstract: The effects of severe acute respiratory syndrome coronavirus-2 (SARS-CoV-2) infection in women on the gestation course and the health of the fetus, particularly in the first and second trimesters, remain very poorly explored. This report describes a case in which the normal development of pregnancy was complicated immediately after the patient had experienced Coronavirus disease 2019 (COVID-19) at the 21st week of gestation. Specific conditions included critical blood flow in the fetal umbilical artery, fetal growth restriction (1st percentile), right ventricular hypertrophy, hydropericardium, echo-characteristics of hypoxic-ischemic brain injury (leukomalacia in periventricular area) and intraventricular hemorrhage at the 25th week of gestation. Premature male neonate delivered at the 26th week of gestation died after 1 day 18 h due to asystole. The results of independent polymerase chain reaction (PCR), mass spectrometry and immunohistochemistry analyses of placenta tissue, umbilical cord blood and child blood jointly indicated vertical transmission of SARS–CoV-2 from mother to the fetus, which we conclude to be the major cause for the development of maternal vascular malperfusion in the studied case.

Keywords: pregnancy; vertical transmission; fetal growth restriction; COVID-19; coronavirus; SARS-CoV-2

1. Introduction

Pregnancy is characterized by physiological immunosuppression with predisposition to respiratory viral infections [1]. In previous years, the severe acute respiratory syndrome coronavirus (SARS-CoV) and the Middle East respiratory syndrome (MERS) coronavirus increased the rate of hospitalization in an intensive care unit and lethal outcomes in pregnant women [2]. The effects of SARS-CoV-2 on maternal and perinatal outcomes remain poorly understood due to the limited research of clinical manifestations and laboratory findings in pregnant women with Coronavirus disease 2019 (COVID-19) [3,4]. Thus, there is as yet no consensus regarding the probability and implications of the vertical transplacental transmission of SARS-CoV-2 [5–7]. Several findings indicate the possibility of vertical

SARS-CoV-2 transmission. First, angiotensin-converting enzyme 2 (ACE2) (the main cellular receptor binding virus) was found to be expressed in the placenta, ovary, uterus and vagina [8]. Second, clinical studies in China revealed immunoglobulin M (IgM) antibodies in neonates from mothers with positive SARS-CoV-2 tests [9,10]. Third, IgM antibodies, representing the acute phase of viral infection, are sufficiently large in size to pass from the mother's blood through the placenta. Finally, viral RNA and protein were found in the placenta [11–14]. The vast majority of SARS-CoV-2 clinical cases of pregnant women have been studied in the third trimester of pregnancy. The systematic review by Alexander M. Kotlyar et al. indicated that vertical transmission of SARS-CoV-2 infection in the third trimester is possible but rare (probability around 2–3.7%) and it is not associated with severe neonatal pathology [15]. Out of 936 neonates from mothers with COVID-19, 27 neonates were detected SARS-CoV-2 positive by the polymerase chain reaction (PCR) test with a nasopharyngeal swab. The results of SARS-CoV-2 viral RNA testing were positive for 1 out of 34 neonatal cord blood samples (2.9%), 2 out of 26 placenta samples (7.7%), 0 out of 51 amniotic fluid samples (0%), 0 out of 17 urine samples (0%), and 3 out of 31 fecal or rectal swab samples (9.7%). The results of serology analysis of the neonates based on the presence of immunoglobulin M were positive for 3 out of 82 samples (3.7%) [15]. However, very little remains known about maternal and neonatal outcomes due to SARS-CoV-2 infection in the first trimester and, particularly, the second trimester of pregnancy [11,12,15]. Unlike the first and the third trimesters, the second trimester is associated with notable attenuation of the mother's immune activity [1]. To the best of our knowledge, only two case reports of second trimester SARS-CoV-2 newborn testing have been published until now [11,12]. In the first case, viral mRNA was found in the placenta and umbilical cord blood of a child born after 22 weeks of gestation [11]. Electron microscopy confirmed the presence of viral capsids on the fetal side of placenta. In the second case, all newborn samples were SARS-CoV-2 negative, except the fetal side of placenta [12]. In both cases, the child did not survive. Acute inflammation in placental tissue was considered to be the main cause of the adverse pregnancy outcome. Further studies are necessary to characterize the effect and potential risks of SARS-CoV-2 infection in the second trimester for fetus development.

Here we report the case of a second trimester pregnancy complicated by SARS-CoV-2 infection at the 21st week of gestation. The complications included fetal growth restriction (1st percentile), right ventricular hypertrophy, hydropericardium, echo-characteristics of hypoxic-ischemic brain injury (leukomalacia in periventricular area) and intraventricular hemorrhage at the 25th week of gestation. The thorough examination of this clinical case indicates the association between SARS-CoV-2 and maternal vascular malperfusion and unambiguously demonstrates vertical SARS-CoV-2 transmission from mother to the fetus associated with severe neonatal pathology.

2. Materials and Methods

Sample Collection and Preparation

All procedures for the collection, transport and preparation of the samples were carried out according to the restrictions and protocols of SR 1.3.3118–13 «Safety procedures for work with microorganisms of the I–II groups of pathogenicity (hazard)». Mothers' nasopharyngeal swabs and blood, umbilical cord blood, amniotic fluid and the sample of placenta were obtained right before and during C-section. Newborn nasopharyngeal samples were obtained within 3 h after birth. Nasopharyngeal swabs were placed in transport media. Nasopharyngeal specimens were stored at +4 °C and analyzed within 24 h. Blood samples were placed in a tube with EDTA, aliquoted in 100 µL and stored at −20 °C. A sample of placental tissue was obtained from the chorionic side. Autopsy tissue samples of lung, brain, intestine, liver and sample of placental tissues were frozen and stored at −20 °C.

For PCR analysis, tissue samples were thawed and homogenized in 500 µL of RNAase-DNAase-free water. Aliquots of blood and 100 µL of tissue homogenates were pretreated with 400 µL QIAzol Lysis Reagent (Kiagen GmbH, Germany). Virus RNA was extracted from 100 µL nasopharyngeal samples and 200 µL purified homogenates with kit PREP-NA (DNA-Technology LLC, Russia) and eluted in 50 µL.

For proteomic analysis (high-performance liquid chromatography with tandem mass spectrometry, HPLC-MS/MS), frozen tissue (100 mg) was homogenized using a glass-glass tissue grinder in lysis buffer (4% SDS, 150 mM TRIS-HCl, 10 mM DTT, protease inhibitors cocktail). Homogenate was heated at 95 °C for 10 min, sonicated three times for 2 min and centrifuged at $10,000 \times g$, +4 °C for 10 min. The supernatant was collected (SDS extract). The pellet was extracted with urea buffer (8 M urea, 50 mM TRIS–HCl) for 30 min at room temperature with constant stirring, centrifuged at $10,000 \times g$, +4 °C. Supernatant was collected (urea extract). The protein concentration was determined by BCA assay. Aliquots of each extract containing 100 µg of total protein were mixed with 8 M urea in 0.1 M Tris-HCl, pH 8.5 in the ultrafiltration unit and were then processed by the filter aided sample preparation (FASP) using Microcon 30 k centrifugal ultrafiltration units according to the previous literature [16].

3. Pathomorphology and Ommunohistochemistry Examination

Macro and microscopic examination of placenta was performed in accordance with the principles adopted by the Amsterdam placental workshop group consensus [17]. The placenta was weighed without extraplacental membranes and umbilical cord. Tissue fragments (ca. 0.5 cm wide) were excised through all parts of the placenta. The fragments were fixed in 10% neutral formalin and embedded in paraffin. Paraffin sections were stained with hematoxylin and eosin for microscopic examination.

The immunohistochemical study included reactions with polyclonal rabbit antibodies against the S1 subunit of the spike protein (SARS-CoV-2 Spike antibody, GTX135356, GeneTex, USA) and against the nucleocapsid protein (SARS-CoV-2 Nucleocapsid, GTX 135357, GeneTex, USA) with working dilution ratio of 1:500. Immunostaining reactions were carried out on a Ventana Benchmark XT automatic immunostainer with an ultraVIEW Universal DAB imaging system (Roche, USA). For positive and negative controls, sections from SARS-CoV-2 Spike FFPE 293T cell pellet block (GTX435640 GeneTex, USA) and SARS-CoV-2 Nucleocapsid FFPE 293T cell pellet block (GTX435641) were used, as recommended by the antibody manufacturer. The second negative control was done using paraffin sections of tissue from the placenta of a patient without SARS-CoV-2.

For the microscopic analysis of histo- and immunohistochemical reactions and photo documentation we used a light microscope NIKON ECLIPS 80i (Nikon, Japan), morphometry program NIS-Elements AR 5.11 and digital color camera DS-Fi1 (Nikon).

4. PCR Analysis

SARS-CoV-2/SARS-CoV Multiplex REAL-TIME-PCR (RT-PCR) detection kit (DNA-Technology LLC, Russia) targeting the N gene and the $\overline{E}$ gene (specific for SARS-CoV-2) the conserved region of the E gene (common for a group of coronaviruses like SARS-CoV, including SARS-CoV and SARS-CoV-2) was used following the manufacturer's protocol. The assay includes an internal positive control to identify possible RT-PCR inhibition and to confirm the integrity of the reagents of the kit. Thermal cycling was performed at 35 °C for 20 min for reverse transcription, followed by: (1) 95 °C for 5 min, (2) 5 cycles of 94 °C for 10 s, (3) 64 °C for 10 s, (4) 42 cycles of 94 °C for 5 s, (5) 64 °C for 10 s, (6) 80 °C for 5 s with a thermocycler RealTime system DTprime 4X1 (DNA-Technology LLC, Russia). Any value of the threshold cycle was interpreted as positive for SARS-CoV-2 RNA. Samples were tested twice, starting with RNA isolation.

5. Proteomic Analysis of Tissue (HPLC-MS/MS)

The tryptic peptides were analyzed in triplicate on a nano-HPLC Dionex Ultimate 3000 system (Thermo Fisher Scientific, USA) coupled to a TIMS TOF Pro (Bruker Daltonics, USA) mass-spectrometer. The sample volume was 2 µL per injection. HPLC separation was carried out using a packed emitter column (C18, 25 cm × 75 µm 1.6 µm) (Ion Optics,

Parkville, Australia) by gradient elution. Mobile phase A was 0.1% formic acid in water; mobile phase B was 0.1% formic acid in acetonitrile. LC separation was achieved at a flow of 400 nL/min using a 40 min gradient from 4% to 90% of phase B.

Mass spectrometry measurements were carried out using the Parallel Accumulation Serial Fragmentation (PASEF™) acquisition method. The electrospray ionization (ESI) source settings were the following: 4500 V capillary voltage, 500 V endplate offset, 3.0 L/min of dry gas at temperature of 180 °C. The measurements were carried out in the m/z range from 100 to 1700 Th. The range of ion mobilities included values from 0.60–1.60 Vs/cm^2 (1/k0). The total cycle time was set at 1.16 s and the number of PASEF MS/MS scans was set to 10. For low sample amounts, the total cycle time was set to 1.88 s.

6. Protein Identification

The obtained data were analyzed using PEAKS Studio 8.5 and MaxQuant version 1.6.7.0 using the following parameters—parent mass error tolerance–20 ppm; fragment mass error tolerance–0.03 Da. Due to the mild denaturation conditions, the absence of reduction and alkylation steps in one of the sample preparation approaches and short hydrolysis time, up to 3 missed cleavages were allowed. However, only the peptides with both trypsin-specific ends were considered for identification purposes. Oxidation of methionine and carbamidomethylation of cysteine residues were set as possible variable modifications. Up to 3 variable modifications per peptide were allowed. The search was carried out using the Swissprot SARS-CoV-2 database with the human one set as the contamination database. FDR thresholds for all stages were set to 0.01 (1%) or lower.

7. Results

A healthy 27-year-old primipara at the 21st week of gestation was diagnosed with a moderate form of SARS-CoV-2 infection. Clinical symptoms included hyperthermia up to 39 °C, cough, anosmia, ageusia and decrease in oxygen saturation (SpO$_2$) to 92%. According to computed tomography (CT) data bilateral polysegmental pneumonia was detected (15% of lung tissue damage). The patient was administered antibiotics (cephalosporin), low molecular weight heparin, antiviral drugs (lopinavir-ritonavir) and dexamethasone. Oxygen therapy was initiated on day 10. Therapy with low molecular weight heparins was continued until delivery. According to the screening test at 12 weeks three days, nuchal translucency was 1.8 mm, crown-rump length was 59 mm. According to the ultrasound scan at the 19th week of gestation, the fetus size was consistent with gestational age. Amniotic fluid index was normal.

At the 23rd week of gestation when a pregnant woman was already COVID-19 negative and had no clinical signs of disease, the ultrasound scan detected fetal growth restriction (3rd percentile), oligohydramnios (AFI was 2.6), intraventricular hemorrhage, changes in the diffusion of lung parenchyma, hydrothorax, relative cardiomegaly, hyperechogenic bowel. The Doppler scan showed absent diastolic flow in the umbilical artery.

Starting from the 23rd week of gestation, the fetus was regularly monitored. According to the Doppler scan at the 25th week of gestation the impaired feto-placental circulation was observed—fetal umbilical artery Doppler pulsatility index was 1.9, absent end-diastolic flow, middle cerebral artery pulsatility index was 1.3, peak systolic velocity was 40 cm/s, decreased cerebroplacental ratio was 0.68, a-wave in ductus venosus was positive. The uteroplacental circulation was normal. The ultrasound scan showed fetal growth restriction (1st percentile), right ventricular hypertrophy, hydropericardium, decrease in global heart contractility (Figure 1). According to neurosonography, echo-characteristics of hypoxic-ischemic brain injury (leukomalacia in periventricular area), intraventricular hemorrhage (blood clots in lateral ventricles) and partial agenesis of the corpus callosum were found.

The main clinical parameters of the pregnant woman when admitting to the hospital are presented in Table 1. Urine test showed absence of protein in urine. All parameters in biochemical blood analysis were normal. Markers of angiogenic/antiangiogenic factors PlGF (placental growth factor) 17.08 pg/mL, sFlt-1 (soluble fms-like tyrosine kinase-1)

1846 pg/mL, sFlt-1/P1GF 166.63 demonstrate placental disorders. Screening showed the presence of SARS-CoV-2 antibodies IgG (ELISA kit S-2382 «DS-EIA-ANTI-SARS-CoV-2-G») with positivity index 13.0. IgM antibodies against cytomegalovirus, herpes simplex virus 1 and 2, Epstein-Barr virus were not detected.

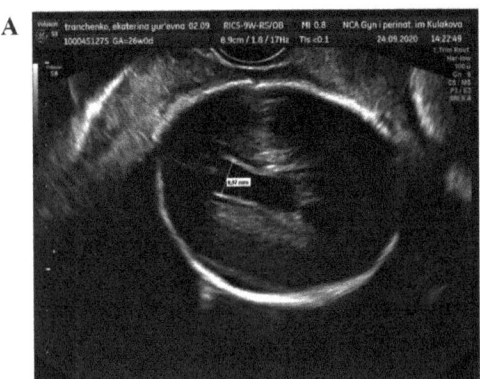
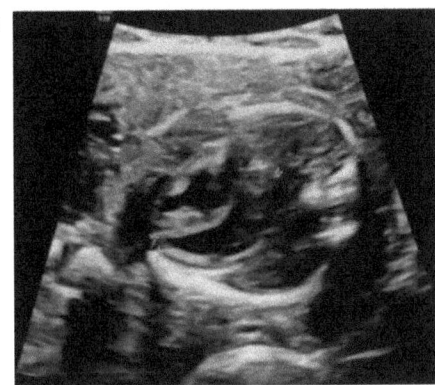

Figure 1. Ultrasound fetal heart scans at the 25th week of gestation: (**A**) intraventricular hemorrhage; (**B**) myocardial hypertrophy.

Table 1. Main laboratory parameters of the pregnant woman.

Parameter, Units	Value	Range
Leukocytes $\times 10^9$/L	1.41	3.53–42.8
Erythrocytes $\times 10^{12}$/L	3.64	2.79–5.26
Haemoglobin g/L	116	75–160
Haematocrit level L/L	0.34	0.34–0.45
Platelets $\times 10^9$/L	333	91–1058
Lymphocytes %	2.7	5–62
CRP mg	1.28	0.08–229
Fibrinogen g/L	3.59	2.02–9.04
Activated partial thromboplastin time s	28.2	20–38
PR sec	11.3	10.2–20.8
Thrombin time s	21.1	11–16
D-dimer ng/L	1253	25–34,280

At the 26th week of gestation characteristics of blood flow centralization were detected. We recorded fetal umbilical artery pulsatility index 1.42, positive end-diastolic flow, middle cerebral artery pulsatility index 0.96, peak systolic velocity 46.3 cm/s, cerebroplacental ratio 0.67 (decreased), reverse blood flow in ductus venosus. Ultrasound scan indicated fetal growth restriction (0.1 percentile) and anhydramnios.

Cesarean section was performed at the 26th week of gestation. Premature male neonate was delivered with the birth weight 397 g and length 27 cm. Apgar score at the 1st min and the 5th min was 5 and 7, accordingly. Delayed cord clamping was performed. The neonate was transferred to the neonatal intensive unit (NICU). Neonate examination revealed the congenital pneumonia, disseminated intravascular coagulation, antenatal intraventricular hemorrhage grade 3 on the right side at the stage of cyst formation, congenital anemia and cardiomegaly. The neonate was small for gestational age. Antibodies IgG against SARS-CoV-2 were detected with positivity index 6.3. According to microbiological culture of feces, blood, throat and rhinopharynx did not demonstrate any growth. Asystole was the cause of neonate death after 1 day 18 h 21 min.

According to morphological examination, the size of the placenta was 12 × 9.5 × 1.5 cm, the weight of the placenta was 114 g after separation of the umbilical cord and membranes (less than 10%). On the fetal and maternal surfaces and the incision, extensive areas of old infarct were determined, occupying 1/2–2/3 of the area Supplementary Materials Figure S1A,B. Microscopic examination of the placenta showed numerous old infarcts and large areas of villi surrounded by fibrin (Figure 2). Plethora and hemolysis were revealed in the vessels of terminal and intermediate villi. Small areas of hemorrhage and lymphocytic-monocytic infiltration were found in the decidual tissue. In some areas, neutrophilic leukocytes were determined. In the decidual tissue of the extraplacental membranes, multiple lymphocytic-monocytic infiltrates were observed (Figure 2). The umbilical cord was normal, without signs of inflammation. Immunohistochemical analysis showed strong positive cytoplasmic expression of SARS-Cov-2 Nucleocapsid and SARS-CoV-2 Spike (S1 subunit) in the cytotrophoblast and syncytiotrophoblast (Figure 3).

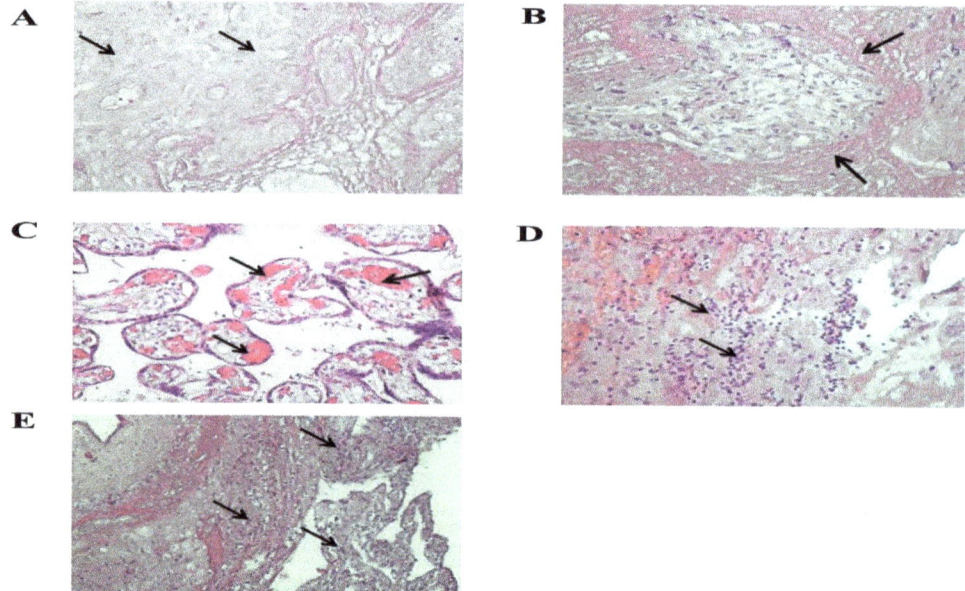

Figure 2. Microscopic changes in the placenta: (**A**)—infarct, ×200; (**B**)—massive deposits of perivillous fibrin, ×200; (**C**)—pronounced plethora of villous vessels, ×200; (**D,E**)—lymphocytic-macrophage infiltrate in the decidual tissue of the placenta and extraplacental membranes, ×200; ×100. Stained with hematoxylin and eosin.

The corpse of the neonate weighed 470 g (normal weight 739 ± 181 g) and was 27 cm long (normal length 32.2 ± 2.4 cm). The meninges were smooth and shiny. The brain weighed 75 g (normal weight 105 ± 21 g). Brain examination revealed hemorrhage in the lateral ventricles, subependymal hemorrhages up to 0.3 cm in bilateral intraventricular hemorrhage of the 3rd grade with areas of periventricular leukomalacia and hemorrhages in the thalamus Supplementary Materials Figures S1C,D and S2C.

Thymus weighed 0.24 g (normal weight 2 ± 1.1 g), with microscopic signs of accidental involution. Punctate hemorrhages were observed on the visceral pleura. The right lung was 7.27 g, the left lung was 5.8 g. The total lung weight was 19.07 g (normal weight 20.6 ± 6.3 g). The lungs were reddish on the cut. Microscopy analysis revealed canalicular-stage structure, areas of atelectasis, extensive fields of intra-alveolar hemorrhages and the presence of hyaline membranes along the walls of the alveoli (Supplementary Materials

Figure S2A,B). The heart was of a cone-shape, size 2.4 × 2 × 1.4 cm, weight 2.77 g (normal weight 5.2 ± 1.3 g). Small punctate hemorrhages were revealed on the epicardium. The valves were formed correctly. The oval window was open with a diameter of 0.3 cm. The thickness of the myocardium of the left and right ventricles was 0.3 cm. Microbiological examination of tissue samples of the lung, liver and blood and intestine revealed no microorganisms.

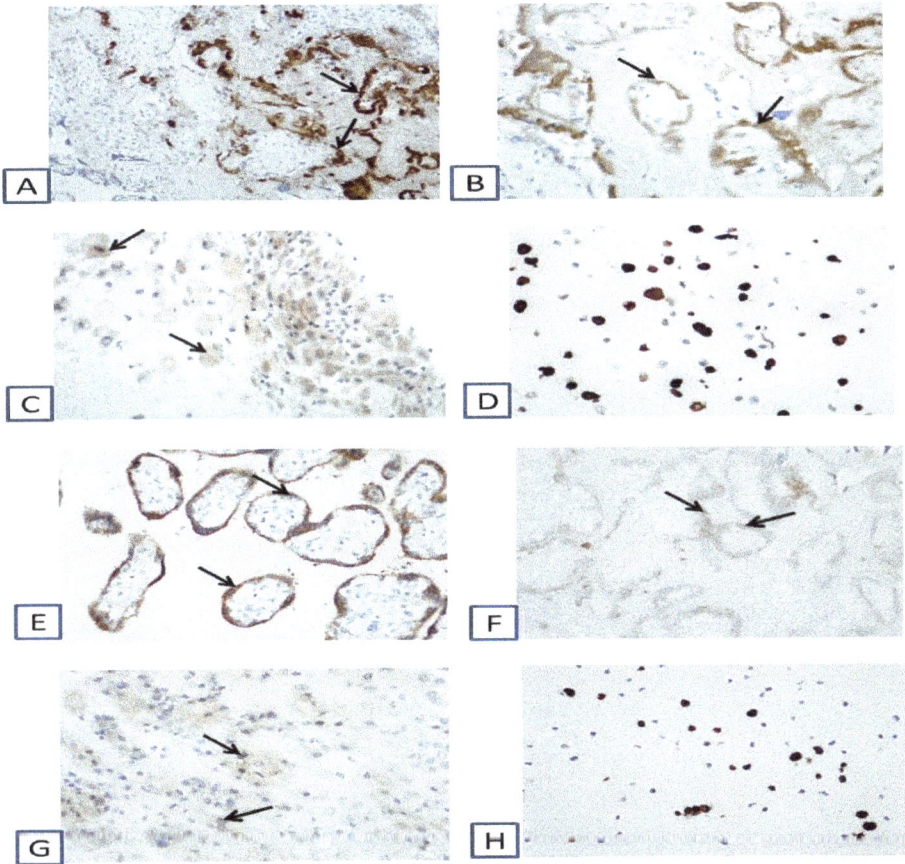

Figure 3. Immunohistochemical changes in the placenta due to the positive immunohistochemical reaction with antibodies against severe acute respiratory syndrome coronavirus-2 (SARS-CoV-2) (Coronavirus disease 2019 (COVID-19)) Nucleocapsid (**A–D**) and against SARS-CoV-2 (COVID-19) Spike (S1 subunit) (**E–H**): (**A,E**)—in the trophoblast of villi, ×200; (**B,F**)—in the trophoblast of the villi in the infarction area, ×200; (**C,G**)—in decidual tissue, ×200; (**D**)—SARS-Cov-2(COVID-19) Nucleocapsid FFPE 293T cell pellet Block, ×200; (**H**)—SARS-CoV-2 (COVID-19) Spike FFPE 293T cell pellet block, ×200.

RT-PCR on the placenta and umbilical cord blood was positive for three SARS-CoV-2 and SARS-CoV-like genes (Supplementary Materials Figure S3).

Over 1000 proteins were identified in the COVID-19 patient placenta sample, among which the P0DTC9 | NCAP-SARS2 Nucleoprotein of SARS-CoV-2 was detected (Figure 4). Nucleocapsid N protein was reliably detected and identified in the COVID-19 patient placenta sample via two unique peptides (Supplementary Materials Table S1 and Figure S4).

```
  1  MSDNGPQNQR NAPRITFGGP SDSTGSNQNG ERSGARSKQR RPQGLPNNTA SWFTALTQHG KEDLKFPRGQ GVPINTNSSP
 81  DDQIGYYRRA TRRIRGGDGK MKDLSPRWYF YYLGTGPEAG LPYGANKDGI IWVATEGALN TPKDHIGTRN PANNAAIVLQ
161  LPQGTTLPKG FYAEGSRGGS QASSRSSSRS RNSSRNSTPG SSRGTSPARM AGNGGDAALA LLLLDRLNQL ESKMSGKGQQ
241  QQGQTVTKKS AAEASKKPRQ KRTATKAYNV TQAFGRRGPE QTQGNFGDQE LIRQGTDYKH WPQIAQFAPS ASAFFGMSRI
321  GMEVTPSGTW LTYTGAIKLD DKDPNFKDQV ILLNKHIDAY KTFPPTEPKK DKKKKADETQ ALPQRQKKQQ TVTLLPAADL
401  DDFSKQLQQS MSSADSTQA
```

Figure 4. Sequence coverage of the P0DTC9 | NCAP-SARS2 Nucleoprotein from SARS CoV-2 in the placenta sample from COVID-19 patient.

8. Discussion

Overall, our experience includes 42 SARS-COV-2 positive pregnant women who delivered in the National Medical Research Center for Obstetrics, Gynecology and Perinatology in the period from April to July 2020 [18]. All newborns were SARS-CoV-2 negative according to the results of PCR analysis of the placenta, amniotic fluid, umbilical cord blood, nasopharyngeal and rectal swabs [18]. However, according to the earlier results by Auriti et al., some newborns become SARS-CoV-2 positive on the 5th day, which suggests the possibility of horizontal transmission of the virus [19]. Our experience also includes 62 women who were SARS-COV-2 positive at different stages of pregnancy but recovered by the time of labor. All newborns were SARS-CoV-2 negative according to the PCR analysis. This indicated the absence of transplacental transmission of the virus from mother to the fetus and the teratogenic effect of the virus to the fetus, in agreement with previous studies [20,21]. Previously reported adverse outcomes of the SARS-CoV-2 infection included an increase in the rate of preterm birth and hospitalization of newborns in the NICU [22].

Most studies have found no evidence of vertical transmission of SARS-CoV-2 from an infected mother to the fetus or newborn [5–7,23]. However, mostly the infection in the 3rd trimester has been studied until now. Data on the possibility of vertical transmission and the effects of SARS-CoV-19 on the fetus in the 1st and 2nd trimesters remain very limited.

Vivanti et al. were the first to describe a case of delivery at the 35th week of gestation in a woman with the symptoms of SARS-CoV-2 infection, positive PCR result in the placenta, amniotic fluid and in the bronchoalveolar secretions of the newborn. The authors also diagnosed the signs of damage of the white matter of the brain [24]. Also, several reports indicate the association between SARS-CoV-2 infection and the levels of certain molecular receptors, such as angiotensin-converting enzyme 2 (ACE-2). Thus, the levels of angiotensin II and ACE-2 in the placental tissue have been recently reported to increase with the gestational age and indicate the risk of the placental damage in the third trimester [25,26].

Unlike earlier studies, our report describes a case of the second trimester COVID-19 associated with SARS-CoV-2 transmission to the placenta and to the fetus in utero. In this case, our patient had no previous risk factors of severe neonatal pathology, the pregnancy developed normally, as confirmed by the screening tests in the first and the second trimesters. However, two weeks after having experienced SARS-CoV-2 infection, the ultrasound scan detected fetal growth restriction (3rd percentile), oligohydramnios (AFI-2.6), intraventricular hemorrhage, changes in the diffusion of lung parenchyma, hydrothorax, relative cardiomegaly, hyperechogenic bowel. The Doppler scan showed absent umbilical artery flow.

Apart from the SARS-CoV-2 infection, there were no other possible reasons and for the development of such severe placental insufficiency in this woman. Within 4 weeks of dynamic observation, the fetal-placental blood flow deteriorated to critical levels, and therefore a surgical delivery was performed. So it can be proposed that in this case the SARS-CoV-2 infection was the independent risk factor for placental insufficiency and severe neonatal pathology.

The changes revealed in the placenta are consistent with the literature data on the development of maternal vascular malperfusion in SARS-CoV-2 positive women [27,28]. Taglauer et al. and Facchetti et al. observed the increased perivillous fibrin in 46.7% and 26.7% of cases, respectively, and placental infarctions in 33.3% and 40% cases, respectively [29,30]. Therefore, we consider SARS-CoV-2 infection to be the major reason for the development of the placental damage in our study. This conclusion is supported by the results of PCR and mass spectrometry indicating the presence of SARS-CoV-2 in placental tissue and umbilical cord blood. Furthermore, the results of our immunohistochemical analysis show the obvious positive cytoplasmic expression of SARS-CoV-2 Nucleocapsid and SARS-CoV-2 Spike (S1 subunit) in the cytotrophoblast and syncytiotrophoblast, which is a strong indication for the vertical transmission of infection from mother to fetus [24]. This conclusion is further confirmed by the positive results of RT-PCR of the placenta and umbilical cord blood for three SARS-CoV-2 and SARS-CoV-like genes.

Several earlier case reports have shown the presence of SARS-CoV-2 viral RNA and protein in the placenta and virions found within the syncytiotrophoblast [11–14]. Few studies have found antibodies against immunoglobulin M (IgM) in neonates born from SARS-CoV-2 positive mothers [9,10]. This raises concerns regarding the possibility of intrauterine transmission, as IgM cannot penetrate the placenta.

Also, the developing lesions of the placenta commonly lead to severe disorders of the placenta and are associated with poor obstetrical outcomes such as fetal growth restriction and fetal death [31,32]. Therefore, fetal damage and its subsequent death observed in our study were very likely due to the placental lesions caused by SARS-CoV-2.

The developments of deposits of perivillous fibrin and extensive infarction of villi are due to disorders of the uterine circulation in the placenta. In turn, the deposits of perivillous fibrin and extensive placental infarctions naturally cause fetal hypoxia, which results in bilateral intraventricular hemorrhage and disease of the hyaline membranes. Histological evaluation of the placenta in mothers infected with SARS-CoV-2 has been described in several studies showing various abnormalities [26]. Those abnormalities shared certain pathological patterns, including vascular perfusion failure, fibrin deposition, and chronic willitis or interillosis. In a pathological study of the placenta from a mother infected with SARS-CoV-2, 12 out of 15 placentas showed signs of maternal vascular malperfusion, with 4 placentas showing central and peripheral villi infarctions [28].

Apart from the clinical and morphological value, our results also present the first confirmation of SARS-CoV-2 proteins in infected placenta by proteomics (HPLC-MS/MS). Tryptic peptides identified in the COVID-19 patient placenta sample coincide with the major peptides from our previous study [33]. The N protein, being the most abundant protein in the virion, is the best candidate for mass-spectrometry detection of the SARS-CoV-2. The obtained results confirmed the potential of mass-spectrometry approaches for the detection of the SARS-CoV-2 in different samples including biological fluids and tissues.

9. Conclusions

The studied case clearly showed that transplacental transmission of SARS-CoV-2 infection is possible not only in the last trimester of pregnancy, but also in earlier stages of pregnancy. Transplacental transmission can cause the inflammation of placenta and neonatal viremia with the damage of various organs and systems. For the first time, the expression of Nucleocapsid N SARS-COV-2 protein in the placenta was confirmed by proteomic method (HPLC-MS/MS).

Supplementary Materials: The following are available online at https://www.mdpi.com/1999-4915/13/3/447/s1, Figure S1: Extensive infarctions of the placenta (A—maternal surface, B—fetal surface, sectional view) and hemorrhages in the brain (C,D), Figure S2: Microscopic changes in the lungs (A,B) and the brain (C): A—hemorrhages in the lumen of the alveoli, g-e ×100; B—hyaline membranes in the alveoli, d ×200; B—hemorrhages in the periventricular region, g-e ×100, Figure S3: Fluorescence cycles in RT-PCR for three SARS-CoV-2 genes (blue, orange and purple color, respectively): 1—the positive control, 2—the placental (A) and umbilical cord blood (B) samples,

Figure S4: MS/MS data of detected peptides of P0DTC9 | NCAP_SARS2 Nucleoprotein, Table S1: Peptides from the P0DTC9 | NCAP_SARS2 Nucleoprotein identified in the placenta sample from COVID-19 patient.

Author Contributions: Conceptualization, G.S., R.G.S., V.F., H.C., E.N. and D.T.; data curation, A.P., N.S., K.C. and E.P.; formal analysis, A.P., N.S., E.P. and A.K.; investigation, A.B. (Anna Bugrova), A.K., O.B., A.B. (Alexander Brzhozovskiy), E.P., G.K. and A.S.; methodology, A.B. (Alexander Brzhozovskiy), O.B., E.P. and G.K.; project administration, G.S., R.G.S., V.F., E.N. and D.T.; software, O.B., A.S., A.B. (Anna Bugrova) and N.S.; writing—original draft, N.S., K.C., R.G.S., E.P. and U.P.; writing—review and editing, V.F., E.N., D.T. and G.S. All authors have read and agreed to the published version of the manuscript.

Funding: The reported study was funded by RFBR according to the research project № 20-04-60093.

Institutional Review Board Statement: All clinical investigations were conducted according to the principles expressed in the Declaration of Helsinki. The research was approved by the Ethical Committee of the National Medical Research Center for Obstetrics, Gynecology, and Perinatology, named after Academician V.I. Kulakov of the Ministry of Healthcare of Russian Federation (Record No. 4 from 23 April 2020).

Informed Consent Statement: Patients who participated in this study had read and signed an informed consent form.

Data Availability Statement: The data presented in this study are available within the article and its supplementary materials at https://www.mdpi.com/1999-4915/13/3/447/s1.

Acknowledgments: The National Natural Science Foundation of China (No.81961138016, No.K20200008).

Conflicts of Interest: The authors declare no conflict of interest. The funders had no role in the design of the study; in the collection, analyses, or interpretation of data; in the writing of the manuscript, or in the decision to publish the results.

References

1. Mor, G.; Aldo, P.; Alvero, A.B. The unique immunological and microbial aspects of pregnancy. *Nat. Rev. Immunol.* **2017**, *17*, 469–482. [CrossRef] [PubMed]
2. Zumla, A.; Hui, D.S.; Perlman, S. Middle East respiratory syndrome. *Lancet* **2015**, *386*, 995–1007. [CrossRef]
3. Liua, H.; Wang, L.-L.; Zhao, S.-J.; Kwak-Kim, J.; Mor, G.; Liao, A.-H. Why are pregnant women susceptible to COVID-19? An immunological viewpoint. *J. Reprod. Immunol.* **2020**, *139*. [CrossRef]
4. Rasmussen, S.A.; Smulian, J.C.; Lednicky, J.A.; Wen, T.S.; Jamieson, D.J. Coronavirus Disease 2019 (COVID-19) and pregnancy: What obstetricians need to know. *Am. J. Obstet. Gynecol.* **2020**, *222*, 415–426. [CrossRef]
5. Fan, C.; Lei, D.; Fang, C.; Li, C.; Wang, M.; Liu, Y.; Bao, Y.; Sun, Y.; Huang, J.; Guo, Y.; et al. Perinatal Transmission of COVID-19 Associated SARS-CoV-2: Should We Worry? *Clin. Infect. Dis.* **2020**, 2019–2021. [CrossRef]
6. Della Gatta, A.N.; Rizzo, R.; Pilu, G.; Simonazzi, G. Coronavirus disease 2019 during pregnancy: A systematic review of reported cases. *Am. J. Obstet. Gynecol.* **2020**, *223*, 36–41. [CrossRef]
7. Yang, Z.; Liu, Y. Vertical Transmission of Severe Acute Respiratory Syndrome Coronavirus 2: A Systematic Review. *Am. J. Perinat.* **2020**, *37*, 1055–1060. [CrossRef]
8. Jing, Y.; Run-Qian, L.; Hao-Ran, W.; Hao-Ran, C.; Ya-Bin, L.; Yang, G.; Fei, C. Potential influence of COVID-19/ACE2 on the female reproductive system. *Mol. Hum. Reprod.* **2020**, *26*, 367–373. [CrossRef] [PubMed]
9. Dong, L.; Tian, J.; He, S.; Zhu, C.; Wang, J.; Liu, C.; Yang, J. Possible Vertical Transmission of SARS-CoV-2 From an Infected Mother to Her Newborn. *JAMA J. Am. Med. Assoc.* **2020**, *323*, 1846–1848. [CrossRef]
10. Zeng, H.; Xu, C.; Fan, J.; Tang, Y.; Deng, Q.; Zhang, W.; Long, X. Antibodies in Infants Born to Mothers With COVID-19 Pneumonia. *JAMA J. Am. Med. Assoc.* **2020**, *323*, 1848–1849. [CrossRef]
11. Hosier, H.; Farhadian, S.F.; Morotti, R.A.; Deshmukh, U.; Lu-Culligan, A.; Campbell, K.H.; Yasumoto, Y.; Vogels, C.B.F.; Casanovas-Massana, A.; Vijayakumar, P.; et al. SARS-CoV-2 infection of the placenta. *J. Clin. Investig.* **2020**, *130*, 4947–4953. [CrossRef] [PubMed]
12. Baud, D.; Greub, G.; Favre, G.; Gengler, C.; Jaton, K.; Dubruc, E.; Pomar, L. Second-Trimester Miscarriage in a Pregnant Woman With SARS-CoV-2 Infection. *JAMA J. Am. Med. Assoc.* **2020**, *323*, 2198–2200. [CrossRef]
13. Patanè, L.; Morotti, D.; Giunta, M.R.; Sigismondi, C.; Piccoli, M.G.; Frigerio, L.; Mangili, G.; Arosio, M.; Cornolti, G. Vertical transmission of coronavirus disease 2019: Severe acute respiratory syndrome coronavirus 2 RNA on the fetal side of the placenta in pregnancies with coronavirus disease 2019–positive mothers and neonates at birth. *Am. J. Obstet. Gynecol. MFM* **2020**, *2*, 100145. [CrossRef]

14. Kirtsman, M.; Diambomba, Y.; Poutanen, S.M.; Malinowski, A.K.; Vlachodimitropoulou, E.; Parks, W.T.; Erdman, L.; Morris, S.K.; Shah, P.S. Probable congenital sars-cov-2 infection in a neonate born to a woman with active sars-cov-2 infection. *Cmaj* **2020**, *192*, E647–E650. [CrossRef]
15. Kotlyar, A.M.; Grechukhina, O.; Chen, A.; Popkhadze, S.; Grimshaw, A.; Tal, O.; Taylor, H.S.; Tal, R. Vertical transmission of coronavirus disease 2019: A systematic review and meta-analysis. *Am. J. Obstet. Gynecol.* **2020**. [CrossRef] [PubMed]
16. Wiśniewski, J.R. Quantitative Evaluation of Filter Aided Sample Preparation (FASP) and Multienzyme Digestion FASP Protocols. *Anal. Chem.* **2016**, *88*, 5438–5443. [CrossRef]
17. Khong, T.Y.; Mooney, E.E.; Ariel, I.; Balmus, N.C.M.; Boyd, T.K.; Brundler, M.A.; Derricott, H.; Evans, M.J.; Faye-Petersen, O.M.; Gillan, J.E.; et al. Sampling and definitions of placental lesions Amsterdam placental workshop group consensus statement. *Arch. Pathol. Lab. Med.* **2016**, *140*, 698–713. [CrossRef] [PubMed]
18. Shmakov, R.G.; Prikhodko, A.; Polushkina, E.; Shmakova, E.; Pyregov, A.; Bychenko, V.; Priputnevich, T.V.; Dolgushin, G.O.; Yarotskaya, E.; Pekarev, O.; et al. Clinical course of novel COVID-19 infection in pregnant women. *J. Matern. Neonatal Med.* **2020**, 1–7. [CrossRef]
19. Auriti, C.; De Rose, D.U.; Tzialla, C.; Caforio, L.; Ciccia, M.; Manzoni, P.; Stronati, M. Vertical Transmission of SARS-CoV-2 (COVID-19): Are Hypotheses More than Evidences? *Am. J. Perinatol.* **2020**, *37*, S31–S38. [CrossRef]
20. Li, Y.; Zhao, R.; Zheng, S.; Chen, X.; Wang, J.; Sheng, X.; Zhou, J.; Cai, H.; Fang, Q.; Yu, F.; et al. Lack of Vertical Transmission of Severe Acute Respiratory Syndrome Coronavirus 2, China. *Emerg. Infect. Dis.* **2020**, *26*, 1335–1336. [CrossRef] [PubMed]
21. Wang, X.; Zhou, Z.; Zhang, J.; Zhu, F.; Tang, Y.; Shen, X. A Case of 2019 Novel Coronavirus in a Pregnant Woman With Preterm Delivery. *Clin. Infect. Dis.* **2020**, *71*, 844–846. [CrossRef] [PubMed]
22. Juan, J.; Gil, M.M.; Rong, Z.; Zhang, Y.; Yang, H.; Poon, L.C. Effect of coronavirus disease 2019 (COVID-19) on maternal, perinatal and neonatal outcome: Systematic review. *Ultrasound Obstet. Gynecol.* **2020**, *56*, 15–27. [CrossRef]
23. Yang, Z.; Wang, M.; Zhu, Z.; Liu, Y. Coronavirus disease 2019 (COVID-19) and pregnancy: A systematic review. *J. Matern. Neonatal Med.* **2020**, 1–4. [CrossRef] [PubMed]
24. Vivanti, A.J.; Vauloup-Fellous, C.; Prevot, S.; Zupan, V.; Suffee, C.; Do Cao, J.; Benachi, A.; De Luca, D. Transplacental transmission of SARS-CoV-2 infection. *Nat. Commun.* **2020**, *11*, 1–7. [CrossRef]
25. Li, M.; Chen, L.; Zhang, J.; Xiong, C.; Li, X. The SARS-CoV-2 receptor ACE2 expression of maternal-fetal interface and fetal organs by single-cell transcriptome study. *PLoS ONE* **2020**, *15*, e0230295. [CrossRef] [PubMed]
26. Mao, L.; Jin, H.; Wang, M.; Hu, Y.; Chen, S.; He, Q.; Chang, J.; Hong, C.; Zhou, Y.; Wang, D.; et al. Neurologic Manifestations of Hospitalized Patients With Coronavirus Disease 2019 in Wuhan, China. *JAMA Neurol.* **2020**, *77*, 683. [CrossRef] [PubMed]
27. Baergen, R.N.; Heller, D.S. Placental Pathology in Covid-19 Positive Mothers: Preliminary Findings. *Pediatr. Dev. Pathol.* **2020**, *23*, 177–180. [CrossRef]
28. Shanes, E.D.; Mithal, L.B.; Otero, S.; Azad, H.A.; Miller, E.S.; Goldstein, J.A. Placental Pathology in COVID-19. *Am. J. Clin. Pathol.* **2020**, *154*, 23–32. [CrossRef] [PubMed]
29. Taglauer, E.; Benarroch, Y.; Rop, K.; Barnett, E.; Sabharwal, V.; Yarrington, C.; Wachman, E.M. Consistent localization of SARS-CoV-2 spike glycoprotein and ACE2 over TMPRSS2 predominance in placental villi of 15 COVID-19 positive maternal-fetal dyads. *Placenta* **2020**, *100*, 69–74. [CrossRef]
30. Facchetti, F.; Bugatti, M.; Drera, E.; Tripodo, C.; Sartori, E.; Cancila, V.; Papaccio, M.; Castellani, R.; Casola, S.; Boniotti, M.B.; et al. SARS-CoV2 vertical transmission with adverse effects on the newborn revealed through integrated immunohistochemical, electron microscopy and molecular analyses of Placenta. *EBioMedicine* **2020**, *59*. [CrossRef]
31. Andres, R.L.; Kuyper, W.; Resnik, R.; Piacquadio, K.M.; Benirschke, K. The association of maternal floor infarction of the placenta with adverse perinatal outcome. *Am. J. Obstet. Gynecol.* **1990**, *163*, 935–938. [CrossRef]
32. Kim, E.N.; Lee, J.Y.; Shim, J.Y.; Hwang, D.; Kim, K.C.; Kim, S.R.; Kim, C.J. Clinicopathological characteristics of miscarriages featuring placental massive perivillous fibrin deposition. *Placenta* **2019**, *86*, 45–51. [CrossRef] [PubMed]
33. Nikolaev, E.N.; Indeykina, M.I.; Brzhozovskiy, A.G.; Bugrova, A.E.; Kononikhin, A.S.; Starodubtseva, N.L.; Petrotchenko, E.V.; Kovalev, G.I.; Borchers, C.H.; Sukhikh, G.T. Mass-Spectrometric Detection of SARS-CoV-2 Virus in Scrapings of the Epithelium of the Nasopharynx of Infected Patients via Nucleocapsid N Protein. *J. Proteome Res.* **2020**, *19*, 4393–4397. [CrossRef] [PubMed]

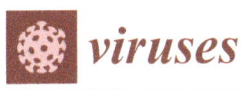

Case Report

Is the First of the Two Born Saved? A Rare and Dramatic Case of Double Placental Damage from SARS-CoV-2

Leonardo Resta [1], Antonella Vimercati [2], Sara Sablone [3], Andrea Marzullo [1], Gerardo Cazzato [1,*], Giuseppe Ingravallo [1], Giulia Mazzia [1], Francesca Arezzo [2], Anna Colagrande [1] and Roberta Rossi [1]

[1] Section of Pathology, Department of Emergency and Organ Transplantation (DETO), University of Bari "Aldo Moro", 70124 Bari, Italy; leonardo.resta@uniba.it (L.R.); andrea.marzullo@uniba.it (A.M.); giuseppe.ingravallo@uniba.it (G.I.); g.mazzia@studenti.uniba.it (G.M.); anna.colagrande@gmail.com (A.C.); roberta.rossi@policlinico.ba.it (R.R.)

[2] Section of Gynecology and Obstretics, Department of Biomedical Sciences and Human Oncology, University of Bari "Aldo Moro", 70124 Bari, Italy; antonella.vimercati@uniba.it (A.V.); francescaarezzo@libero.it (F.A.)

[3] Section of Legal Medicine, Department of Interdisciplinary Medicine, University of Bari, 70124 Bari, Italy; sarasabloneml@gmail.com

* Correspondence: gerycazzato@hotmail.it; Tel.: +39-340-5203641

Abstract: The current coronavirus pandemic has affected, in a short time, various and different areas of medicine. Among these, the obstetric field has certainly been touched in full, and the knowledge of the mechanisms potentially responsible for placental damage from SARS-CoV-2 occupy a certain importance. Here we present here a rare case of dichorionic twins born at 30 weeks and 4 days of amenorrhea, one of whom died in the first few hours of life after placental damages potentially related to SARS-CoV-2. We also propose a brief review of the current literature giving ample emphasis to similar cases described.

Keywords: SARS-CoV-2; placenta; COVID-19; fetus; autopsy

Citation: Resta, L.; Vimercati, A.; Sablone, S.; Marzullo, A.; Cazzato, G.; Ingravallo, G.; Mazzia, G.; Arezzo, F.; Colagrande, A.; Rossi, R. Is the First of the Two Born Saved? A Rare and Dramatic Case of Double Placental Damage from SARS-CoV-2. *Viruses* 2021, *13*, 995. https://doi.org/10.3390/v13060995

Academic Editors: David Baud and Leó Pomar

Received: 27 April 2021
Accepted: 25 May 2021
Published: 26 May 2021

Publisher's Note: MDPI stays neutral with regard to jurisdictional claims in published maps and institutional affiliations.

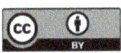

Copyright: © 2021 by the authors. Licensee MDPI, Basel, Switzerland. This article is an open access article distributed under the terms and conditions of the Creative Commons Attribution (CC BY) license (https://creativecommons.org/licenses/by/4.0/).

1. Introduction

The SARS-CoV-2 pandemic (Severe Acute Respiratory Syndrome Coronavirus-2) has had a global impact that has affected all different and distinct areas of medicine [1,2]. Among these, a place of great importance is occupied by the study and analysis of the effects of the virus on pregnant women. Although at the beginning of the pandemic there were few and anecdotal case reports or case series concerning these obstetric areas, an increasing number of scientific papers have tried to shed light on the mechanisms of etiopathogenesis and possible maternal–fetal transmission of the infection [3–5]. We present here a rare case of a COVID-positive woman, pregnant at 30 weeks + 4 days of amenorrhea, with a bi-chorial, bi-amniotic twin pregnancy, and with the birth of the first living and viable fetus and the birth of the second fetus with severe intra-partum distress and death after few minutes. We conducted morphological, immunophenotypic, electron microscopy and real-time polymerase chain reaction (RT-PCR) studies in order to confirm the presence of SARS-CoV-2 in placental tissues.

2. Materials and Methods

The patient was a 32-year-old woman with an early miscarriage previously suffering from mild hypothyroidism, 165 cm tall and 57 kg in weight. Approximately 2 weeks before labor, she contracted SARS-CoV-2, confirmed with a GeneXpert Dx Xpress SARS-CoV-2 RT-PCR assay (Cepheid). The analytical sensitivity and specificity are reported by the manufacturer as 100% (87/87 samples) and 100% (30/30 samples), with a limit of detection of 250 copies/mL or 0.0100 plaque-forming units per milliliter) [6], and she was experiencing modest symptoms, including cough, fatigue, headache, generalized malaise, and mild dyspnea without the need for mechanical ventilation. She was afebrile, heart rate (HR) = 100/min, respiratory rate (RR) = 14/min, blood pressure (BP) = 98 × 60 mmHg, oxygen saturation (SpO2) = 98% on room air, fetal heart rate (FHR) = 147/min and 113/min. She had been given antibiotic therapy for premature rupture of membranes (Prom) after a few days from maternal SARS-CoV-2 infection and prophylactic administration of corticosteroids for prematurity. Despite the administration of tocolytics, unstoppable labor was experienced at 30 weeks and 4 days of amenorrhea. Thus, preterm vaginal delivery occurred, and the first infant proved viable (weight 1295 g), while the second showed hypotonia and cyanosis and died after few minutes (weight 1340 g).

Placentas underwent routine clinical examination consisting of storage at 4 °C prior to fixation, fixation in 10% buffered formalin, photographs of the maternal and fetal surface, measurement, trimmed weight, sectioning, and examination of the cut surface. Sections submitted included 2 of membrane rolls, at least 2 of umbilical cord, 3 maternal surface biopsies, 2 full thickness sections, and representative sampling of any lesions present. Sections underwent routine processing, embedding, sectioning at 5 µm and staining with H&E. Histologic examination was performed by subspecialty perinatal pathologists who were aware of the COVID-19 status. Cases were reviewed by 2 pathologists to confirm the diagnoses. They were observed using an Olympus BX-51 optical microscope equipped with the Olympus DP80 image acquisition system. Anti-SARS-CoV-2 spike S1 glycoprotein monoclonal antibody, Thermo Fisher, Rabbit, was added, at pH 6, diluted 1:800, and the antigen was demonstrated by heat-induced citrate buffer epitope retrieval for enzymatic immunohistochemical (IHC) analysis. In addition, electronic microscopy analysis was made from villi samples of both the chorial discs. At the moment of delivery, samples were immediately fixed in 2.5% gluteraldehyde for 4 hours at 4 °C, and after overnight immersion in phosphate buffer, post-fixed with osmium tetroxide in PBS for 2 h at a temperature of 4 °C. The prepared samples were processed for inclusion in Araldite epoxy resin (M) CY212 (TAAB, Aldermason, UK). Semithin sections 0.5 µm thick were stained with toluidine blue for microscopic analysis. Ultrathin sections were mounted on nickel grilles with uranium acetate and lead citrate contrast. The semithin sections were observed with a Nikon photomicroscope equipped with a Nikon Coolpix DS-U1 digital camera (Nikon Instruments SpA, Calenzano, Italy). The ultrathin sections were observed with a Morgagni 268 electron transmission microscope (FEI Company, Naples, Italy).

3. Results

The first placental disc weighed 240 grams, measured 14 × 12 × 1.5 cm, had smooth and shiny membranes, and had a 31 cm umbilical cord, normospiralized, with paracentric insertion. The second disc weighed 340 g, measured 15 × 10 × 1.5 cm, had smooth and shiny membranes, and had a 15 cm, normospiralized funiculus with central insertion.

The first chorionic disc corresponded to the gestational age and presented very large areas of intervillous fibrinous deposition (Figure 1) with the presence of numerous perivillary histiocytes. Minor recent infarct foci were also described, while umbilical cord and amnio–chorionic membranes were completely normal. The immunohistochemical reaction for the SARS-CoV-2 protein S1 was strongly expressed both in the syncytiotrophoblast cells and in the perivillary histiocytes described in H&E (Figure 2).

Electron microscopy showed signs of circular formations with a 100–130 nm diameter, with peripheral electron dense spicules, which are likely viral particles in the cytoplasm of the perivillary histiocytes (Figure 3).

Additionally, in the second case, developmental characteristics corresponding to gestational age, large areas of intervillous fibrinous deposition (Figure 4A), and the presence of numerous perivillary histiocytes (Figure 4B) were described. Immunostaining for anti-SARS-CoV-2 S1 protein was strongly positive at the level of syncytiotrophoblast and perivillary histiocytes (Figure 4C).

Following the birth, the baby was subjected to a nasopharyngeal swab, which was positive, but which, when repeated after a few minutes, gave a negative result for SARS-

CoV-2. Four days after death, a complete autopsy on the newborn was performed. On external examination, no malformations were detected. All-natural orifices were probed and appeared patent. Weight (1322 g) and anthropometric parameters were consistent with gestational age (30 w+ 4 d) in a twin pregnancy. External genitalia were normal and indicative of a male phenotype. By a skin and subcutaneous tissue Y-shaped incision, the thoracic and abdominal cavities were explored, noting that umbilical arteries normally extended on either side of the urinary bladder, along the inner abdominal wall, and the umbilical vein normally coursed towards the liver in the falciform ligament and patent. The domes of the diaphragm were inspected, and their positions were at the fourth rib interspaces bilaterally. After removing the chest plate, it was observed with a diaphanoscope, and four ossification nuclei were detected. Mild pleural, pericardial, and peritoneal effusions were noted. Lungs appeared hypo-expanded and crouched in their natural cavities. The heart only exhibited some subepicardial petechial spots on the anterior ventricular surfaces, and its opening in situ showed no congenital anomalies. After evisceration by the Rokitansky technique, all organs were carefully separated, dissected, and subjected to tissue sampling. At skull examination, normal tension of fontanels was appreciated. After their dissection, the brain was inspected in situ and then removed, revealing reduced tissue consistency due to decomposition and no focal lesions. Tissue samples were also taken from the brain. Histologically, all the organs removed, including the lung (Figure 4D), showed congestive and sometimes hemorrhagic phenomena. A focal epicardial lympho-monocytic infiltrate was also detected. A circumscribed area of coagulative necrosis was in the spleen beneath the capsule. For suspicion of the first positive swab, a histological lung sample was submitted to immunostaining for anti-SARS-CoV-2 S1 spike protein, which was totally negative. The data are summarized in Table 1.

Table 1. Features of twin pregnancy.

Characteristics	Fetus 1	Fetus 2
Condition	Born alive	Death after few minutes
Birth weight	1295 g	1340 g
APGAR score 1'–5'	9–10	1–1
Sex	Female	Male
First nasopharyngeal swab	positive	positive
Second nasopharyngeal swab	negative	negative
Placental Findings	Perivillous fibrin deposition Perivillous histiocytes	Perivillous fibrin deposition Perivillous histiocytes
Anti-SARS-CoV-2 S1 spike protein	positive	positive

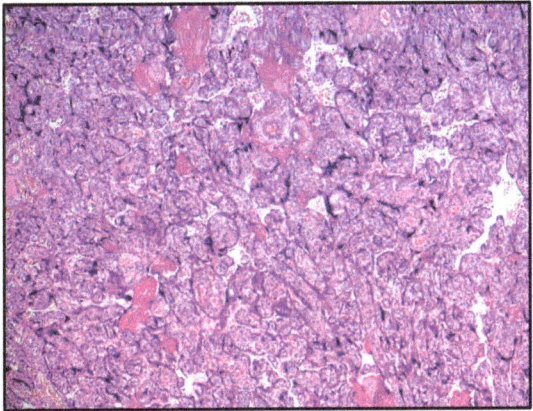

Figure 1. Histological features of the first chorionic disc: deposition of intervillous fibrin and chorionic villi corresponding to the gestational age (30 weeks). Hematoxylin-Eosin, 10×.

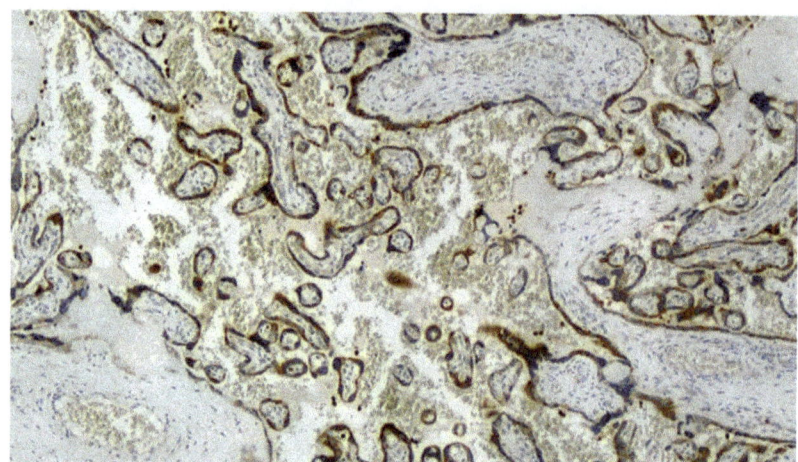

Figure 2. Immunostaining for anti-SARS-CoV-2 spike protein S1 positive at the level of the syncytiotrophoblast and perivillary histiocytes. (IHC, Original Magnification: 10×).

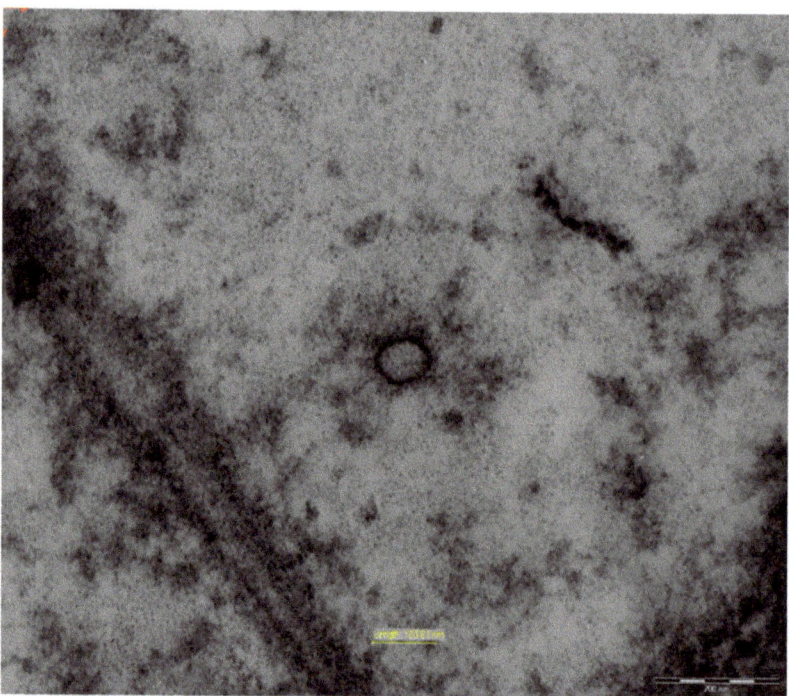

Figure 3. Circular formations with a 100–130 nm diameter were observed, with peripheral electron dense spicules, which are likely viral particles in the cytoplasm of the perivillary histiocytes. (Electron microscopy, 71,000×).

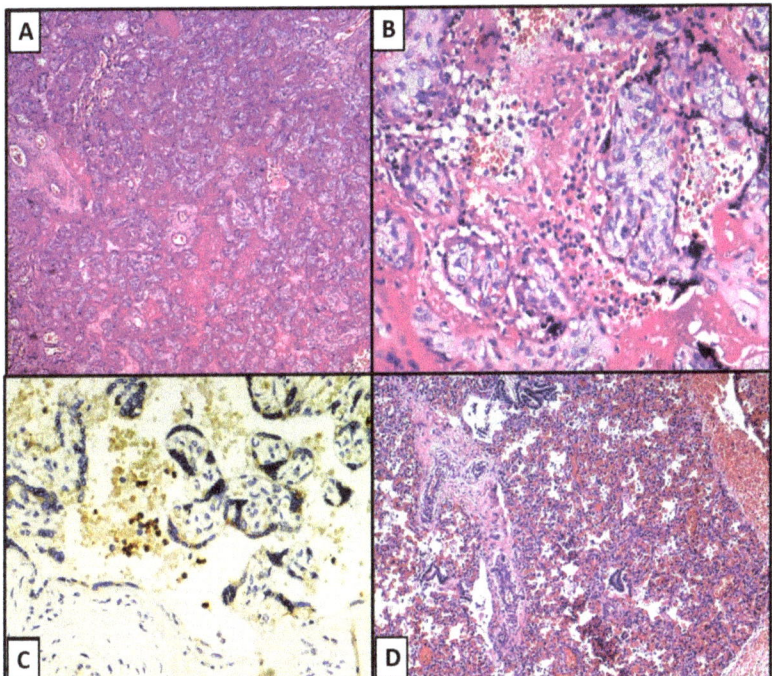

Figure 4. (**A**) Histology of the second chorionic disc with extensive and massive deposition of intervillous fibrin and presence of histiocytes available perivillary. (Hematoxylin–eosin, 4×). (**B**) Histological detail of the chorionic villi corresponding to the gestational age (30 weeks) with the presence of numerous histiocytes available perivillary (Hematoxylin–eosin, 20×). (**C**) Immunostaining for anti-SARS-CoV-2 S1 protein antibody strongly positive at the level of syncytiotrophoblast and perivillary histiocytes (brown staining, immunohistochemistry antiSARS-CoV-2 S1 spike protein, original magnification: 20×). (**D**) Histological examination of lung parenchyma of stillborn fetus with marked congestive phenomena and areas of peribronchial and interstitial hemorrhagic infiltration (hematoxylin–eosin, original magnification: 10×).

4. Discussion

The new coronavirus-2 (COVID-19) pandemic has assumed a global importance that has affected various and distinct sectors of medicine [1,2]. Among these, the role of SARS-CoV-2 in placental pathology and the analysis of the risk of maternal–fetal transmission are of some importance [3–5]. In these months of the pandemic, different case reports and case series have tried to shed light on the placental histopathological alterations linked to the virus, and we ourselves have recently published a paper that reported the data of over 70 pregnancies of COVID-positive mothers [5]. The most significant finding is an increase in the rate of features of maternal vascular malperfusion (MVM), most prominently decidual arteriopathy including atherosis and fibrinoid necrosis and mural hypertrophy of membrane arterioles [5,7,8]. MVM, previously known as maternal vascular underperfusion, has been associated with oligohydramnios, fetal growth restriction, preterm birth, and stillbirth [9,10]. On the other hand, maternal–fetal transmission of the virus is a very rare event, with about 0.34% of cases described in the literature in COVID-positive mothers [7,11]. Our case is very important because it demonstrates once more how fetal discharge can be counted among the outcomes of SARS-CoV-2 infection. In this regard, recently, Poisson et al. [12] reported a rare case of fetal demise in a positive SARS-CoV-2 patient whose placental characteristics indicated extensive fetal vascular malperfusion with large infarct areas resulting in a rather substantial loss of the surface of the chorionic villi. Additionally, Baud et al. reported [13] a pregnant woman with symptomatic coronavirus disease who experienced a second-trimester miscarriage in association with documented placental SARS-CoV-2 infection. Richtmann et al. [14] reported their experience in Brazil of five SARS-CoV-2 positive women whose fetuses had died. Analysis of the placentas showed mainly moderate/severe chorionamniotitis, fetal thrombi, intervillous fibrin deposition, and intervillositis. More specifically, two cases had massive deposition of intervillous fibrin associated with mixed intervillitis and villitis, and intense neutrophil and lymphocyte T infiltration. Pulinx et al. [15] reported a more than rare case of vertical transmission of SARS-CoV-2 in a young 30-year-old woman from whose fetus had been collected various amniotic fluid samples at various times of pregnancy. Histological examination of placental tissues showed presence of extensive intervillous fibrin depositions and ischemic necrosis of the surrounding villi, together with aggregates of histiocytes and cytotoxic T lymphocytes in the intervillous space. In our case we observed severe placental alterations in a twin pregnancy. While in the first fetus these alterations did not compromise the viability, in the second, perhaps due to the prolongation of the expulsive phase and the ischemia of the contractions, the placental lesions (especially the intervillar fibrin and the activity of intervillar histiocytic cells) caused severe intra-partum suffering that irreversibly compromised the viability of the fetus. The relationship between COVID-related placental damage and neonatal death is possible, but this neonatal death can also result from other causes and factors.

5. Conclusions

Our case represents a rarity for two reasons: there was not the very rare maternal–fetal transmission of SARS-CoV-2 despite the placental parenchyma being strongly positive for immunostaining for the spike protein, but at the same time the damage to both placental discs did not allow the second fetus to be able to be adequately oxygenated in the intrapartum, leading to a disastrous outcome. We could sum it all up with "died of COVID without COVID".

Author Contributions: Conceptualization, G.C. and LR.; methodology, S.S.; validation, A.M., L.R., and A.V.; formal analysis, G.M.; investigation, A.C.; resources, A.V.; data curation, G.C.; writing—original draft preparation, G.C. and G.M.; writing—review and editing, L.R, A.M., F.A., and R.R.; visualization, G.I.; supervision, L.R. All authors have read and agreed to the published version of the manuscript.

Funding: This research received no external funding.

Informed Consent Statement: Informed consent was obtained from all subjects involved in the study.

Conflicts of Interest: The authors declare no conflict of interest.

References

1. Jin, Y.; Yang, H.; Ji, W.; Wu, W.; Chen, S.; Zhang, W.; Duan, G. Virology, Epidemiology, Pathogenesis, and Control of COVID-19. *Viruses* **2020**, *12*, 372. [CrossRef] [PubMed]
2. Khan, M.; Adil, S.F.; Alkhathlan, H.Z.; Tahir, M.N.; Saif, S.; Khan, M.; Khan, S.T. COVID-19: A Global Challenge with Old History, Epidemiology and Progress So Far. *Molecules* **2020**, *26*, 39. [CrossRef] [PubMed]
3. Schwartz, D.A. An analysis of 38 pregnant women with COVID-19, their newborn infants, and maternal-fetal transmission of SARS-CoV-2: Maternal coronavirus infections and pregnancy outcomes. *Arch. Pathol. Lab. Med.* **2020**, *144*, 799–805. [CrossRef] [PubMed]
4. Menter, T.; Mertz, K.D.; Jiang., S.; Chen, H.; Monod, C.; Tzankov, A.; Waldvogel, S.; Schulzke, S.M.; Hösli, I.; Bruder, E. Placental Pathology Findings during and after SARS-CoV-2 Infection: Features of Villitis and Malperfusion. *Pathobiology* **2020**, *88*, 69–77. [CrossRef] [PubMed]
5. Resta, L.; Vimercati, A.; Cazzato, G.; Mazzia, G.; Cicinelli, E.; Colagrande, A.; Fanelli, M.; Scarcella, S.V.; Ceci, O.; Rossi, R. SARS-CoV-2 and Placenta: New Insights and Perspectives. *Viruses* **2021**, *13*, 723. [CrossRef] [PubMed]
6. Cepheid. Xpert®Xpress SARS-CoV-2 Instructions for Use for Labs. 2020. Available online: https://www.fda.gov/media/136314/download (accessed on 1 February 2021).

7. Shanes, E.D.; Mithal, L.B.; Otero, S.; Azad, H.A.; Miller, E.S.; Goldstein, J.A. Placental Pathology in COVID-19. *Am. J. Clin. Pathol.* **2020**, *154*, 23–32. [CrossRef] [PubMed]
8. Zhou, Y.Y.; Ravishankar, S.; Luo, G.; Redline, R.W. Predictors of High Grade and Other Clinically Significant Placental Findings by Indication for Submission in Singleton Placentas From Term Births. *Pediatr. Dev. Pathol.* **2020**, *23*, 274–284. [CrossRef] [PubMed]
9. Khong, T.Y.; Mooney, E.E.; Ariel, I.; Balmus, N.C.M.; Boyd, T.K.; Brundler, M.-A.; Derricott, H.; Evans, M.J.; Faye-Petersen, O.M.; Gillan, J.E.; et al. Sampling and Definitions of Placental Lesions: Amsterdam Placental Workshop Group Consensus Statement. *Arch. Pathol. Lab. Med.* **2016**, *140*, 698–713. [CrossRef] [PubMed]
10. Redline, R.W. Severe fetal placental vascular lesions in term infants with neurologic impairment. *Am. J. Obstet. Gynecol.* **2005**, *192*, 452–457. [CrossRef] [PubMed]
11. Hosier, H.; Farhadian, S.F.; Morotti, R.A.; Deshmukh, U.; Lu-Culligan, A.; Campbell, K.H.; Yasumoto, Y.; Vogels, C.B.; Casanovas-Massana, A.; Vijayakumar, P.; et al. SARS-CoV-2 infection of the placenta. *J. Clin. Investig.* **2020**, *1*, 4947–4953. [CrossRef] [PubMed]
12. Poisson, T.M.; Pierone, G. Placental pathology and fetal demise at 35 weeks of gestation in a woman with SARS-CoV-2 infection: A case report. *Case Rep. Womens Health* **2021**, *30*, e00289. [CrossRef] [PubMed]
13. Baud, D.; Greub, G.; Favre, G.; Gengler, C.; Jaton, K.; Dubruc, E.; Pomar, L. Second-Trimester Miscarriage in a Pregnant Woman With SARS-CoV-2 Infection. *JAMA* **2020**, *2*, 2198–2200. [CrossRef] [PubMed]
14. Richtmann, R.; Torloni, M.R.; Oyamada Otani, A.R.; Levi, J.E.; Crema Tobara, M.; de Almeida Silva, C.; Dias, L.; Miglioli-Galvão, L.; Martins Silva, P.; Macoto Kondo, M. Fetal deaths in pregnancies with SARS-CoV-2 infection in Brazil: A case series. *Case Rep. Womens Health* **2020**, *12*, e00243. [CrossRef] [PubMed]
15. Pulinx, B.; Kieffer, D.; Michiels, I.; Petermans, S.; Strybol, D.; Delvaux, S.; Baldewijns, M.; Raymaekers, M.; Cartuyvels, R.; Maurissen, W. Vertical transmission of SARS-CoV-2 infection and preterm birth. *Eur. J. Clin. Microbiol. Infect. Dis.* **2020**, *39*, 2441–2445. [CrossRef] [PubMed]

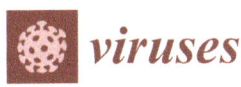

Article

SARS-CoV-2 and Placenta: New Insights and Perspectives

Leonardo Resta [1], Antonella Vimercati [2], Gerardo Cazzato [1,*], Giulia Mazzia [1], Ettore Cicinelli [2], Anna Colagrande [1], Margherita Fanelli [3], Sara Vincenza Scarcella [1], Oronzo Ceci [1] and Roberta Rossi [1]

[1] Section of Pathology, Department of Emergency and Organ Transplantation (DETO), University of Bari "Aldo Moro", 70124 Bari, Italy; leonardo.resta@uniba.it (L.R.); giulia.mazzia1@gmail.com (G.M.); anna.colagrande@gmail.com (A.C.); vincenza.scarcella@policlinico.ba.it (S.V.S.); oronzoruggiero.ceci@uniba.it (O.C.); roberta.rossi@policlinico.ba.it (R.R.)
[2] Department of Biomedical Sciences and Human Oncology, Gynecologic and Obstetrics Clinic, University of Bari "Aldo Moro", 70124 Bari, Italy; antonella.vimercati@uniba.it (A.V.); ettore.cicinelli@uniba.it (E.C.)
[3] Medical Statistic, Department of Interdisciplinary Medicine, University of Bari "Aldo Moro", 70124 Bari, Italy; margherita.fanelli@uniba.it
* Correspondence: gerycazzato@hotmail.it; Tel.: +39-340-5203641

Abstract: The study of SARS-CoV-2 positive pregnant women is of some importance for gynecologists, obstetricians, neonatologists and women themselves. In recent months, new works have tried to clarify what happens at the fetal–placental level in women positive for the virus, and different pathogenesis mechanisms have been proposed. Here, we present the results of a large series of placentas of Coronavirus disease (COVID) positive women, in a reference center for COVID-positive pregnancies, on which we conducted histological, immunohistochemical and electron microscopy investigations. A case–control study was conducted in order to highlight any histopathological alterations attributable to SARS-CoV-2. The prevalence of maternal vascular malperfusion was not significantly different between cases and controls (54.3% vs. 43.7% $p = 0.19$), whereas the differences with regard to fetal vascular malperfusion (21.1% vs. 4.2% $p < 0.001$) were significant. More frequent in cases with respect to controls were decidual arteriopathy (40.9% vs. 1.4% $p < 0.0001$), decidual inflammation (32.4% vs. 0.7% $p < 0.0001$), perivillous fibrin deposition (36.6% vs. 3.5% $p < 0.0001$) and fetal vessel thrombi (22.5% vs. 0.7% $p < 0.0001$). No significant differences in the percentage of terminal villous hyperplasia and chorioamnionitis were observed between the two groups. As the pandemic continues, these studies will become more urgent in order to clarify the possible mechanism of maternal–fetal transmission of the virus.

Keywords: SARS-CoV-2; pregnancy; COVID-19; placenta; transmission; outcomes; viruses

1. Introduction

At the end of December 2019, Chinese doctors in Wuhan, in the province of Hubei, China, started to report the first cases of an anomalous pulmonary infection not directly attributable to known infectious agents [1]. By the start of January 2020, the World Health Organization (WHO) had confirmed that the etiological agent in the cases of pneumonia was a new strain of Coronavirus, denominated SARS-CoV-2 (Severe Acute Respiratory Syndrome due to Coronavirus-2), and within just a few months, the pandemic still unfolding today had developed [1,2]. Despite the morphological and genomic resemblances to SARS-CoV-1, responsible for the Asiatic SARS epidemic in 2002–2004, and to MERS-CoV, associated with the Middle East Coronavirus respiratory syndrome, SARS-CoV-2 is much more contagious, although the mortality rate is actually lower [1–4]. In Italy, the first confirmed cases date back to the end of January, when two Chinese tourists from the province of Hubei, traveling to Rome, were found positive for SARS-CoV-2 [5]. Then, in February, after the first infections that developed in Codogno (Lombardy), many other infection foci emerged, firstly mainly in northern Italy, in the Lombard provinces of Brescia, Bergamo and Milan, but then spreading all over the peninsula [5,6]. By 11 February 2021,

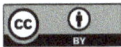

all the Italian regions had been infected by COVID-19 and more than two million positive cases had been recorded [7].

As regards placental disease in virus-positive pregnant women, only case reports or small, limited case series were reported in the first months of the pandemic [4,8–10]. However, as time passed, more and more cases of placental infection by SARS-CoV-2 were described, and there can be no doubt that with the progressive reduction in age of patients affected, the question of placental involvement and of potential maternal–fetal transmission has become an important matter of debate [10–12].

A study of the current literature seems to show that neonatal transmission is very rare, and that there are no specific SARS-CoV-2 histopathologic placental modifications observed in adverse perinatal outcomes, nor is there any evident greater risk of spontaneous abortion, preeclampsia, pre-term delivery or stillbirth [4,11,12]. However, few large case series have yet been reported owing to the obvious technical instrumental difficulties [13]. The present case–control study aimed to report the analysis of a large series of placentas from SARS-CoV-2-positive mothers observed at a COVID-19 reference center during the pandemic, and to compare them with a control group in order to highlight any histopathological alterations attributable to SARS-CoV-2. The research is documented by histopathological, ultrastructural and immunohistochemical findings, which are compared with other literature data.

2. Materials and Methods

2.1. Patients

The study was made of 83 placentas from 81 pregnant mothers (2 twin pregnancies) followed at the Gynecology and Obstetrics Operative Unit from 15 September 2020 to 31 January 2021, identified through electronic clinical records. All the women who presented during labor and delivery underwent testing with GeneXpert Dx Xpress SARS-CoV-2 RT-PCR (Cepheid) [14]. The analytical sensitivity and specificity of this test are reported by the manufacturers as 100% (87/87 samples) and 100% (30/30 samples), respectively, with a detection limit of 250 copies/mL or 0.0100 plaque-forming units per milliliter [15]. Positivity to the SARS-CoV-2 test was an independent criterion for the histopathologic analysis of the placentas. Among the positive SARS-CoV-2 group, twelve cases were excluded because they were related to unavoidable abortions due to maternal pathologies, which occurred in the 2nd trimester of the pregnancy, and to endo-uterine fetal deaths (EUFD) unrelated to SARS-CoV-2 positivity. The final sample included 71 placentas.

2.2. Controls

The SARS-CoV-2 group was compared with a control group of 142 placentas (1:2), selected from a population of pregnancy with physiological outcome, matched by gestational age and maternal age. Historical controls were selected from an archive of 500 placentas of women who had given birth between 2013 and 2018, of which 214 had a physiological fetal outcome. In accordance with the Amsterdam criteria, the parameters considered were: early maternal malperfusion, late maternal malperfusion, fetal malperfusion, placental infection/inflammation, villitis of unknown origin, delayed maturation of the villi; in addition, placental alterations (excluded from the Amsterdam criteria), including intravenous and chorangiotic hemorrhage, were taken into account. All records were retrieved from the electronic archives of our laboratory.

2.3. Procedure

The placentas were fixed in Formalin buffered at 10%, and photographs of the maternal and fetal surfaces were taken; they were then weighed, sampled and examined along the cut surface. The samples obtained included 2 rolls of amnio-chorial membrane, at least 2 samples from the umbilical cord, 3 from the maternal surface, 2 full-thickness sections and representative samples of any lesions presents. All samples were subjected to routine treatment, inclusion, 5 µm sectioning and hematoxylin–eosin staining (H&E). They were observed with an Olympus BX-51 Optical Microscope equipped with the Olympus DP80 image acquisition system. To randomly chosen sections of 51 placentas, the anti-SARS-CoV-2 spike S1 glycoprotein monoclonal antibody, Thermofisher, Rabbit, was added, at pH 6, diluted 1:800, and the antigenic unmasking heat-induced citrate buffer epitope retrieval, for enzymatic immunohistochemical (IHC) analysis. In addition, electronic microscopy analysis was performed for 30 of the 83 placentas. At the moment of delivery, random placental parenchyma samples were immediately fixed in 2.5% Gluteraldehyde for 4 h at 4 °C, and after overnight immersion in phosphate buffer, post-fixed with Osmium Tetroxide in PBS for 2 h at a temperature of 4 °C. The prepared samples were processed for inclusion in araldite epoxy resin (M) CY212 (TAAB, Aldermason, UK). Semifine sections 0.5 µm thick were stained with Toluidine Blue for microscopic analysis. Ultrafine sections were mounted on nickel grilles with uranium acetate and lead citrate contrast. The semifine sections were observed with a Nikon photomicroscope equipped with a Nikon Coolpix DS-U1 Digital Camera (Nikon Instruments SpA, Calenzano, Italy). The ultrafine sections were observed with a Morgagni 268 electron transmission microscope (FEI Company, Naples, Italy). All cases were examined independently under double-blind conditions by two pathologists with expertise in the field of perinatal pathology, to confirm the diagnoses.

2.4. Statistical Analysis

A preliminary description of maternal features in the SARS-CoV-2 group and control group was made, comparisons between means were performed with Student's t test for independent groups, and comparisons between percentages were made via chi-square test. The placental findings were compared by chi-square test. To correct for the potential presence of type I errors induced by multiple testing, all results were false discovery rate (FDR) corrected with alpha = 0.05. Quantities are reported as mean ± standard deviation. Categorical data are reported as frequencies and percentages. Statistical analysis was performed by means of SAS Software 9.4 (https://support.sas.com/software/94/index.html).

3. Results

All the SARS-CoV-2-positive pregnant women who presented to the Gynecologic and Obstetrics Clinic in the period between 15 September 2020 and 16 January 2021 were enrolled in the study. Of the 83 placentas in the SARS-CoV-2 -positive group, 6 were from unavoidable abortions due to maternal disease that developed in the second trimester of pregnancy and 6 from endo-uterine fetal deaths (EUFD) in the third trimester; all these placentas were excluded from the statistical analyses. The final sample included 71 placentas; 62 women had delivered at term (37–42 weeks) and 7 preterm (≤37 weeks). The mean gestational period was 38.5 ± 2.9 (20–42) weeks. The gravidae were aged 19 to 46 years, with a mean age 33.1 ± 6.1 years; 37 had a spontaneous vaginal delivery, 32 underwent cesarian section, urgent or elective; 31 were primiparous, 25 at their second pregnancy and 13 multiparous. No prior disease before or during pregnancy was reported by 54 women, while 3 were carriers of the methylenetetrahydrofolate-reductase gene (MTHFR), 1 of which was in association with a PAI-1 deficit, 4 were in treatment for hypothyroidism, 5 were affected by gestational diabetes treated with a special diet (in 1 case the metabolic disease was associated with hypertension and in 1 with allergic asthma), and 6 women were affected by hypertension; finally, 2 women had developed hepatogestosis. All these women were positive for SARS-CoV-2 at the moment of delivery; 42 patients (60.9%) were asymptomatic while 24 (34.8%) had a flu-like syndrome with one or more of the following symptoms: slight fever, headache, cough, myalgia, anosmia and ageusia. Of these, 13% required treatment. Finally, three (4.3%) patients had moderate/severe symptoms (two patients needed oxygen in cannula ventilation and one patient mechanical non-invasive ventilation). The Apgar scores of liveborn infants at 1 min were 8 or 9. All Apgar scores at 5 min were 9 or 10. No neonatal deaths occurred. All the infants were negative for SARS-CoV-2 at nasopharyngeal and/or pharyngeal swab.

The 71 placentas from SARS-CoV-2 -positive mothers were compared with 142 control placentas matched by gestational age and maternal age. The maternal and pregnancy features are reported in Table 1.

Table 1. Maternal and pregnancy features in SARS-COV-2 and control groups.

Maternal and Pregnancy Features	SARS-COV-2 Group	Control Group	Uncorrected p Values	FDR Corrected p Values
Maternal age (years), means ± sd (range)	33.1 ± 6.1 (19–46)	33.1 ± 5.7 (16–46)	0.97	0.97
Gestational age (week), means ± sd (range)	38.5 ± 2.9 (20–42)	38.9 ± 1.8 (32–42)	0.24	0.83
Apgar score 1 min, mean (sd)	9 (0.7)	9 (0.9)	0.62	0.83
Apgar score 5 min, mean (sd)	10 (0.5)	10 (0.4)	0.54	0.83
Primiparous, n (%)	31 (44.9)	97 (68.3)	0.0021	0.008
Cesarean Section, n (%)	32 (46.4)	124 (87.3)	<0.0001	0.0001
Diabetes, n (%)	5 (7)	11 (7.7)	0.55	0.61
Hypertension, n (%)	6 (8.6)	15 (10.6)	0.63	0.63
Thyroid dysfunction, n (%)	4 (5.8)	7 (4.9)	0.53	0.61
Other pathology, n (%)	3 (4.3)	2 (1.4)	0.20	0.37
PROM, n (%)	6 (8.6)	34 (23.9)	0.0063	0.017
IUGR, n (%)	0 (0)	18 (12.7)	0.0005	0.003
Polyhydramnios, n (%)	1 (1.4)	4 (2.8)	0.46	0.61
Oligohydramnios, n (%)	1 (1.4)	13 (9.2)	0.02	0.05

FDR correction was performed separately for means comparisons and for proportion comparisons. n = number of cases; sd = standard deviation.

In accordance with the matching, there were no significant differences in maternal and gestational age between SARS-CoV-2-positive and control mothers ($p > 0.05$). Maternal diseases were equally distributed in the two groups. PROMs were significantly less prevalent in the cases than the controls (8.4% vs. 23.9% $p = 0.017$), as were IUGR (0% vs. 12.7% $p = 0.003$) and oligohydramnios (1.4 vs. 9.2 $p = 0.05$). There were no differences for polyhydramnios ($p = 0.61$). Apgar scores at 1 min and 5 min were not significantly different ($p = 0.83$).

The mean placental weight was not significantly different between the two groups ($p = 0.48$). No differences in the percentage of maternal vascular malperfusion were observed in the cases compared to controls (54.3% vs. 43.7% $p = 0.19$), whereas the differences with regard to fetal vascular malperfusion (21.1% vs. 4.2% $p < 0.001$) were significant. The same applied for decidual arteriopathy (40.9% vs. 1.4% $p < 0.0001$), decidual inflammation (32.4% vs. 0.7% $p < 0.0001$), perivillous fibrin deposition (36.6% vs. 3.5% $p < 0.0001$) and fetal vessel thrombi (22.5% vs. 0.7% $p < 0.0001$). In contrast, a lower percentage of villous hypervascularization (12.7% vs. 34.5% $p < 0.001$) was observed in the SARS-CoV-2-positive group compared to controls (Figures 1–5). No significant differences in the percentage of terminal villous hyperplasia and chorioamnionitis were observed between the two groups (Table 2). The anti-SARS-CoV-2 spike-S1 glycoprotein antibody's results were significantly different, with 33/51 cases (65%) of diffuse positivity throughout the examined section and 18/51 cases (35%) of localized positivity, the expression being prevalent in the cytoplasm of the villi trophoblasts. We also observed positivity in 13/51 (25%) cases in the endothelium of the villi capillaries in sites of thrombosis; 14/51 cases (28%) showed positivity in the maternal decidual cells and in the intervillous histiocytes from maternal blood (Figures 6–9).

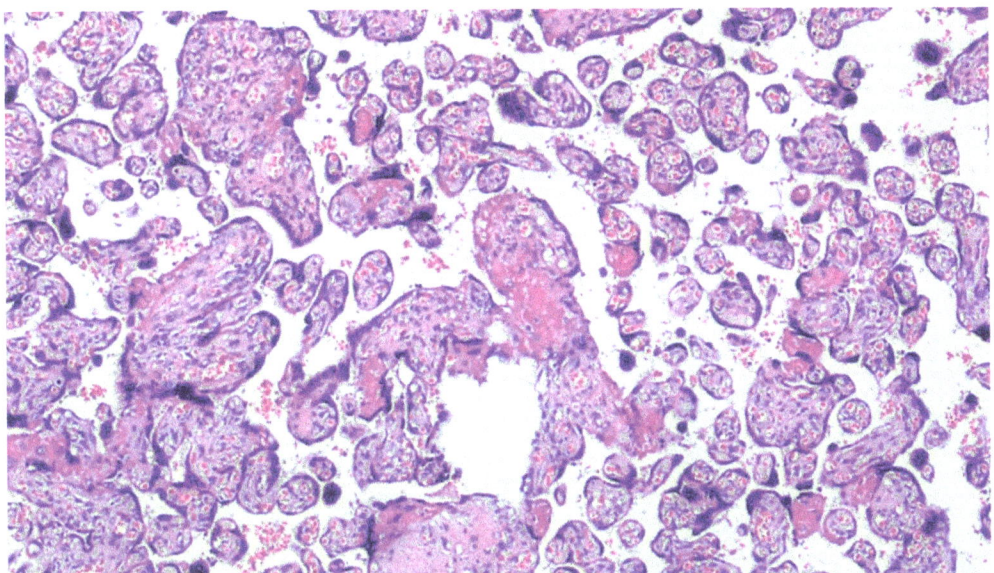

Figure 1. COVID-19-positive mother placenta. Terminal chorionic villi with poor vascular component (distal hypoplasia of the villi due to early maternal malperfusion) with increased syncytial nodes. Some villi show a deposition of fibrin in the intervillar space with progressive reduction of the villi (H&E, Hematoxylin and Eosin, 100×).

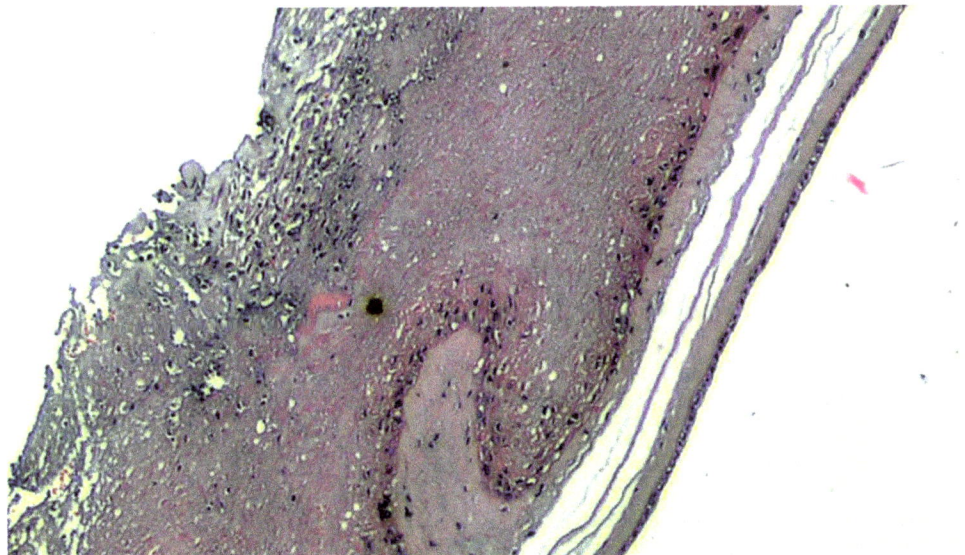

Figure 2. Amnio-chorionic membranes characterized by the presence of maternal neutrophilic granulocytes that infiltrate the sub-amniotic chorion starting from the maternal blood (H&E, 100×).

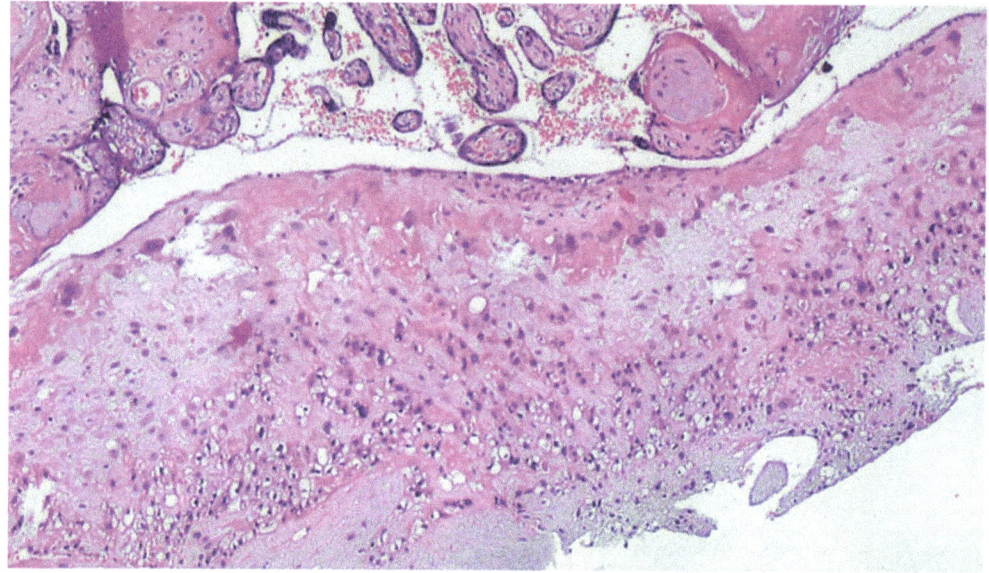

Figure 3. Basal deciduitis with a little trophoblastic component (superficial implant) and with few inflammatory cells (H&E, 200×).

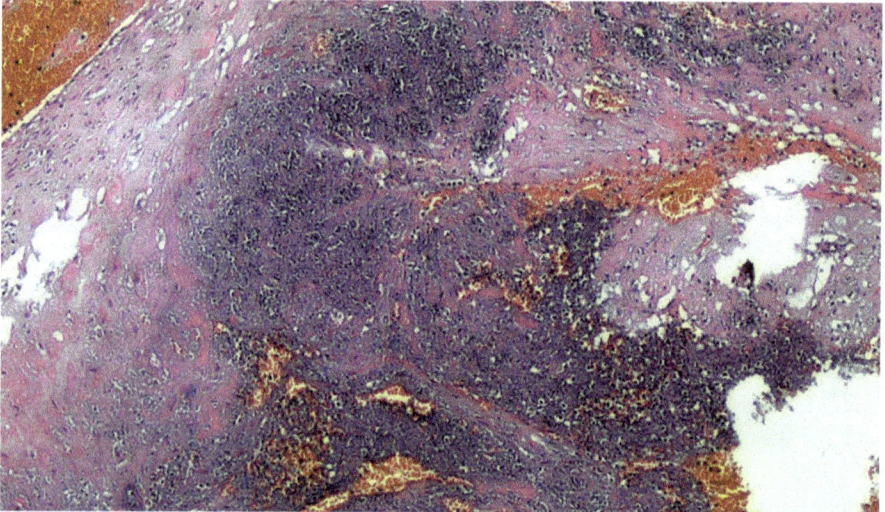

Figure 4. Deciduitis with large foci of necrosis and massive infiltration of mainly granulocytic inflammatory elements (acute deciduous, H&E, 200×) in the placenta of a COVID-positive mother.

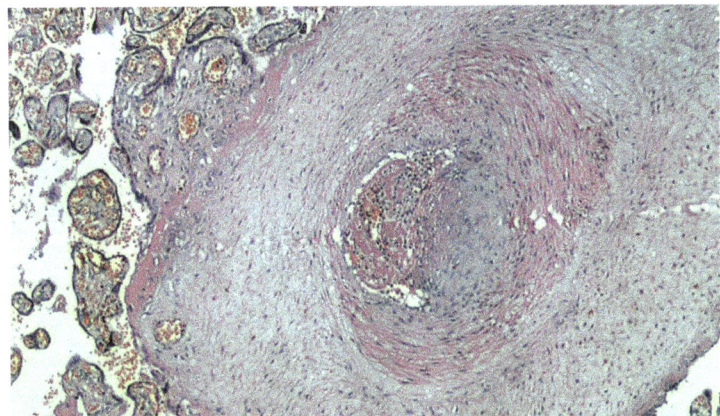

Figure 5. Histological section of the main villus: the artery has a thickened muscular wall, marked intimal fibrous thickening (probable organization of arterial thrombus), clear reduction of the lumen, and recent thrombosis of the residual lumen. H&E, 200×.

Table 2. Placental findings in SARS-COV-2 and control groups.

Placental Finding	SARS-COV-2 Group (71 Cases)	Control Group (142 Cases)	Uncorrected p Values	FDR-Corrected p Values
Weight (grams), means ± sd (range)	515 ± 84 (240–760)	499.2 ± 176.6 (130–1020)	0.48	0.48
Maternal malperfusion, n (%)	38 (54.3)	62 (43.7)	0.15	0.19
Decidual arteriopathy, n (%)	29 (40.9)	2 (1.4)	<0.0001	<0.0001
Fetal malperfusion, n (%)	15 (21.1)	6 (4.2)	<0.0001	<0.0001
Decidual inflammation, n (%)	23 (32.4)	1 (0.7)	<0.0001	<0.0001
Perivillous fibrin deposition, n (%)	26 (36.6)	5 (3.5)	<0.0001	<0.0001
Terminal villous hyperplasia n (%)	14 (19.7)	30 (21.1)	0.81	0.81
Villous hypervascularization, n (%)	9 (12.7)	49 (34.5)	0.0007	0.0011
Thrombi in fetal vessels, n (%)	16 (22.2)	1 (0.7)	<0.0001	<0.0001
Chorioamnionitis, n (%)	5 (7)	7 (4.9)	0.37	0.41

FDR correction was performed separately for means comparisons and for proportion comparisons. n = number of cases.

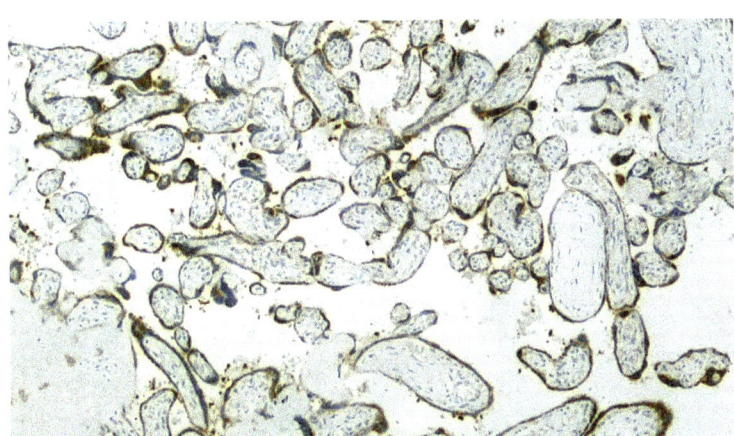

Figure 6. Section set up for immunohistochemistry investigation using the Sars-CoV-2 anti-spikes glycoprotein antibody. Note the widespread involvement of brown-colored syncytiotrophoblast (Immunohistochemistry, IHC, 100×).

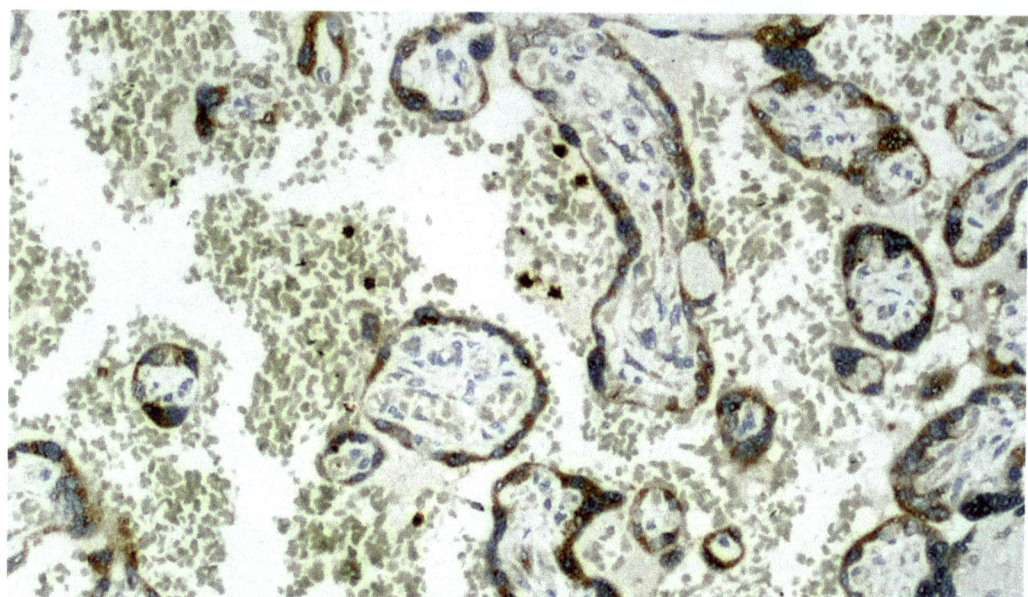

Figure 7. Detail of the previous image. In addition to the positivity expressed by the trophoblast, a very intense positivity is observed in the leukocytes of the maternal blood (IHC, 400×).

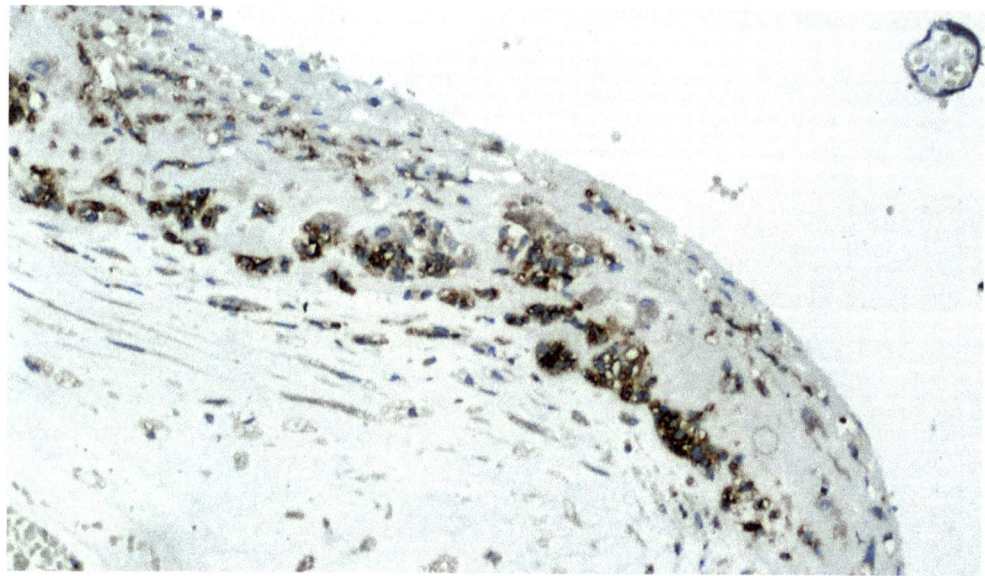

Figure 8. Expression of viral antigen in stromal cells of the basal decidua (IHC, 400×).

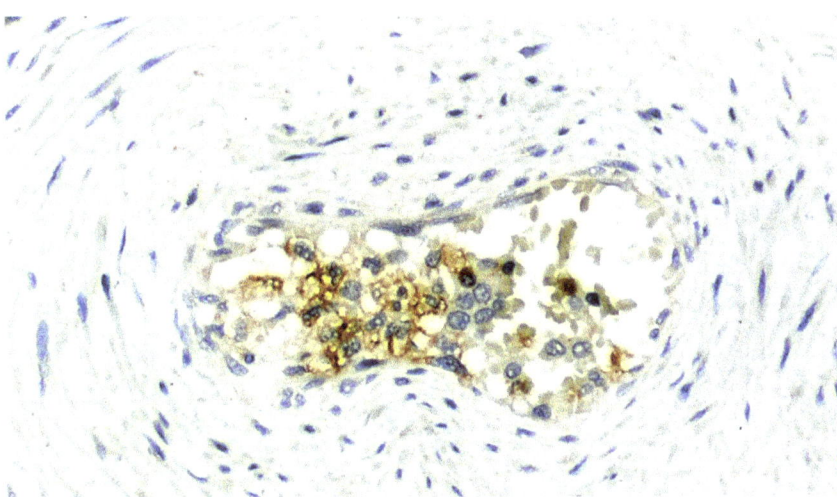

Figure 9. Detail of a small vessel of an 8th order main villus characterized by the expression of a spike glycoprotein antigen on endothelial cells degenerated during thrombosis (IHC, 400×).

Electron microscopy showed signs of endothelial damage in the fetal vessels, with endothelial hypertrophy and a reduced lumen. In the cytoplasm of the trophoblasts of some cells, circular formations with a 100–130 nm diameter were observed, with peripheral electron dense spicules, which are likely viral particles (Figures 10 and 11).

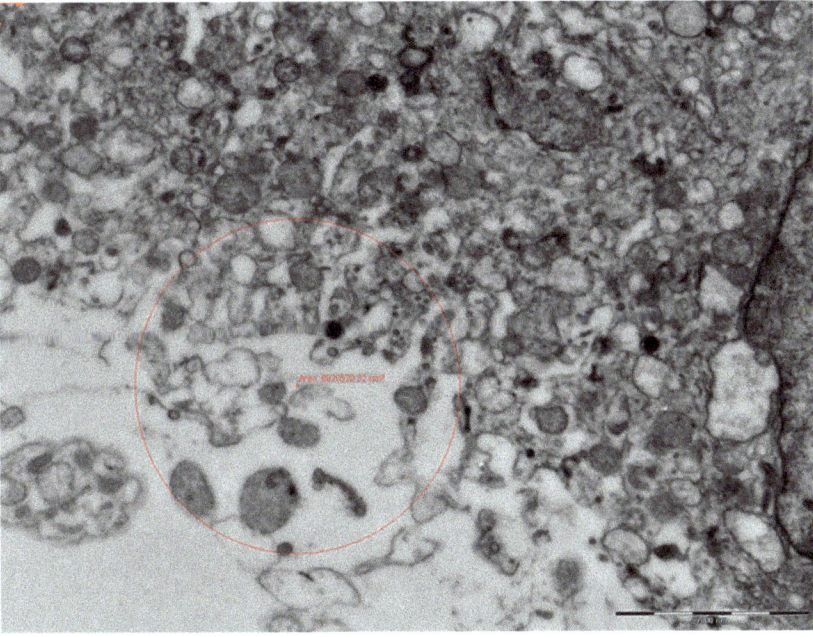

Figure 10. Photomicrograph of syncytium trophoblast cytoplasm. In addition to the microvillary projections, the cell has numerous secretory vacuoles, mitochondria and electrondense lysosomes (11,000×).

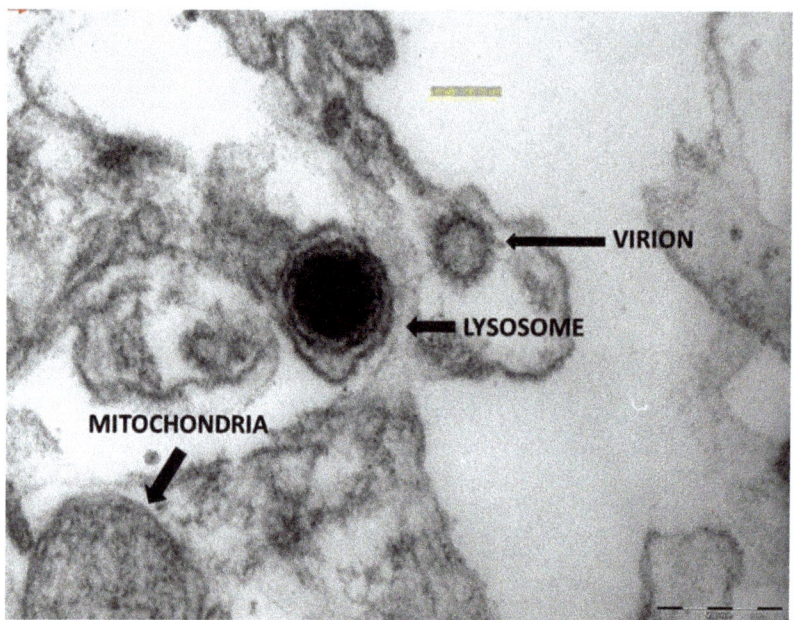

Figure 11. Strong magnification of a spherical particle of 106,720 nm with spicular electron-dense projections next to a strongly electrondense lysosomal formation (71,000×).

4. Discussion

In recent months, various reports have been published describing studies of the placentas of mothers affected by SARS-CoV-2. Some case reports and case series have aimed to throw light on the pathophysiologic aspects of SARS-CoV-2 infection in pregnant women [11–13,16]. These studies were focused in particular on the maternal outcomes of patients with symptomatic disease; maternal death, stillbirth and neonatal death were reported to occur in about 1% of the cases [17]. The risk of SARS-CoV-2 positivity in a newborn from a mother admitted to hospital with symptomatic disease is about 2.5% [17]. Few works in the literature have reported solid evidence of vertical transplacental transmission [12,13,16,18].

Allotey J et al. suggest that pregnant women with symptomatic SARS-CoV-2 infection are less likely to present with fever and myalgia, but are more likely to need intensive care, ventilation, and have a higher risk of pre-term delivery [19,20]; moreover, death occurs in a small number of cases that are COVID-related [21–24]. Among the 71 placentas we analyzed, there were no cases of the maternal–fetal transmission of SARS-CoV-2, and all the newborns were in good health at birth, with similar APGAR scores at 1 min and 5 min to those of the controls ($p = 0.83$). The cases of unavoidable abortion in the second trimester ($n = 6$) were linked to diseases not correlated with a viral infection in course, such as chromosomal alterations and maternal conditions such as systemic lupus erythematosus (SLE) and diabetes, which are in themselves often associated with a greater spontaneous abortion rate [25]. In the same way, the six endouterine fetal deaths were attributable to maternal conditions (pre-eclampsia and diabetes) that, in our opinion, could not be correlated with the infection [25,26]. As can be seen in Table 1, the placental alterations we observed are only partially comparable to those in the control population, with signs of maternal vascular malperfusion (MVM) being observed in both cohorts. In this sense, despite what was declared by Shanes [27] and Menter [13], we believe that the vascular modifications of villi considered to be signs of MVM can also be seen as functional adaptation phenomena in many cases, leading to a favorable neonatal outcome [28]. It is easier to correlate some of the alterations in the patients group to SARS-CoV-2 infection, such as the presence of thrombi in the utero–placental arteries, of deciduitis foci with tissue necrosis, and of an inflammatory infiltrate, which are likely correlated to virus-mediated damage, as pointed out by Baergen [29]; these were more frequent in the virus-infected patients than the controls. These latter findings were also confirmed by Prabhu et al. [30]. Phenomena such as fetal vascular malperfusion (FVM) and thrombosis, particularly of small caliber vessels of the main sixth or eighth order villi, can be correlated to SARS-CoV-2. Intervillous fibrin deposits are reported to be a very common observation in SARS-CoV-2-positive women, as described by Chen et al. [31]. This finding seems to be related more to an immuno-mediated outcome of maternal origin, rather than being a sign of true maternal malperfusion. [27,29]. It is possible that immunological stimulation of the mother, as well as trophoblasts damage, may be the underlying cause of the greater intervillous fibrin deposits in SARS-CoV-2-positive placentas. Some authors [12,21,22,24] have described the presence of intervillous histiocytes, interpreted as a sign of perivillitis. In our experience, perivillitis with a significantly elevated number of histiocytes was observed in only three cases, whereas the immunohistochemistry studies showed strong positivity for the anti-SARS-CoV-2 spike glycoprotein antibody in maternal white blood cells. It is important to note that several patients showed alterations normally attributable to maternal diseases that have nothing to do with viral infection, such as diabetes or latent hypertension, aspecific inflammatory reactions of the membranes, and non-specific unreactive villitis. However, the immunohistochemical studies showed the presence of the viral antigen in many maternal cells, particularly deciduous stromal and endothelial cells, and in perivillous inflammatory cells. This issue has already been pointed out by Patanè et al. [23]; indeed, the positivity observed in syncytiotrophoblasts could be interpreted as a barrier effect of these cells between the maternal and the fetal compartments. Only in rare cases was endothelial positivity in the fetal capillaries associated with thrombosis. The vascular damage that can occur is demonstrated by the frequent aspects of endothelial hyperplasia of the fetal capillaries and the reduced lumen that we observed. The finding, through electron microscopy, of structures compatible with the virus in syncytial cells, associated with gross vacuolization of the cytoplasm, confirms the positivity of this cell layer in terms of immunohistochemistry, as well as justifying the trophoblast necrosis phenomena described by some authors, and has been indicated as the cause of maternal–fetal transmission of the virus [32,33].

5. Conclusions

Our study, conducted on a large number of placentas, shows that in cases of SARS-CoV-2-positive pregnant women without transmission of the disease to the fetus, the placentas are largely unaffected by the inflammatory process. However, there are some more frequent characteristics in the placentas of infected women, in particular, maternal thrombosis and deciduous, increased intervillous fibrin, and, in rare cases, fetal thrombosis. The immunohistochemical investigation demonstrates positivity for the anti-SARS-CoV-2 spike glycoprotein antibody both among maternal cells (including inflammatory intervillary cells) and in the trophoblast, and rarely in the endothelium. The ultrastructural investigation demonstrated both the suffering of fetal endothelia and the presence of particles attributable to SARS-CoV-2 in the trophoblast, in conjunction with its degeneration.

As the pandemic continues, these studies will become more urgent for clarifying the possible mechanism of the maternal–fetal transmission of the virus.

Author Contributions: Conceptualization, G.C. and L.R.; methodology, L.R. and M.F.; software, M.F.; validation, G.C., G.M. and L.R.; formal analysis, A.V.; investigation, R.R.; resources, E.C.; data curation, A.C. and M.F.; writing—original draft preparation, G.C. and G.M.; writing—review and editing, G.C., G.M., S.V.S., M.F. and L.R.; visualization, O.C.; supervision, L.R. All authors have read and agreed to the published version of the manuscript.

Funding: This research received no external funding.

Institutional Review Board Statement: The study was conducted according to the guidelines of the Declaration of Helsinki, and approved by the Institutional Review Board of Policlinico di Bari (deliberation number 261, 11 February 2021).

Informed Consent Statement: Informed consent was obtained from all subjects involved in the study.

Conflicts of Interest: The authors declare no conflict of interest.

References

1. Yüce, M.; Filiztekin, E.; Özkaya, K.G. COVID-19 diagnosis-A review of current methods. *Biosens. Bioelectron.* **2021**, *172*, 112752. [CrossRef] [PubMed]
2. Harrison, A.G.; Lin, T.; Wang, P. Mechanisms of SARS-CoV-2 Transmission and Pathogenesis. *Trends Immunol.* **2020**, *41*, 1100–1115. [CrossRef]
3. Kirtipal, N.; Bharadwaj, S.; Kang, S.G. From SARS to SARS-CoV-2, insights on structure, pathogenicity and immunity aspects of pandemic human coronaviruses. *Infect. Genet. Evol.* **2020**, *85*, 104502. [CrossRef] [PubMed]
4. Di Mascio, D.; Khalil, A.; Saccone, G.; Rizzo, G.; Buca, D.; Liberati, M.; Vecchiet, J.; Nappi, L.; Scambia, G.; Berghella, V.; et al. Outcome of coronavirus spectrum infections (SARS, MERS, COVID-19) during pregnancy: A systematic review and meta-analysis. *Am. J. Obstet. Gynecol.* **2020**, *2*, 100107. [CrossRef]
5. Zehender, G.; Lai, A.; Bergna, A.; Meroni, L.; Riva, A.; Balotta, C.; Tarkowski, M.; Gabrieli, A.; Bernacchia, D.; Rusconi, S.; et al. Genomic characterization and phylogenetic analysis of SARS-COV-2 in Italy. *J. Med. Virol.* **2020**, *92*, 1637–1640. [CrossRef] [PubMed]
6. Giovanetti, M.; Angeletti, S.; Benvenuto, D.; Ciccozzi, M. A doubt of multiple introduction of SARS-CoV-2 in Italy: A preliminary overview. *J. Med. Virol.* **2020**, *92*, 1634–1636. [CrossRef]
7. Available online: https://covid19.who.int/region/euro/country/it (accessed on 11 February 2021).
8. Algarroba, G.N.; Rekawek, P.; Vahanian, S.A.; Khullar, P.; Palaia, T.; Peltier, M.R.; Chavez, M.R.; Vintzileos, A.M. Visualization of severe acute respiratory syndrome coronavirus 2 invading the human placenta using electron microscopy. *Am. J. Obstet. Gynecol.* **2020**, *223*, 275–278. [CrossRef]
9. Hosier, H.; Farhadian, S.F.; Morotti, R.A.; Deshmukh, U.; Lu-Culligan, A.; Campbell, K.H.; Yasumoto, Y.; Vogels, C.B.; Casanovas-Massana, A.; Vijayakumar, P.; et al. SARS-CoV-2 infection of the placenta. *J. Clin. Investig.* **2020**, *130*, 4947–4953. [CrossRef]
10. Gujski, M.; Humeniuk, E.; Bojar, I. Current State of Knowledge About SARS-CoV-2 and COVID-19 Disease in Pregnant Women. *Med. Sci. Monit.* **2020**, *26*, e924725. [CrossRef]
11. Sisman, J.; Jaleel, M.A.; Moreno, W.; Rajaram, V.; Collins, R.R.J.; Savani, R.C.; Rakheja, D.; Evans, A.S. Intrauterine Transmission of SARS-COV-2 Infection in a Preterm Infant. *Pediatr. Infect. Dis. J.* **2020**, *39*, e265–e267. [CrossRef]
12. Schwartz, D.A. An analysis of 38 pregnant women with COVID-19, their newborn infants, and maternal-fetal transmission of SARS-CoV-2: Maternal coronavirus infections and pregnancy outcomes. *Arch. Pathol. Lab. Med.* **2020**, *144*, 799–805. [CrossRef]
13. Menter, T.; Mertz, K.D.; Jiang, S.; Chen, H.; Monod, C.; Tzankov, A.; Waldvogel, S.; Schulzke, S.M.; Hösli, I.; Bruder, E. Placental Pathology Findings during and after SARS-CoV-2 Infection: Features of Villitis and Malperfusion. *Pathobiology* **2020**, *88*, 69–77. [CrossRef]
14. CDC 2019-Novel Coronavirus (2019-nCoV) Real-Time RT-PCR Diagnostic Panel. 2020. Available online: https://www.fda.gov/media/134922/download.
15. Cepheid. Xpert® Xpress SARS-CoV-2 Instructions for Use for Labs 2020. Available online: https://www.fda.gov/media/136314/download (accessed on 5 February 2021).
16. Baergen, R.N.; Heller, D.S. Placental Pathology in Covid-19 Positive Mothers: Preliminary Findings. *Pediatric Dev. Pathol.* **2020**, *23*, 177–180. [CrossRef]
17. Knight, M.; Bunch, K.; Vousden, N.; Morris, E.; Simpson, N.; Gale, C.; O'Brien, P.; Quigley, M.; Brocklehurst, P.; Kurinczuk, J. Characteristics and outcomes of pregnant women admitted to hospital with confirmed SARS-CoV-2 infection in UK: National population based cohort study. *BMJ* **2020**, *369*, m2107. [CrossRef]
18. Vivanti, A.J.; Vauloup-Fellous, C.; Prevot, S.; Zupan, V.; Suffee, C.; Do Cao, J.; Benachi, A.; De Luca, D. Transplacental transmission of SARS-CoV-2 infection. *Nat. Commun.* **2020**, *11*, 3572. [CrossRef]
19. Allotey, J.; Stallings, E.; Bonet, M.; Yap, M.; Chatterjee, S.; Kew, T.; Debenham, L.; Llavall, A.C.; Dixit, A.; Zhou, D.; et al. Clinical manifestations, risk factors, and maternal and perinatal outcomes of coronavirus disease 2019 in pregnancy: Living systematic review and meta-analysis. *BMJ* **2020**, *370*, m3320. [CrossRef]
20. Mullins, E.; Hudak, M.L.; Banerjee, J.; Getzlaff, T.; Townson, J.; Barnette, K.; Playle, R.; Bourne, T.; Lees, C. PAN-COVID Investigators and the National Perinatal COVID-19 Registry Study Group. Pregnancy and neonatal outcomes of COVID-19: Co-reporting of common outcomes from PAN-COVID and AAP SONPM registries. *medRxiv* **2021**. [CrossRef]
21. Facchetti, F.; Bugatti, M.; Drera, E.; Tripodo, C.; Sartori, E.; Cancila, V.; Papaccio, M.; Castellani, R.; Casola, S.; Boniotti, M.B.; et al. SARS-CoV2 vertical transmission with adverse effects on the newborn revealed through integrated immunohistochemical, electron microscopy and molecular analyses of Placenta. *EBioMedicine* **2020**, *59*, 102951. [CrossRef] [PubMed]
22. Karimu, A.L.; Burton, G.J. The effects of maternal vascular pressure on the dimensions of the placental capillaries. *BJOG* **1994**, *101*, 57–63. [CrossRef] [PubMed]

23. Patanè, L.; Morotti, D.; Giunta, M.R.; Sigismondi, C.; Piccoli, M.G.; Frigerio, L.; Mangili, G.; Arosio, M.; Cornolti, G. Vertical transmission of coronavirus disease 2019: Severe acute respiratory syndrome coronavirus 2 RNA on the fetal side of the placenta in pregnancies with coronavirus disease 2019-positive mothers and neonates at birth. *Am. J. Obstet. Gynecol.* **2020**, *2*, 100145. [CrossRef] [PubMed]
24. Kaufmann, P.; Senn, D.K.; Schweikhart, G. Classification of Human placental villi. I. histology and scanning electron microscopy. *Cell Tissue Res.* **1979**, *200*, 409–423. [CrossRef]
25. Galang, R.R.; Chang, K.; Strid, P.; Snead, M.C.; Woodworth, K.R.; House, L.D.; Perez, M.; Barfield, W.D.; Meaney-Delman, D.; Jamieson, D.J.; et al. Severe Coronavirus Infections in Pregnancy: A Systematic Review. *Obstet. Gynecol.* **2020**, *136*, 262–272. [CrossRef]
26. Takemoto, M.; Menezes, M.O.; Andreucci, C.B.; Knobel, R.; Sousa, L.; Katz, L.; Fonseca, E.B.; Magalhães, C.G.; Oliveira, W.K.; Rezende-Filho, J.; et al. Maternal mortality and COVID-19. *J. Matern. Fetal Neonatal Med.* **2020**, 1–7. [CrossRef]
27. Shanes, E.D.; Mithal, L.B.; Otero, S.; Azad, H.A.; Miller, E.S.; Goldstein, J.A. Placental Pathology in COVID-19. *Am. J. Clin. Pathol.* **2020**, *154*, 23–32. [CrossRef]
28. Loverro, M.T.; Damiani, G.R.; Di Naro, E.; Schonauer, L.M.; Laforgia, N.; Loverro, M.; Capursi, T.; Muzzupapa, G.; Resta, L. Analysis of relation between placental lesions and perinatal outcome according to Amsterdam criteria: A comparative study. *Acta Biomed.* **2020**, *91*, e2020061.
29. Wastnedge, E.A.N.; Reynolds, R.M.; van Boeckel, S.R.; Stock, S.J.; Denison, F.C.; Maybin, J.A.; Critchley, H.O.D. Pregnancy and COVID-19. *Physiol. Rev.* **2021**, *101*, 303–318. [CrossRef]
30. Prabhu, M.; Cagino, K.; Matthews, K.C.; Friedlander, R.L.; Glynn, S.M.; Kubiak, J.M.; Yang, Y.J.; Zhao, Z.; Baergen, R.N.; DiPace, J.I.; et al. Pregnancy and postpartum outcomes in a universally tested population for SARS-CoV-2 in New York City: A prospective cohort study. *BJOG* **2020**, *127*, 1548–1556. [CrossRef] [PubMed]
31. Chen, S.; Huang, B.; Luo, D.J.; Li, X.; Yang, F.; Zhao, Y.; Nie, X.; Huang, B.X. Pregnancy with new coronavirus infection: Clinical characteristics and placental pathological analysis of three cases. *Chin. J. Pathol.* **2020**, *49*, 418–423.
32. Kirtsman, M.; Diambomba, Y.; Poutane, S.M.; Malinowski, A.K.; Vlachodimitropoulou, E.; Parks, W.T.; Erdman, L.; Morris, S.K.; Shah, P.S. Probable congenital SARS-CoV-2 infection in a neonate born to a woman with active SARS-CoV-2 infection. *CMAJ* **2020**, *192*, E647–E650. [CrossRef] [PubMed]
33. Smithgall, M.C.; Liu-Jarin, X.; Hamele-Bena, D.; Cimic, A.; Mourad, M.; Debelenko, L.; Chen, X. Third Trimester Placentas of SARS-CoV-2-Positive Women: Histomorphology, including Viral Immunohistochemistry and in Situ Hybridization. Short running title: Placentas in SARS-CoV-2-Positive Women. *Histopathology* **2020**, *77*, 994–999. [CrossRef]

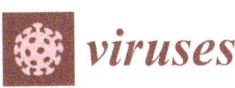

Article

SARS-CoV-2 Vaccine Willingness among Pregnant and Breastfeeding Women during the First Pandemic Wave: A Cross-Sectional Study in Switzerland

Sarah Stuckelberger [1], Guillaume Favre [1], Michael Ceulemans [2,3], Hedvig Nordeng [4,5], Eva Gerbier [1], Valentine Lambelet [1], Milos Stojanov [1], Ursula Winterfeld [6], David Baud [1], Alice Panchaud [7,8,*,†] and Léo Pomar [1,9,*,†]

1. Department Woman-Mother-Child, Lausanne University Hospital and University of Lausanne, 1011 Lausanne, Switzerland; Sarah.Stuckelberger@chuv.ch (S.S.); guillaume.favre@chuv.ch (G.F.); Eva.Gerbier@chuv.ch (E.G.); valentine.lambelet@gmail.com (V.L.); Milos.Stojanov@chuv.ch (M.S.); David.Baud@chuv.ch (D.B.)
2. Department of Pharmaceutical and Pharmacological Sciences, KU Leuven, 3000 Leuven, Belgium; michael.ceulemans@kuleuven.be
3. Teratology Information Service, Pharmacovigilance Centre Lareb, 5237 MH 's-Hertogenbosch, The Netherlands
4. Pharmacoepidemiology and Drug Safety Research Group, Department of Pharmacy, PharmaTox Strategic Initiative, Faculty of Mathematics and Natural Sciences, University of Oslo, 0315 Oslo, Norway; h.m.e.nordeng@farmasi.uio.no
5. Department of Child Health and Development, Norwegian Institute of Public Health, 0403 Oslo, Norway
6. Swiss Teratogen Information Service, Service de Pharmacologie Clinique, Lausanne University Hospital and University of Lausanne, 1011 Lausanne, Switzerland; Ursula.Winterfeld@chuv.ch
7. Institute of Primary Health Care (BIHAM), University of Bern, 3012 Bern, Switzerland
8. Service of Pharmacy, Lausanne University Hospital and University of Lausanne, 1011 Lausanne, Switzerland
9. School of Health Sciences (HESAV) Midwifery Department, University of Applied Sciences and Arts Western Switzerland, 1011 Lausanne, Switzerland
* Correspondence: alice.panchaud@chuv.ch (A.P.); leo.pomar@chuv.ch (L.P.)
† Similar contribution as senior authors.

Abstract: As pregnant women are at high risk of severe SARS-CoV-2 infection and COVID-19 vaccines are available in Switzerland, this study aimed to assess the willingness of Swiss pregnant and breastfeeding women to become vaccinated. Through a cross-sectional online study conducted after the first pandemic wave, vaccination practices and willingness to become vaccinated against SARS-CoV-2 if a vaccine was available were evaluated through binary, multi-choice, and open-ended questions. Factors associated with vaccine willingness were evaluated through univariable and multivariable analysis. A total of 1551 women responded to questions related to the primary outcome. Only 29.7% (153/515) of pregnant and 38.6% (400/1036) of breastfeeding women were willing to get vaccinated against SARS-CoV-2 if a vaccine had been available during the first wave. Positive predictors associated with SARS-CoV-2 vaccine acceptance were an age older than 40 years, a higher educational level, history of influenza vaccination within the previous year, having an obstetrician as the primary healthcare practitioner, and being in their third trimester of pregnancy. After the first pandemic wave, Switzerland had a low SARS-CoV-2 vaccination acceptance rate, emphasizing the need to identify and reduce barriers for immunization in pregnant and breastfeeding women, particularly among the youngest and those with a lower educational level.

Keywords: SARS-CoV-2; coronavirus; COVID-19; pregnancy; breastfeeding; vaccine willingness

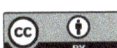

1. Introduction

In 2020, the outbreak of a novel coronavirus, the severe acute respiratory syndrome coronavirus 2 (SARS-CoV-2), was declared a pandemic with more than 166 million confirmed cases worldwide. In Switzerland, more than 680,000 people tested positive with more than 10,000 deaths reported [1].

Pregnant women are considered a vulnerable population for SARS-CoV-2 infection. Current evidence suggests that they are up to 70% more susceptible to infection. If infected, they are also at greater risk of developing complications [2–4] such as admission to an intensive care unit, mechanical ventilation, and death [5,6]. Increased risk of caesarian section, iatrogenic prematurity, post-partum hemorrhage, preeclampsia, and miscarriage have also been reported [7–11].

Currently, two SARS-CoV-2 mRNA vaccines approved by Swissmedic (the Swiss authority for the utilization and surveillance of therapeutic products) are used in the vaccine campaign in Switzerland [12]. However, vaccines cannot curb epidemics without widespread acceptance. The World Health Organization (WHO) has listed vaccine hesitancy as one of the top ten threats to global health [13], especially for populations at risk. In Switzerland, as in many countries, vaccination programs have already been established to protect pregnant women and their infants from serious infections such as influenza and pertussis. Both influenza and pertussis vaccines have proven to be effective in protecting mothers and their newborns [14,15]. However, immunization rates for influenza and pertussis have been disappointingly low in Switzerland [16] mainly due to a lack of adequate promotion and compliance [17]. Low uptake of vaccination in pregnancy has been reported worldwide [18,19] with several studies identifying inadequate knowledge about the disease threat; doubts about vaccine safety, efficacy, and benefits; and the lack of recommendations from vaccine providers, as the main obstacles among pregnant women [20–22]. Maternal characteristics may also play a role. Unemployment, younger age (<25 years old), and high perceived stress have been associated with lower vaccination rates during pregnancy, whereas a history of depression increased the likelihood of being vaccinated [23].

SARS-CoV-2 vaccination has recently been recommended in Switzerland for pregnant women who have additional risk factors or are at high risk of exposure through their work. This vaccination strategy may represent a barrier to the successful vaccination of all members of this high-risk group, especially when compared to some countries where pregnant women are routinely vaccinated or considered a priority group. This is a glaring example of the need to better understand the many factors influencing the acceptance of and access to vaccination, especially among more vulnerable populations such as pregnant women to develop targeted information campaigns.

Thus, in a cross-sectional survey during the first wave of the pandemic, we investigated COVID-19 vaccine willingness among Swiss pregnant and breastfeeding women if a vaccine was available, as well as the factors contributing to their acceptance or hesitancy.

2. Materials and Methods

2.1. Study Population and Data Collection

This Swiss cross-sectional online study is part of a European multi-center study conducted in several countries (Belgium, Ireland, Norway, The Netherlands, United Kingdom) and approved by the Ethics Committee Research of UZ/KU Leuven (id: S63966). The questionnaire used in Switzerland was available in German, French, and Italian. The goal was to examine the overall impact of the SARS-CoV-2 pandemic on pregnant and breastfeeding women (i.e., pregnancy/breastfeeding experience, life and professional habits, mental health status, relationship with the healthcare system, medication use, and vaccine perceptions during pregnancy/breastfeeding) [24]. The COVID-19 vaccine willingness of pregnant and breastfeeding women included in the multi-center study has already been published [25], and the Swiss rate was among the lowest, hence the need to investigate the factors associated with vaccine acceptance in a Swiss-specific study.

In Switzerland, the online questionnaire was accessible from 18 June to 12 July 2020 through websites, forums, and social media (www.letsfamily.ch, www.swissmom.ch, www.medela.ch, www.chuv.ch). All data were collected and processed anonymously. All participants provided online informed consent prior to survey initiation.

2.2. Study Population

To be eligible, Swiss women needed to be at least 18 years old and be pregnant at the time of the survey or have breastfed within the past three months.

2.3. Variables

We collected information on sociodemographic characteristics (i.e., age, primary language, marital status, working status, education level), medical history (i.e., gravidity, parity, co-morbidities, smoking during pregnancy, main practitioner for the pregnancy follow-up, clinical course of the neonate for breastfeeding mothers), exposure to SARS-CoV-2 or presence in an at-risk setting (i.e., symptoms potentially related to COVID-19, hospitalization related to COVID-19, testing by RT-PCR, serology or computed tomography, living with someone who tested positive, co-habiting with an elderly person (>65 years old)). The negative impact of the SARS-CoV-2 pandemic on the pregnancy/breastfeeding experience, life habits, and work was assessed through participants graded answers: "yes" or "rather yes", grouped as "negative impact of the SARS-CoV-2 pandemic"; and "rather no" or "no", grouped as "no negative impact of the SARS-CoV-2 pandemic". Mental health status was assessed using validated screening tests including the Edinburgh Postnatal Depression Scale for depression [26,27], the Generalized Anxiety Disorder 7-item Scale for anxiety [28], and the Perceived Stress Scale for stress [29,30]. Information on vaccination practices was obtained through a dichotomic question on vaccination against influenza within the past year (yes or no) and multi-choice questions assessing their opinion on influenza vaccine usefulness during pregnancy and breastfeeding, the fear of maternal and fetal/neonatal side effects, and overall vaccination acceptance.

2.4. Main Outcomes

COVID-19 vaccine willingness of pregnant and breastfeeding women if a vaccine had been available was evaluated through participants' graded answers: "fully agree", "rather agree", "rather disagree", or "fully disagree". Participants who "fully agree" or "rather agree" were grouped as "willing to get vaccinated against SARS-CoV-2" and those who "rather disagree" or "fully disagree" were grouped as "not willing to get vaccinated against SARS-CoV-2" in the analysis.

2.5. Statistical Analysis

Baseline and medical characteristics, SARS-CoV-2 exposure (SARS-CoV-2 testing, symptoms, and hospitalization), fears, impacts of the pandemic, mental health symptoms, and vaccination habits were presented using descriptive statistics for both pregnant and breastfeeding women. The prevalence of participants willing to get vaccinated against COVID-19 was calculated.

The associations between variables of interest and the willingness to get vaccinated against SARS-CoV-2 was measured by univariate and multivariate logistic regression and were presented as crude odds ratios (OR) and adjusted odds ratios (aORs) with 95% confidence intervals (95% CI). Variables with $p > 0.10$ in the univariate analysis were not included in the multivariate model. The variables of interest were maternal age >40 years old, educational level (dichotomized as higher than high school or not), professional activity (dichotomized as active or not), primary language (French, German, Italian), maternal co-morbidities (grouped into a single "any maternal co-morbidity" variable), testing positive for SARS-CoV-2 infection (either by RT-PCR, serology, or CT-scan, grouped into a single "tested positive for SARS-CoV-2" variable), living with someone >65 years old, having a negative impact by the pandemic on the pregnancy/breastfeeding experience, life habits, and work, experiencing symptoms of severe depression (EDS ≥ 13), anxiety (GAD-7 ≥ 15), or high stress perceived (PSS ≥ 27) (grouped into a single variable), being vaccinated against influenza in the past year, previous history of declining vaccination, and fear of side effects related to vaccines (for the mother and the fetus/neonate). Variables specific to pregnant women (pregnancy practitioner, current trimester of gestation, and fear of an adverse fetal outcome in case of maternal SARS-CoV-2 infection) were studied in a supplementary multivariate model including only pregnant participants.

2.6. Missing Values

Maternal comorbidities were considered as absent if not reported, based on the assumption that severe comorbidities are normally documented. Based on the hypothesis of missing variables completely at random (MCAR), multiple imputations with chained equations (10 replications) were performed to increase the power of comparisons for missing values.

3. Results

A total of 2064 respondents participated in the survey (1161 using the French questionnaire, 868 using the German questionnaire, and 35 using the Italian questionnaire) including 1501 breastfeeding and 563 pregnant women. Among them, 513 (24.9%) did not answer the question relating to whether they were willing to get vaccinated against SARS-CoV-2 if a vaccine was available. Thus, 75.1% (n = 1551) contributed to the analyses addressing the primary aim of the study (1036 breastfeeding mothers and 515 pregnant women) (Figure 1).

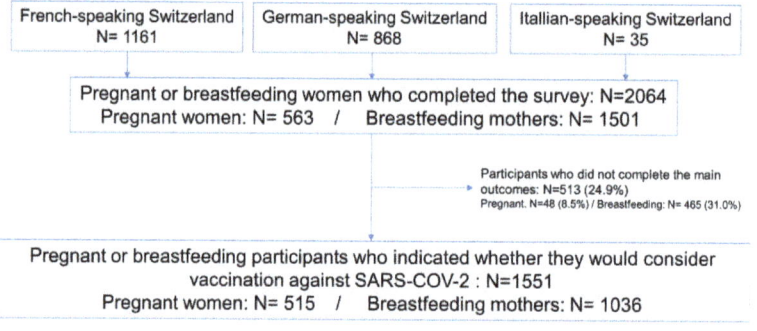

Figure 1. Flow chart.

3.1. Baseline Characteristics

Baseline characteristics are presented in Table 1. The median age of respondents was 33 years and the majority were married or cohabiting (79.8%; 1237/1551). A significant proportion of women were healthcare providers (20.4%; 317/1551) or homemakers (9.0%; 139/1551). A high proportion of participants (46.5%; 721/1551) had an education level above high school. Overall, 9.7% (151/1551) reported having co-morbidities.

Among the pregnant participants, the median gestational age was 28 weeks' gestation at the time of survey completion. Half of them were multigravida (275/515), among which 74.4% (204/274) and 18.2% (50/274) had one or more previous children respectively. More than 90% (468/515) were under the care of an obstetrician. Among the breastfeeding participants, 2.8% (29/1036) had their neonates hospitalized in an intensive care unit.

3.2. SARS-CoV-2 Exposure, Fears, and Beliefs

Data on SARS-CoV-2 exposure, fears, and beliefs are presented in Table 2. Almost 55% (850/1551) of participants reported having experienced symptoms potentially related to SARS-CoV-2 within the 3 months preceding the survey. Only 10.9% (170/1551) of the women had been tested for SARS-CoV-2 infection, among which 10.5% had a positive result (18/170) through a PCR-based nasopharyngeal swab, serology, or CT-scan. Less than 1.0% (9/1551) reported having been hospitalized due to COVID-19. Only 1.2% (18/1551) of participants reported living with someone older than 65 years old. Participants reported that the COVID-19 pandemic had a negative impact on their pregnancy or breastfeeding experience in 35.3% (97/275) and 8.0% (41/512) of cases, respectively. According to their responses, 11.0% (170/1551) of them experienced symptoms of severe depression (EDS ≥ 13), anxiety (GAD-7 ≥ 15), or high stress (PSS ≥ 27) over the last four weeks. More than half of pregnant women (53.4%; 275/515) declared that they feared an adverse fetal outcome in case of maternal infection.

Table 1. Baseline characteristics and medical history of participants. Abbreviations: ENT, ear nose throat; IQR, interquartile range; NICU, neonatal intensive care unit, HCP, healthcare provider.

		Pregnant Women		Breastfeeding Mothers		Total	
		n = 515	(%)	n = 1036	(%)	n = 1551	(%)
Baseline characteristics							
Maternal age (years)—median (IQR)		33	(31–35)	33	(31–35)	33	(31–35)
	>40 years	19	(3.7)	63	(6.1)	82	(5.3)
Marital status							
	Married/cohabiting	422	(81.9)	815	(78.7)	1237	(79.8)
	Single/divorced/others	4	(0.8)	9	(0.9)	13	(0.8)
	Unknown	89	(17.3)	212	(20.5)	301	(19.4)
Working status							
	Health care provider	122	(23.7)	195	(18.8)	317	(20.4)
	Employed other than HCP	257	(49.9)	465	(44.9)	722	(46.6)
	Student	3	(0.6)	7	(0.7)	10	(0.6)
	Housewife	21	(4.1)	118	(11.4)	139	(9.0)
	Job seeker	12	(2.3)	23	(2.2)	35	(2.3)
	Unknown	100	(19.4)	228	(22.0)	328	(21.1)
Educational level							
	Less than high school	9	(1.8)	20	(1.9)	29	(1.9)
	High school	75	(14.6)	212	(20.5)	287	(18.5)
	More than high school	257	(49.9)	464	(44.8)	721	(46.5)
	Unknown	174	(33.8)	340	(32.8)	514	(33.0)
Primary language							
	French	217	(42.1)	418	(40.4)	635	(40.9)
	German	183	(35.5)	322	(31.1)	505	(32.6)
	Italian	8	(1.6)	23	(2.2)	31	(2.0)
	Other	18	(3.5)	61	(5.8)	79	(5.1)
	Unknown	89	(17.3)	212	(20.5)	301	(19.4)
Maternal co-morbidities							
Any comorbidity		51	(9.9)	100	(9.7)	151	(9.7)
	Pulmonary	14	(2.7)	28	(2.7)	42	(2.7)
	Cardio-vascular	6	(1.2)	11	(1.1)	17	(1.1)
	Pregestational diabetes	5	(1.0)	9	(0.9)	14	(0.9)
	Thyroid dysfunction	12	(2.3)	27	(2.6)	39	(2.5)
	Oncologic	1	(0.2)	2	(0.2)	3	(0.2)
	Hematologic	2	(0.4)	0	(0.0)	2	(0.1)
	Auto-immune	2	(0.4)	4	(0.4)	6	(0.4)
	Neurologic	3	(0.6)	4	(0.4)	7	(0.5)
	Psychic	3	(0.6)	6	(0.6)	9	(0.6)
	Digestive	3	(0.6)	7	(0.7)	10	(0.7)
	Uro-genital tract	6	(1.2)	15	(1.4)	21	(1.4)
	Cutaneous	2	(0.4)	4	(0.4)	6	(0.4)
	ENT	0	(0.0)	1	(0.1)	1	(0.1)
Smoking		69	(13.4)	149	(14.4)	218	(14.1)

Table 1. Cont.

		Pregnant Women		Breastfeeding Mothers		Total	
		n = 515	(%)	n = 1036	(%)	n = 1551	(%)
Actual pregnancy or breastfeeding							
Practitioner:	Obstetrician	468	90.9				
	Midwife	13	8.3				
	Family physician	4	0.8				
Gestation	1	240	46.6	/			
	>1	275	53.4				
Parity	0	20/274	7.3	/			
	1	204/274	74.4				
	>1	50/274	18.2				
Planned pregnancy		483	93.8	/			
Gestational age—median (IQR)		28	(18-34)	/			
	1st Trimester	79	(15.0)				
	2nd Trimester	194	(40.7)				
	3rd Trimester	241	(44.3)				
Neonate hospitalized in NICU		/		29	(2.8)		

Table 2. SARS-CoV-2 exposure, fears, and beliefs. Abbreviations: PCR, polymerase chain reaction.

			Pregnant Women		Breastfeeding Mothers		Total	
			n = 515	(%)	n = 1036	(%)	n = 1551	(%)
SARS-COV-2 exposure								
Symptoms during the 3 last months			296	(57.5)	554	(53.5)	850	(54.8)
Hospitalized for COVID-19			2	(0.4)	7	(0.7)	9	(0.6)
Tested for SARS-CoV-2 infection			48	(9.3)	122	(11.8)	170	(10.9)
	PCR on nasopharyngeal swab		39	(7.6)	112	(108.0)	151	(9.7)
		positive	5/39	(12.8)	6/112	(5.3)	11/151	(7.3)
		negative	33/39	(84.6)	103/112	(92.0)	136/151	(90.1)
		unknown	1/39	(2.6)	3/112	(2.7)	4/151	(2.7)
	Serology		7	(1.4)	21	(2.0)	28	(1.8)
		positive	3/7	(42.9)	2/21	(9.5)	5/28	(17.9)
		negative	3/7	(42.9)	16/21	(76.2)	19/28	(67.9)
		unknown	1/7	(14.2)	3/21	(14.3)	4/28	(14.3)
	Scanner		2	(0.4)	2	(0.2)	4	(2.6)
		positive	2/2	(100.0)	0/2	(0.0)	2/4	(50.0)
		negative	0/2	(0.0)	2/2	(100.0)	2/4	(50.0)
Living with someone with symptoms			82	(15.9)	220	(21.2)	302	(19.5)
Living with someone tested positive			4	(0.8)	10	(1.0)	14	(0.9)
Living with someone > 65 years old			6	(1.2)	12	(1.2)	18	(1.2)
Negative impact of the COVID-19 pandemic on:								
Pregnancy or breastfeeding experience			97	(18.8)	41	(4.0)	138	(8.9)
	unknown		240	(46.6)	524	(50.6)	764	(49.3)
Life habits			350	(68.2)	700	(67.6)	1050	(67.7)
	unknown		8	(1.6)	25	(2.4)	33	(2.1)
Work			295	(57.3)	394	(38.0)	689	(44.4)
	unknown		100	(19.4)	320	(30.9)	420	(27.1)
Fear of an adverse fetal outcome			275	(53.4)	/			
Symptoms of severe depression, anxiety or high stress perceived during the 1st wave			53	(10.3)	117	(11.3)	170	(11.0)

3.3. Vaccination Practices and Beliefs

Only 19.3% (85/440) of pregnant and 28.0% (249/891) of breastfeeding women were vaccinated against influenza in the past year. Among the participants, 10.5% (163/1551) and 0.1% (2/1551) mentioned fear of potential consequences for their fetus/infant or themselves respectively resulting from vaccination during pregnancy or breastfeeding. More than 20% (324/1551) of them indicated usually declining influenza vaccination, and 7.5% (117/1551) think the influenza vaccine is not needed during pregnancy or breastfeeding (Figure 2).

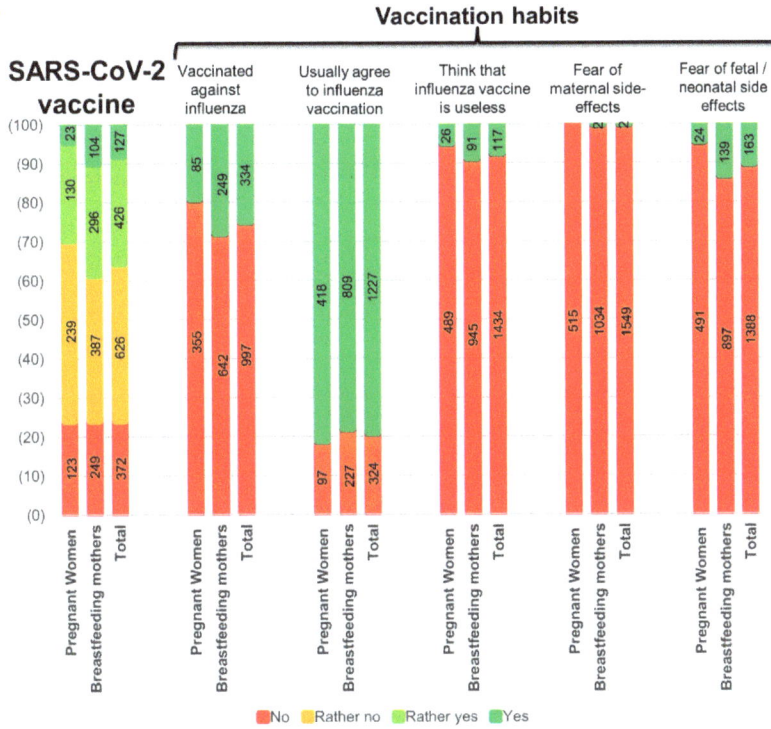

Figure 2. SARS-CoV-2 vaccine willingness among Swiss pregnant and breastfeeding women, and vaccination habits.

3.4. Willingness to Get the SARS-CoV-2 Vaccine

Only 29.7% (153/515) of pregnant and 38.6% (400/1036) of breastfeeding women were willing to get vaccinated against SARS-CoV-2 if a vaccine had been available during the first wave. More specifically, 8.1% (127/1551) fully agreed, 27.5% (426/1551) somewhat agreed, 40.4% (626/1551) somewhat disagreed, and 24% (372/1551) fully disagreed to get vaccinated (Figure 2 and Table S1).

3.5. Factors Associated with SARS-CoV-2 Vaccine Willingness

Potential predictors of SARS-CoV-2 vaccine acceptance are shown in Table 3. Sociodemographic factors such as a maternal age above 40 years old (aOR 1.8 [1.1–3.2]), an educational level higher than high school (aOR 1.5 [1.2–2.0]), and Italian as a primary language (aOR 3.3 [1.4–8.0]) were associated with a higher rate of vaccine acceptance. On the other hand, German-speaking participants were less likely to get vaccinated (aOR 0.7 [0.5–0.9]).

Table 3. Factors associated with SARS-CoV-2 vaccine willingness among Swiss pregnant and breastfeeding women. Abbreviations: aOR, adjusted odds ratio; CI, confidence interval; CT, computed tomography; OR, odds ratio; RT-PCR, reverse-transcriptase polymerase chain reaction; T, trimester of gestation.

		Participants Willing to Get Vaccinated against COVID-19		Participants Not Willing to Get Vaccinated against COVID-19		OR	(95 % CI)	p	aOR	(95% CI)	p
		N	(%)	N	(%)						
		553	(35.7)	998	(64.3)						
Baseline characteristics											
Maternal age >40 years		42	(7.6)	40	(4.0)	2.0	(1.3–3.0)	0.003	1.8	(1.1–3.2)	0.028
Educational level > highschool		300 *	(75.9)	421 *	(65.6)	1.7	(1.3–2.2)	<0.001	1.5	(1.1–2.0)	0.017
Professionally active		387 *	(87.4)	652 *	(83.6)	1.4	(1.0–1.9)	0.007	1.0	(0.7–1.5)	0.919
Primary language	French	238	(52.8)	397	(49.7)	1.1	(0.9–1.4)	0.295			
	German	159 *	(35.3)	346 *	(43.3)	0.7	(0.6–0.9)	0.005	0.7	(0.5–0.9)	0.015
	Italian	19 *	(4.2)	12 *	(1.5)	2.9	(1.4–6.0)	0.005	3.3	(1.4–8.0)	0.007
Any maternal co-morbidity		58	(10.5)	93	(9.3)	1.1	(0.8–1.6)	0.457			
Impact of the SARS-COV-2 pandemic											
Tested positive for SARS-CoV-2 (RT-PCR, serology and/or CT)		9	(1.6)	3	(0.3)	5.5	(1.5–20.4)	0.011	3.3	(0.8–13.7)	0.095
Living with someone >65 years old		10	(1.8)	8	(0.8)	2.3	(0.8–6.7)	0.076	2.0	(0.7–6.1)	0.094
Negative impact of the pandemic on	Pregnancy	52	(19.9)	86	(16.3)	1.1	(1.0–1.2)	0.215			
	Life habits	398 *	(72.8)	652 *	(67.2)	1.3	(1.0–1.7)	0.023	1.0	(0.8–1.4)	0.822
	Work	244	(60.1)	445	(61.4)	1.0	(0.7–1.2)	0.672			
Symptoms of severe depression, anxiety or high stress		68	(12.3)	102	(10.2)	1.2	(0.9–1.7)	0.211			
Vaccination habits and beliefs											
Vaccinated against Influenza last year		197 *	(41.1)	137 *	(16.1)	3.6	(2.8–4.7)	<0.001	2.1	(1.5–2.8)	<0.001
Usually decline vaccination		30	(5.4)	294	(29.5)	0.1	(0.1–0.2)	<0.001	0.2	(0.1–0.3)	<0.001
Fear of side effects related to vaccines		51	(9.2)	114	(11.4)	0.8	(0.6–1.1)	0.179			
Supplementary model including pregnancy-related variables (tested only in pregnant women, N = 515)	N	N	(%)	N	(%)	OR	(95%CI)	p	aOR	(95%CI)	p
		153	(29.7)	362	(60.3)						
Follow-up by an obstetrician		144	(94.1)	324	(89.5)	1.9	(0.9–4.0)	0.101	3.6	(1.2–11.2)	0.027
Gestational age	T1	25	(16.3)	54	(15.0)	1.1	(0.7–1.9)	0.691			
	T2	47	(30.7)	147	(40.7)	0.6	(0.4–1.0)	0.033	0.6	(0.4–0.9)	0.015
	T3	81	(52.9)	160	(44.3)	1.4	(1.0–2.0)	0.074	1.8	(1.1–2.7)	0.018
Fear of an adverse fetal outcome in case of infection		75	(49.0)	200	(55.3)	0.9	(0.8–1.0)	0.196			

* Multiple imputations on missing values.

Having had the influenza vaccination in the past year was a positive predictor for SARS-CoV-2 vaccine acceptance (aOR 2.1 [1.5–2.8]). Women who usually declined influenza vaccination were less likely to be willing to get the SARS-CoV-2 vaccine (aOR 0.2 [0.1–0.3]).

When assessing the impact of the SARS-CoV-2 pandemic, none of the variables showed statistically significant influence on the willingness to get vaccinated. However, a trend toward COVID-19 vaccine willingness can be observed among women having a positive diagnosis of SARS-CoV-2 (aOR 3.3 [0.8–13.7] and living with someone older than 65 years old (aOR 2.0 [0.7–6.1]).

Among the pregnant participants, those who had an obstetrician following their pregnancy (aOR 3.6 [1.2–11.2]) and who were in their third trimester of pregnancy (aOR 1.8 [1.1–2.7]) were more likely to be willing to receive the SARS-CoV-2 vaccine. On the other hand, being in their second trimester of pregnancy was associated with a higher SARS-CoV-2 vaccination refusal (aOR 0.6 [0.4–0.9]).

4. Discussion

Our results demonstrate that in Switzerland, only one-third (35.7%; 553/1551) of pregnant and breastfeeding women that participated in the survey were willing to get a SARS-CoV-2 vaccine during the first wave of the pandemic if one had been available. The positive predictors for SARS-CoV-2 vaccine acceptance among all participants were an age older than 40 years, a higher educational level, speaking Italian as their primary language, and having been vaccinated against influenza in the previous year. On the other hand, speaking German and usually declining influenza vaccination were negative predictors. Regarding pregnant participants, having an obstetrician following their pregnancy and being in their third trimester of pregnancy were two positive factors associated with the willingness to be vaccinated against SARS-CoV-2, whereas being in their second trimester of pregnancy was a negative predictor. No association was found between maternal co-morbidities and the participants' willingness to get vaccinated.

4.1. Interpretation

Our study shows that despite Switzerland being among SARS-CoV-2 high incidence countries during the first wave with a particularly negative impact on pregnancy and breastfeeding experience [24], it has a low rate of SARS-CoV-2 vaccination acceptance. The results from our survey of Swiss women were among the lowest when compared to a recent survey conducted in 16 countries that showed a SARS-CoV-2 vaccine acceptance rate among pregnant women of 52.0%, with responses varying substantially between countries (28.8–84.4%) [31]. An American cross-sectional survey showed a rate of 41% of SARS-CoV-2 vaccine acceptance among pregnant women [32]. The low percentage of Swiss pregnant women willing to get the SARS-CoV-2 vaccine that we observed is consistent with the rather low influenza and pertussis immunization rates in Switzerland previously mentioned [16]. We also identified variability in SARS-CoV-2 vaccine acceptance between different regions of Switzerland. This has already been observed with Swiss-German women being more reluctant to get their children vaccinated [33,34]. In contrast, the part of Switzerland most affected by SARS-CoV-2, the Italian part, seems to have a higher rate of vaccine acceptance than the other parts of Switzerland, although fewer Italian speaking women were included, and these results should be interpreted with caution.

In this Swiss sub-analysis, the proportion of breastfeeding women willing to be vaccinated was higher than that of pregnant women (38.6% vs. 29.7%). This difference was also found in all countries included in the European study of which these data are a part, with a difference of up to +25% for the UK [25]. These results support that "vaccine hesitancy" may be even more common during pregnancy, which may be related to an overall greater reluctance to use medicines during pregnancy.

When assessing factors influencing SARS-CoV-2 vaccine willingness among pregnant women, our results are consistent with another study identifying older age and higher educational level as positive predictors [31]. The same observations have been made for acceptance of the pertussis and influenza vaccines [23,31]. The positive correlation that we observed between SARS-CoV-2 vaccine willingness and having received the influenza vaccine during the previous season has also been found in a recent study evaluating pregnant women [32]. In addition, we identified that being in the second trimester of pregnancy might be a negative predictor for SARS CoV 2 vaccine acceptance, suggesting a potential fear for induced fetal malformations. This is consistent with several studies identifying fear for any potential harmful side effects of the vaccine on their fetus or infant as well as concerns regarding safety and effectiveness as major reasons for vaccine reluctance [22,31,32]. Concerns about teratogenicity would be more likely in the first trimester, as second trimester exposures do not cause embryopathy. Here, patients who responded to the survey as being in the second trimester correspond to those who were in the first trimester at the time of the first wave, so our results may suggest that their fear of teratogenicity may be higher in early pregnancy and not necessarily in the second trimester. In contrast, we did not find an association between having experienced symptoms of severe depression, anxiety, or high stress in the weeks prior to the survey and the willingness to get the SARS-CoV-2 vaccine. This is not in line with a previous study where pregnant women with a history of major depressive disorder and moderate anxiety were significantly more likely to get influenza and pertussis vaccines [23]. However, at the time of the survey, no SARS-CoV-2 vaccine was yet available, and thus, no information was available regarding its safety or effectiveness in general and in the pregnant population, which may explain the reluctance of anxious or depressed women who may need safety information before accepting the vaccine. This might also have influenced participants who did not answer the question about SARS-CoV-2 vaccination acceptance, as the ambivalence toward this vaccine is still very strong. It is also interesting to note that while most participants showed acceptance of influenza vaccines, a much smaller percentage actually received it. This might question the access of Swiss breastfeeding and pregnant women to vaccines and how healthcare workers might play a role in it.

Our observations suggest that more than a specific reluctance toward the SARS-CoV-2 vaccine, it is one's personal opinion on vaccination during pregnancy in general that might prevent Swiss pregnant and breastfeeding women from getting vaccinated. Hence, it is our hypothesis that SARS-CoV-2 and influenza or pertussis vaccines are avoided for similar reasons: mainly the lack of recommendation by healthcare professionals and the lack of compliance by pregnant women. Until the end of May 2021, Switzerland has made access to vaccines challenging, even for women that might want to be vaccinated, which could represent a barrier for vaccine acceptance. Furthermore, the ongoing debates over SARS-CoV-2 vaccines may have a negative influence on the willingness of pregnant women to become vaccinated. This emphasizes the need to improve access to vaccination for pregnant women as well as knowledge and acceptance of immunization during pregnancy among healthcare workers and pregnant/breastfeeding women.

4.2. Strengths and Limitations

In terms of temporality, our study explored the experience of Swiss pregnant women during the first wave of the SARS-CoV-2 pandemic. Our study included a large number of participants from different parts of Switzerland, was conducted in three official languages, and is the first to address the question of SARS-CoV-2 vaccine willingness in the country. Selection bias might have occurred as the proportion of participants who are professionally active and highly educated was higher than the general population of Swiss pregnant women [35,36]. This could have led to an increased vaccination acceptance rate, as highly educated women tend to have a higher acceptance of vaccination, which would mean that the vaccine willingness in the overall perinatal population might be even lower than that reported here. The survey was conducted online and, although most Swiss women have good access to the internet, those that rely more on online resources may have come across the online survey more often when looking for information about their pregnancy or breastfeeding. Women hospitalized or severely ill might not have had the opportunity to participate. This could have biased the association between SARS-CoV-2 exposure and the participants' willingness to get vaccinated toward the null. In addition, as only 5% of women declared speaking another language in our survey, we might have an under representation of the immigrant population.

Another limitation might be the overrepresentation of French-speaking participants, which could be explained by the CHUV (Centre Hospitalier Universitaire Vaudois, university hospital of the largest French-speaking canton) leading the present study. Since some studies have shown an increased vaccination acceptance among the French-speaking part of Switzerland, this could have overestimated the rate of SARS-CoV-2 vaccine willingness in our study. Overestimation of SARS-CoV-2 vaccination acceptance could have also happened since a high percentage of participants were healthcare workers, more likely to be exposed to SARS-CoV-2 positive patients, and thus, more prone to being immunized.

Factors reported to be associated with SARS-CoV-2 vaccine willingness, considered in other studies, were not measured [31,32]. Those include socioeconomic status; perceived risk of SARS-CoV-2 (likelihood of infection, self or infant); opinion on the importance to public health to get a vaccine and for the majority of people to get vaccinated; compliance with preventive measures; monitoring of SARS-CoV-2 news and updates; trust and satisfaction with health authorities; as well as trust in science. Further surveys including those variables would be needed to better specify the factors influencing SARS-CoV-2 vaccination acceptance among Swiss pregnant women.

Finally, this survey was conducted at a time when no SARS-CoV-2 vaccine had yet been accepted by Swissmedic nor recommended for pregnant women. This could represent an important bias, since participants were asked if they would accept a potential vaccine without information about its efficiency and safety. Since this survey, the first randomized controlled trial of SARS-CoV-2 vaccination in pregnancy has been initiated [37]. Additionally, following the example of several other countries, the Swiss Society for Gynecology and Obstetrics (SSGO) along with the Federal Public Health Office (OFSP) has recommended, up until the end of May 2021, SARS-CoV-2 vaccination during the second and third trimester for pregnant women at high risk of developing complications or at high risk of exposure [38]. Recent studies also showed robust immune responses and efficient passage of antibodies to newborns after SARS-CoV-2 vaccination of pregnant women [39,40], unlike transplacental immunization through infected mothers, which seems to be less effective [41]. As new guidelines and more data on vaccinated pregnant women become available every day [42], willingness to become vaccinated might evolve, and new studies are urgently needed.

5. Conclusions

Our study suggests disappointing SARS-CoV-2 vaccine willingness among Swiss pregnant and breastfeeding women, emphasizing the need to identify and reduce barriers toward immunization. Inclusion of pregnant women in clinical trials, improving access to vaccines, and providing tailored information for pregnant and breastfeeding women, especially for those of younger age with a lower educational level, are crucially needed to protect them from SARS-CoV-2 and other viral threats ahead.

Supplementary Materials: The following are available online at https://www.mdpi.com/article/10.3390/v13071199/s1, Table S1: Raw data presented in Figure 2.

Author Contributions: M.C., H.N. and A.P. conceived and designed the study. M.S., U.W., D.B. and A.P. translated and promoted the study in Switzerland. S.S., G.F., E.G., V.L., A.P. and L.P. wrote the first version of the report and did the literature review. All authors have read and agreed to the published version of the manuscript.

Funding: This research received no external funding.

Institutional Review Board Statement: The study was conducted according to the guidelines of the Declaration of Helsinki, and approved by EC Research UZ/KU Leuven; S63966; 10 April 2020.

Informed Consent Statement: All participants provided online informed consent prior to survey initiation.

Data Availability Statement: The data presented in this study are available on request from the corresponding author.

Conflicts of Interest: The authors declare no conflict of interest.

References

1. FOPH. Status Report, Switzerland and Liechtenstein. Available online: https://www.covid19.admin.ch/ (accessed on 1 May 2021).
2. Favre, G.; Pomar, L.; Baud, D. Coronavirus Disease 2019 during Pregnancy: Do not Underestimate the Risk of Maternal Adverse Outcomes. *Am. J. Obstet. Gynecol. MFM* **2020**, *2*, 100160. [CrossRef]
3. Jering, K.S.; Claggett, B.L.; Cunningham, J.W.; Rosenthal, N.; Vardeny, O.; Greene, M.F.; Solomon, S.D. Clinical Characteristics and Outcomes of Hospitalized Women Giving Birth With and Without COVID-19. *JAMA Intern. Med.* **2021**, *181*, 714. [CrossRef]
4. Lokken, E.M.; Taylor, G.G.; Huebner, E.M.; Vanderhoeven, J.; Hendrikson, S.; Coler, B.; Sheng, J.S.; Walker, C.L.; McCartney, S.A.; Kretzer, N.M.; et al. Higher SARS-CoV-2 Infection Rate in Pregnant Patients. *Am. J. Obstet. Gynecol.* **2021**. [CrossRef] [PubMed]
5. Zambrano, L.D.; Ellington, S.; Strid, P.; Galang, R.R.; Oduyebo, T.; Tong, V.T.; Woodworth, K.R.; Nahabedian, J.F., III; Azziz-Baumgartner, E.; Gilboa, S.M.; et al. Update: Characteristics of Symptomatic Women of Reproductive Age with Laboratory-Confirmed SARS-CoV-2 Infection by Pregnancy Status-United States, January 22–October 3, 2020. *MMWR Morb. Mortal. Wkly. Rep.* **2020**, *69*, 1641–1647. [CrossRef]
6. Allotey, J.; Stallings, E.; Bonet, M.; Yap, M.; Chatterjee, S.; Kew, T.; Debenham, L.; Llavall, A.C.; Dixit, A.; Zhou, D.; et al. Clinical Manifestations, Risk Factors, and Maternal and Perinatal Outcomes of Coronavirus Disease 2019 in Pregnancy: Living Systematic Review and Meta-Analysis. *BMJ* **2020**, *370*, m3320. [CrossRef] [PubMed]

7. Khalil, A.; Kalafat, E.; Benlioglu, C.; O'Brien, P.; Morris, E.; Draycott, T.; Thangaratinam, S.; Doare, K.L.; Heath, P.; Ladhani, S.; et al. SARS-CoV-2 Infection in Pregnancy: A Systematic Review and Meta-Analysis of Clinical Features and Pregnancy Outcomes. *EClinicalMedicine* **2020**, *25*, 100446. [CrossRef] [PubMed]
8. Martínez-Perez, O.; Vouga, M.; Melguizo, S.C.; Acebal, L.F.; Panchaud, A.; Muñoz-Chápuli, M.; Baud, D. Association Between Mode of Delivery Among Pregnant Women With COVID-19 and Maternal and Neonatal Outcomes in Spain. *JAMA* **2020**, *324*, 296–299. [CrossRef] [PubMed]
9. Khalil, A.; Von Dadelszen, P.; Draycott, T.; Ugwumadu, A.; O'Brien, P.; Magee, L. Change in the Incidence of Stillbirth and Preterm Delivery During the COVID-19 Pandemic. *JAMA* **2020**, *324*, 705. [CrossRef] [PubMed]
10. Hcini, N.; Maamri, F.; Picone, O.; Carod, J.F.; Lambert, V.; Mathieu, M.; Carles, G.; Pomar, L. Maternal, Fetal and Neonatal Outcomes of Large Series of SARS-CoV-2 Positive Pregnancies in Peripartum Period: A Single-Center Prospective Comparative Study. *Eur. J. Obstet. Gynecol. Reprod. Biol.* **2021**, *257*, 11–18. [CrossRef]
11. Baud, D.; Greub, G.; Favre, G.; Gengler, C.; Jaton, K.; Dubruc, E.; Pomar, L. Second-Trimester Miscarriage in a Pregnant Woman With SARS-CoV-2 Infection. *JAMA* **2020**, *323*, 2198–2200. [CrossRef]
12. Swissmedic. Available online: https://www.swissmedic.ch/swissmedic/fr/home/news/coronavirus-covid-19/dritten-impfstoff-gegen-covid-19-erkrankung.html (accessed on 1 May 2021).
13. WHO. Ten Threats. Available online: https://www.who.int/news-room/spotlight/ten-threats-to-global-health-in-2019 (accessed on 1 May 2021).
14. Blanchard-Rohner, G.; Siegrist, C.-A. Vaccination during Pregnancy to Protect Infants Against Influenza: Why and Why Not? *Vaccine* **2011**, *29*, 7542–7550. [CrossRef] [PubMed]
15. Reuman, P.D.; Ayoub, E.M.; Small, P.A. Effect of Passive Maternal Antibody on Influenza Illness in Children: A Prospective Study of Influenza A in Mother-Infant Pairs. *Pediatr. Infect. Dis. J.* **1987**, *6*, 398–403. [CrossRef] [PubMed]
16. Blanchard-Rohner, G.; Eberhardt, C. Review of Maternal Immunisation during Pregnancy: Focus on Pertussis and Influenza. *Swiss Med. Wkly.* **2017**, *147*, w14526. [PubMed]
17. Erb, M.L.; Erlanger, T.E.; Heininger, U. Child-Parent Immunization Survey: How Well are National Immunization Recommendations Accepted by the Target Groups? *Vaccine X* **2019**, *1*, 100013. [CrossRef]
18. Healy, C.M.; Rench, M.A.; Montesinos, D.P.; Ng, N.; Swaim, L.S. Knowledge and Attitiudes of Pregnant Women and their Providers Towards Recommendations for Immunization during Pregnancy. *Vaccine* **2015**, *33*, 5445–5451. [CrossRef] [PubMed]
19. Abu-Raya, B.; Maertens, K.; Edwards, K.M.; Omer, S.B.; Englund, J.A.; Flanagan, K.L.; Snape, M.D.; Amirthalingam, G.; Leuridan, E.; Van Damme, P.; et al. Global Perspectives on Immunization During Pregnancy and Priorities for Future Research and Development: An International Consensus Statement. *Front. Immunol.* **2020**, *11*, 1282. [CrossRef]
20. MacDougall, D.M.; Halperin, S.A. Improving Rates of Maternal Immunization: Challenges and Opportunities. *Hum. Vaccines Immunother.* **2016**, *12*, 857–865. [CrossRef] [PubMed]
21. Wilson, R.J.; Paterson, P.; Jarrett, C.; Larson, H.J. Understanding Factors Influencing Vaccination Acceptance during Pregnancy Globally: A Literature Review. *Vaccine* **2015**, *33*, 6420–6429. [CrossRef]
22. Lutz, C.S.; Carr, W.; Cohn, A.; Rodriguez, L. Understanding Barriers and Predictors of Maternal Immunization: Identifying gaps through an Exploratory Literature Review. *Vaccine* **2018**, *36*, 7445–7455. [CrossRef]
23. Mohammed, H.; Roberts, C.T.; Grzeskowiak, L.E.; Giles, L.; Leemaqz, S.; Dalton, J.; Dekker, G.; Marshall, H.S. Psychosocial Determinants of Pertussis and Influenza Vaccine Uptake in Pregnant Women: A Prospective Study. *Vaccine* **2020**, *38*, 3358–3368. [CrossRef]
24. Ceulemans, M.; Foulon, V.; Ngo, E.; Panchaud, A.; Winterfeld, U.; Pomar, L.; Lambelet, V.; Cleary, B.; O'Shaughnessy, F.; Passier, A.; et al. Mental Health Status of Pregnant and Breastfeeding Women during the COVID-19 Pandemic-A Multinational Cross-Sectional Study. *Acta Obstet. Gynecol. Scand.* **2021**. [CrossRef] [PubMed]
25. Ceulemans, M.; Foulon, V.; Panchaud, A.; Winterfeld, U.; Pomar, L.; Lambelet, V.; Cleary, B.; O'Shaughnessy, F.; Passier, A.; Richardson, J.; et al. Vaccine Willingness and Impact of the COVID-19 Pandemic on Women's Perinatal Experiences and Practices—A Multinational, Cross-Sectional Study Covering the First Wave of the Pandemic. *Int. J. Environ. Res. Public Health* **2021**, *18*, 3367. [CrossRef] [PubMed]
26. Cox, J.L.; Holden, J.M.; Sagovsky, R. Detection of Postnatal Depression. Development of the 10-Item Edinburgh Post-Natal Depression Scale. *Br. J. Psychiatry* **1987**, *150*, 782–786. [CrossRef] [PubMed]
27. Bergink, V.; Kooistra, L.; Berg, M.P.L.-V.D.; Wijnen, H.; Bunevicius, R.; van Baar, A.; Pop, V. Validation of the Edinburgh Depression Scale during Pregnancy. *J. Psychosom. Res.* **2011**, *70*, 385–389. [CrossRef]
28. Spitzer, R.L.; Kroenke, K.; Williams, J.B.; Löwe, B. A Brief Measure for Assessing Generalized Anxiety Disorder: The GAD-7. *Arch. Intern. Med.* **2006**, *166*, 1092–1097. [CrossRef] [PubMed]
29. Cohen, S.; Kamarck, T.; Mermelstein, R. A Global Measure of Perceived Stress. *J. Health Soc. Behav.* **1983**, *24*, 385–396. [CrossRef]
30. Taylor, J.M. Psychometric Analysis of the Ten-Item Perceived Stress Scale. *Psychol. Assess.* **2015**, *27*, 90–101. [CrossRef]
31. Skjefte, M.; Ngirbabul, M.; Akeju, O.; Escudero, D.; Hernandez-Diaz, S.; Wyszynski, D.F.; Wu, J.W. COVID-19 Vaccine Acceptance among Pregnant Women and Mothers of Young Children: Results of a Survey in 16 Countries. *Eur. J. Epidemiol.* **2021**, *36*, 197–211. [CrossRef]

32. Ashley, N.; Battarbee, M.S.S.; Varner, M.; Newes-Adeyi, G.; Daugherty, M.; Gyamfi-Bannerman, C.; Tita, A.; Vorwaller, K.; Vargas, C.; Subramaniam, A.; et al. Attitudes Toward COVID-19 Illness and COVID-19 Vaccination among Pregnant Women: A Cross-Sectional Multicenter Study during August–December 2020. Pre-print.2021. Available online: https://www.medrxiv.org/content/10.1101/2021.03.26.21254402v1 (accessed on 1 May 2021).
33. Lang, P.; Zimmermann, H.; Piller, U.; Steffen, R.; Hatz, C. The Swiss National Vaccination Coverage Survey, 2005–2007. *Public Health Rep.* **2011**, *126*, 97–108. [CrossRef] [PubMed]
34. Les Suisses Sceptiques à L'égard des Vaccins. Available online: https://www.pharmapro.ch/news/les-suisses-sceptiques-a-l-egard-des-vaccins-0222.htm (accessed on 1 May 2021).
35. Niveau de Formation de la Population-Données de L'indicateur. Available online: https://www.bfs.admin.ch/bfs/fr/home/statistiques/situation-economique-sociale-population/egalite-femmes-hommes/formation/niveau-formation.assetdetail.12527179.html (accessed on 1 May 2021).
36. Situation Professionnelle Selon le Sexe et la Situation Familiale. Available online: https://www.bfs.admin.ch/bfs/fr/home/statistiques/catalogues-banques-donnees/tableaux.assetdetail.13108456.html (accessed on 1 May 2021).
37. Pfizer-BioNTech. Study to Evaluate the Safety, Tolerability, and Immunogenicity of SARS CoV-2 RNA Vaccine Candidate (BNT162b2) Against COVID-19 in Healthy Pregnant Women 18 Years of Age and Older. U.S in National Library of Medicine. 2021. Available online: https://clinicaltrials.gov/ct2/show/NCT04754594 (accessed on 1 May 2021).
38. SGGG. Available online: https://www.sggg.ch/fr/nouvelles/detail/1/infection-a-coronavirus-covid-19-et-grossesse/ (accessed on 1 May 2021).
39. Harvard Gazette. Available online: https://news.harvard.edu/gazette/story/2021/03/study-shows-covid-19-vaccinated-mothers-pass-antibodies-to-newborns/ (accessed on 1 May 2021).
40. Gilbert, P.D.; Rudnick, C.A. Newborn Antibodies to SARS-CoV-2 Detected in Cord Blood after Maternal Vaccination. *medRxiv* **2021**. [CrossRef]
41. Atyeo, C.; Pullen, K.M.; Bordt, E.A.; Fischinger, S.; Burke, J.; Michell, A.; Slein, M.D.; Loos, C.; Shook, L.L.; Boatin, A.A.; et al. Compromised SARS-CoV-2-Specific Placental Antibody Transfer. *Cell* **2021**, *184*, 628–642.e10. [CrossRef]
42. Shimabukuro, T.T.; Kim, S.Y.; Myers, T.R.; Moro, P.L.; Oduyebo, T.; Panagiotakopoulos, L.; Marquez, P.L.; Olson, C.K.; Liu, R.; Chang, K.T.; et al. Preliminary Findings of mRNA Covid-19 Vaccine Safety in Pregnant Persons. *N. Engl. J. Med.* **2021**. [CrossRef]

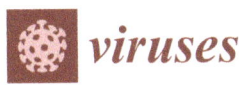

Comment

Data of the COVID-19 mRNA-Vaccine V-Safe Surveillance System and Pregnancy Registry Reveals Poor Embryonic and Second Trimester Fetal Survival Rate. Comment on Stuckelberger et al. SARS-CoV-2 Vaccine Willingness among Pregnant and Breastfeeding Women during the First Pandemic Wave: A Cross-Sectional Study in Switzerland. *Viruses* 2021, *13*, 1199

Serge Stroobandt [1] and Roland Stroobandt [2,*]

1 Independent Researcher, Kolonel Dusartplein 10, 3500 Hasselt, Belgium; serge@stroobandt.com
2 Vaccination Center Oostende-Bredene, 8400 Oostende, Belgium
* Correspondence: roland@stroobandt.com

Citation: Stroobandt, S.; Stroobandt, R. Data of the COVID-19 mRNA-Vaccine V-Safe Surveillance System and Pregnancy Registry Reveals Poor Embryonic and Second Trimester Fetal Survival Rate. Comment on Stuckelberger et al. SARS-CoV-2 Vaccine Willingness among Pregnant and Breastfeeding Women during the First Pandemic Wave: A Cross-Sectional Study in Switzerland. *Viruses* 2021, *13*, 1199. *Viruses* 2021, *13*, 1545. https://doi.org/10.3390/v13081545

Academic Editor: Kenneth Lundstrom

Received: 13 July 2021
Accepted: 30 July 2021
Published: 5 August 2021

Publisher's Note: MDPI stays neutral with regard to jurisdictional claims in published maps and institutional affiliations.

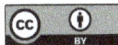

Copyright: © 2021 by the authors. Licensee MDPI, Basel, Switzerland. This article is an open access article distributed under the terms and conditions of the Creative Commons Attribution (CC BY) license (https://creativecommons.org/licenses/by/4.0/).

Dr. Sarah Stuckelberger and her colleagues should be commended for their cross-sectional study assessing the willingness of Swiss pregnant and breastfeeding women to be vaccinated against SARS-CoV-2 [1]. They emphasise the need to identify and reduce barriers towards immunisation. Furthermore, they express the hope that when more data become available about vaccinated pregnant women, willingness to be vaccinated will increase. Moreover, the authors refer to a study [2] that has been unequivocally heralded as a proof of safety for the use of COVID-19 mRNA vaccines in pregnant women.

Regardless, we would like to advise readers that the referenced article contains a serious error regarding the interpretation of the data presented in Table 4. Prospective cohort studies are routinely performed to establish the safety of novel obstetric interventions. Such studies typically compare, at the same gestational age, the wellbeing of a cohort that underwent the intervention to that of a comparable control cohort (or, in the absence of this, the pertaining population) without the intervention. Nonetheless, the cited study compared the control population's incidence rate of spontaneous abortions of 10 to 26% prior to week 20 to the incidence among the 827 study participants of which 700 received their first dose only in the third trimester, i.e., after week 26. However, a correct comparison with the remaining 127 participants sets the 104 spontaneous abortions recorded prior to week 20 at an alarming incidence of 82%, i.e., 3 to 8 times higher than in the control population. This observation suggests that obstetric vaccine safety is severely compromised during pregnancy and may lead to decreased willingness among pregnant women to be vaccinated.

Author Contributions: Both authors contributed equally to this paper. All authors have read and agreed to the published version of the manuscript.

Funding: The authors received no external funding.

Institutional Review Board Statement: Not applicable.

Informed Consent Statement: Not applicable.

Data Availability Statement: Not applicable.

Conflicts of Interest: The authors declare no conflict of interest.

References

1. Stuckelberger, S.; Favre, G.; Ceulemans, M.; Nordeng, H.; Gerbier, E.; Lambelet, V.; Stojanov, M.; Winterfeld, U.; Baud, D.; Panchaud, A.; et al. SARS-CoV-2 Vaccine Willingness among Pregnant and Breastfeeding Women during the First Pandemic Wave: A Cross-Sectional Study in Switzerland. *Viruses* **2021**, *13*, 1199. [CrossRef] [PubMed]
2. Shimabukuro, T.T.; Kim, S.Y.; Myers, T.R.; Moro, P.L.; Oduyebo, T.; Panagiotakopoulos, L.; Marquez, P.L.; Olson, C.K.; Liu, R.; Chang, K.T.; et al. Preliminary Findings of mRNA COVID-19 Vaccine Safety in Pregnant Persons. *N. Engl. J. Med.* **2021**, *384*, 2273–2282. [CrossRef] [PubMed]

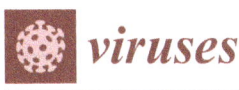

Reply

Current Data on COVID-19 mRNA-Vaccine Safety during Pregnancy Might Be Subject to Selection Bias. Reply to Stroobandt, S.; Stroobandt, R. Data of the COVID-19 mRNA-Vaccine V-Safe Surveillance System and Pregnancy Registry Reveals Poor Embryonic and Second Trimester Fetal Survival Rate. Comment on "Stuckelberger et al. SARS-CoV-2 Vaccine Willingness among Pregnant and Breastfeeding Women during the First Pandemic Wave: A Cross-Sectional Study in Switzerland. *Viruses* 2021, *13*, 1199"

Sarah Stuckelberger [1], Guillaume Favre [1], Michael Ceulemans [2,3], Eva Gerbier [1], Valentine Lambelet [1], Milos Stojanov [1], Ursula Winterfeld [4], David Baud [1], Alice Panchaud [5,6,†] and Léo Pomar [1,7,*,†]

1. Department Woman-Mother-Child, Lausanne University Hospital, University of Lausanne, 1011 Lausanne, Switzerland; Sarah.Stuckelberger@chuv.ch (S.S.); guillaume.favre@chuv.ch (G.F.); Eva.Gerbier@chuv.ch (E.G.); valentine.lambelet@gmail.com (V.L.); Milos.Stojanov@chuv.ch (M.S.); David.Baud@chuv.ch (D.B.)
2. Department of Pharmaceutical and Pharmacological Sciences, KU Leuven, 3000 Leuven, Belgium; michael.ceulemans@kuleuven.be
3. Teratology Information Service, Pharmacovigilance Centre Lareb, 5237 MH 's Hertogenbosch, The Netherlands
4. Swiss Teratogen Information Service, Service de Pharmacologie Clinique, Lausanne University Hospital, University of Lausanne, 1011 Lausanne, Switzerland; Ursula.Winterfeld@chuv.ch
5. Institute of Primary Health Care (BIHAM), University of Bern, 3012 Bern, Switzerland; alice.panchaud@chuv.ch
6. Service of Pharmacy, Lausanne University Hospital, University of Lausanne, 1011 Lausanne, Switzerland
7. School of Health Sciences (HESAV), University of Applied Sciences and Arts Western Switzerland, 1011 Lausanne, Switzerland
* Correspondence: leo.pomar@chuv.ch
† These authors contributed equally to this work.

We would like to thank Stroobandt, S. and Stroobandt, R. for showing interest in our paper [1] and for sharing their concerns regarding COVID-19 vaccine safety in pregnant women [2]. Although not being the main focus of our article, it is a key component of COVID-19 vaccine acceptance in the pregnant woman population.

Both authors are warning the readership of *Viruses* about the safety of COVID-19 mRNA vaccines, suggesting an interpretation error in the results of Shimabukuro et al.'s study which was considered as the first evidence of the safety of the COVID-19 vaccine in pregnancy [3]. Stroobandt, S. and Stroobandt, R.'s interpretation leads to an 82% risk of spontaneous abortion (104 spontaneous abortions for 127 participants exposed to the first dose of the COVID-19 vaccine during the first trimester and who have completed their pregnancy) instead of the 12.6% calculated by Shimabukuro and colleagues (104 spontaneous abortions for 807 participants with a pregnancy outcome at the time of analysis). As we totally disagree with their interpretation of these data, we would like to take the opportunity to respond to their letter.

Shimabukuro et al. decided to include in their analysis all women exposed to a COVID-19 mRNA vaccine during pregnancy and who had the chance to complete their pregnancy (i.e., live birth, spontaneous abortion, stillbirth, induced abortion and ectopic

Publisher's Note: MDPI stays neutral with regard to jurisdictional claims in published maps and institutional affiliations.

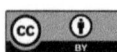

Copyright: © 2021 by the authors. Licensee MDPI, Basel, Switzerland. This article is an open access article distributed under the terms and conditions of the Creative Commons Attribution (CC BY) license (https://creativecommons.org/licenses/by/4.0/).

pregnancy). This conservative approach has led to a larger contribution to the study population of both patients with exposure occurring later in pregnancy and those with a short-term outcome, such as spontaneous abortion, as the available time to follow up was short. To our understanding, this study population might not have fairly represented the population at risk for spontaneous abortion and might have led to a selection of women ending with a spontaneous abortion. Spontaneous abortion incidence rates are sensitive to gestational age at enrollment as the risk decreases over gestation, with later enrollees carrying a lower risk, or no risk of the outcome as mentioned by Stroobandt, S. and Stroobandt, R. Thus, a dedicated analysis estimating the rate of spontaneous abortion by considering all women vaccinated during the first trimester who either had or were at risk of having a spontaneous abortion (i.e., beyond 20 weeks of amenorrhea at the time of the analysis), even if still with an ongoing pregnancy, would probably have provided a fairer estimate. With the information available in the paper by Shimabukuro et al., the spontaneous abortion risk would have probably been around 10% (104 spontaneous abortion for 1132 women vaccinated during the first trimester), which is even lower than the previously published estimate.

In our opinion, the debated data, along with other published data [4,5] show very reassuring results when evaluating the SARS-CoV-2 vaccination safety among pregnant women to date. This is of paramount importance as pregnant women are considered a vulnerable population for SARS-CoV-2 infection [6].

Conflicts of Interest: The authors declare no conflict of interest.

References

1. Stuckelberger, S.; Favre, G.; Ceulemans, M.; Nordeng, H.; Gerbier, E.; Lambelet, V.; Stojanov, M.; Winterfeld, U.; Baud, D.; Panchaud, A.; et al. SARS-CoV-2 Vaccine Willingness among Pregnant and Breastfeeding Women during the First Pandemic Wave: A Cross-Sectional Study in Switzerland. *Viruses* **2021**, *13*, 1199. [CrossRef] [PubMed]
2. Stroobandt, S.; Stroobandt, R. Data of the COVID-19 mRNA-Vaccine V-Safe Surveillance System and Pregnancy Registry Reveals Poor Embryonic and Second Trimester Fetal Survival Rate. Comment on Stuckelberger et al. SARS-CoV-2 Vaccine Willingness among Pregnant and Breastfeeding Women during the First Pandemic Wave: A Cross-Sectional Study in Switzerland. *Viruses* 2021, *13*, 1199. *Viruses* **2021**, *13*, 1545. [CrossRef]
3. Shimabukuro, T.T.; Kim, S.Y.; Myers, T.R.; Moro, P.L.; Oduyebo, T.; Panagiotakopoulos, L.; Marquez, P.L.; Olson, C.K.; Liu, R.; Chang, K.T.; et al. Preliminary Findings of mRNA Covid-19 Vaccine Safety in Pregnant Persons. *N. Engl. J. Med.* **2021**, *384*, 2273–2282. [CrossRef] [PubMed]
4. Bookstein Peretz, S.; Regev, N.; Novick, L.; Nachshol, M.; Goffer, E.; Ben-David, A.; Asraf, K.; Doolman, R.; Sapir, E.; Regev Yochay, G.; et al. Short-term outcome of pregnant women vaccinated by BNT162b2 mRNA COVID-19 vaccine. *Ultrasound Obs. Gynecol.* **2021**. [CrossRef] [PubMed]
5. Goldshtein, I.; Nevo, D.; Steinberg, D.M.; Rotem, R.S.; Gorfine, M.; Chodick, G.; Segal, Y. Association Between BNT162b2 Vaccination and Incidence of SARS-CoV-2 Infection in Pregnant Women. *JAMA* **2021**. [CrossRef] [PubMed]
6. Vouga, M.; Favre, G.; Martinez-Perez, O.; Pomar, L.; Acebal, L.F.; Abascal-Saiz, A.; Hernandez, M.R.V.; Hcini, N.; Lambert, V.; Carles, G.; et al. Maternal outcomes and risk factors for COVID-19 severity among pregnant women. *Sci. Rep.* **2021**, *11*, 13898. [CrossRef] [PubMed]

MDPI
St. Alban-Anlage 66
4052 Basel
Switzerland
Tel. +41 61 683 77 34
Fax +41 61 302 89 18
www.mdpi.com

Viruses Editorial Office
E-mail: viruses@mdpi.com
www.mdpi.com/journal/viruses

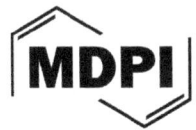